MODULE ON PREVENTIVE STRATEGIES FOR NON-COMMUNICABLE DISEASES

FOR NURSING AND ALLIED HEALTH SCIENCE

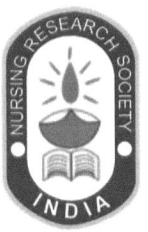

NURSING RESEARCH SOCIETY OF INDIA

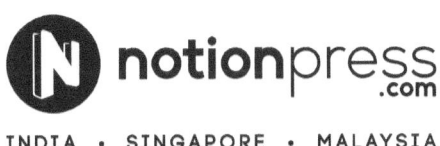

INDIA · SINGAPORE · MALAYSIA

Notion Press

Old No. 38, New No. 6
McNichols Road, Chetpet
Chennai - 600 031

First Published by Notion Press 2019
Copyright © Nursing Research Society of India 2019
All Rights Reserved.

ISBN 978-1-64546-746-5

This book has been published with all efforts taken to make the material error-free after the consent of the author. However, the author and the publisher do not assume and hereby disclaim any liability to any party for any loss, damage, or disruption caused by errors or omissions, whether such errors or omissions result from negligence, accident, or any other cause.

No part of this book may be used, reproduced in any manner whatsoever without written permission from the author, except in the case of brief quotations embodied in critical articles and reviews.

Contents

Foreword   9

Preface   11

Chapter I	Overview of Non-Communicable Diseases (NCDs)	13
Chapter II	Monitoring and Surveillance of the Risk Factors of Non-Communicable Diseases	33
Chapter III	Risk Reduction Strategies for Non-Communicable Diseases	53
Chapter IV	Strengthening Health System Infrastructure for Combating Non-Communicable Diseases	91
Chapter V (A)	Preventive Strategies for Cardiovascular Diseases	132
Chapter V (B)	Preventive Strategies for Cancer	166
Chapter V (C)	Respiratory Diseases: Management and Preventive Strategies	235
Chapter V (D)	Preventive Strategies in Diabetes	263

Chapter V (E)	Preventive Strategies for Osteoporosis	321
Chapter V (F)	Preventive Strategies for Alzheimer's Disease	353
Chapter V (G)	Preventive Strategies for Mental Health Disorder	387
Chapter VI	A Comprehensive Approach to the Prevention and Control of NCDs	435
Chapter VII	Trajectory Model for Chronic Diseases	452
Chapter VIII	A Survey Study to Determine the Risk Factors Associated with Chronic Diseases	460

Foreword   **Dr. Usha Ukande**
President
NRSI

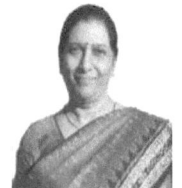

Preface   **Dr. Usha Ukande**   **Dr. Anil Sharma**
President, NRSI   Jt. Secretary, NRSI
Principal   Principal
Choithram College   MTIN, CHARUSAT
of Nursing, Indore   Changa, Gujarat

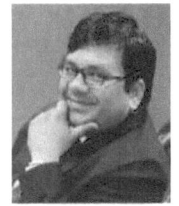

Chapters	Title
Chapter I	**Overview of NCDs** **Mr. Janarthanan B** Senior Tutor College of Nursing JIPMER Puducherry jenu.bcc@gmail.com
Chapter II	**Monitoring and surveillance of Risk Factors of NCDS** **Mr. Janarthanan B** Senior Tutor College of Nursing JIPMER Puducherry jenu.bcc@gmail.com

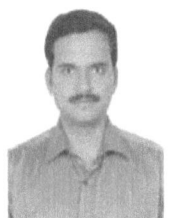

Chapter III   **Interventions for Non-Communicable Diseases Risk Reduction**

Dr. Assuma Beevi
Vice President, NRSI
Director, MIMS Academy
Principal, MIMS College of Nursing
Calicut, Kerala
asmameeran@gmail.com

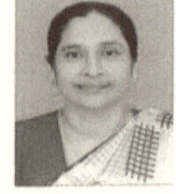

Chapter IV   **Strengthening Health system infrastructure for combating NCDs**

Dr. Jogindravati
Professor cum Principal
SGHS College of Nursing
Sohana, Mohali
Punjab
vati.jogindra@gmail.com

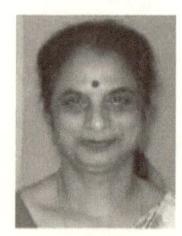

Chapter V   **Preventive Strategies for specific NCDs**

Chapter V(A)   **Cardiovascular Diseases**

Ms. Shweta Pattnaik
Associate Professor
Choithram College of Nursing
Indore (M.P)
shweta.pattnaik24@gmail.com

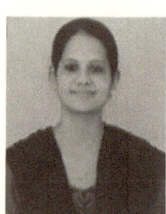

Chapter V(B)   **Cancer**

Dr. T Sivabalan
Professor and Dean
Pravara Institute of Medical Science – DU
College of Nursing, Loni(BK)
Ahmednagar, MH
sivavimal.guru@gmail.com

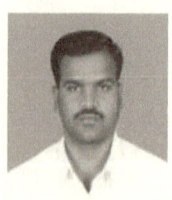

Chapter V(C) **Respiratory Diseases**

Ms. Shweta Pattnaik
Associate Professor
Choithram College of Nursing
Indore (M.P)
shweta.pattnaik24@gmail.com

Chapter V(D) **Diabetes**

Dr. Nancy Fernandes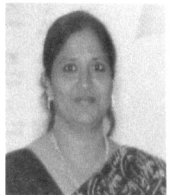
Principal
Leelabai Thackersey College of Nursing
S.N.D.T Women's University
Mumbai (MH)
nancyfernandesltcn64@gmail.com

Chapter V(E) **Osteoporosis**

Dr. Nancy Fernandes
Principal
Leelabai Thackersey College of Nursing
S.N.D.T Women's University
Mumbai (MH)
nancyfernandesltcn64@gmail.com

Chapter V(F) **Alzheimer's Disease**

Dr. T Sivabalan
Professor and Dean
Pravara Institute of Medical Science – DU
College of Nursing, Loni(BK)
Ahmednagar, MH
sivavimal.guru@gmail.com

Chapter V(G)   **Mental Health Disorders**

Dr. K. Lalitha
Director Nursing Services
Sri Balaji Vidyapeeth
Puducherry
<u>lalithakrishnasamy@gmail.com</u>

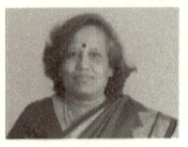

Prof. R. Rajalakshmi
Lecturer
College of Nursing
NIMHANS
Bengaluru, Karnataka

Chapter VI   **A comprehensive approach to the prevention of NCDs**

Mr. Janarthanan B

Chapter VII   **Trajectory Model for Chronic Diseases**

Dr. Usha Ukande
Mrs. Shweta Pattnaik

Chapter VIII   **Research Article:**

A Survey Study to Determine the Risk Factors Associated with Chronic Diseases

Mrs. Shweta Pattnaik
Dr. Usha Ukande

Peer Reviewed By

Dr. Elizabeth Simon
R.N., A.N.P., B.C., Ph.D
Professor
New York Institute of Technology
New York

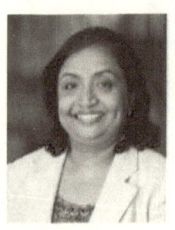

Foreword

Chronic diseases have become a major public health problem in the present times. Non-communicable chronic diseases (NCDs) account for 48% of the global disability (WHO 2011) and 60% of all deaths worldwide. Chronic diseases affect people of all ages, with at least one quarter of deaths occurring in those under the age of 60 years, making it a major concern in health care. In India, the projected number of deaths due to chronic diseases was around 5.21 million in 2008 and is expected to rise to 7.63 million in 2020. Chronic non-communicable diseases such as heart disease, cancer and diabetes are the biggest killers worldwide. While the global chronic disease lifestyle burden is enormous, common risk factors related to chronic diseases are largely modifiable and action can be taken to reduce the relevant morbidity and mortality. India is undergoing rapid epidemiological transition as a consequence of social, economic and ongoing lifestyle changes.

Health disease and disability are dynamic processes which begin before individuals realize they are affected. Disease prevention, therefore, relies on anticipatory actions that can be categorized as primary, secondary or tertiary prevention.

Nursing Research Society of India (NRSI) did a nationwide survey in the year 2013 to assess the distribution of selected NCDs and the common risk factors associated with them. The survey aimed at preparing evidence-based guidelines and strategies for prevention of chronic diseases and promotion of health of people living with chronic diseases.

Foreword

The publication of this multi-author book, "Preventive Strategies for Non-Communicable Diseases" by NRSI, is a step towards contributing to the health promotion of people of India. It is based on the result of the survey done and recommendations submitted by the NRSI members from the 4 regional centers.

The authors, who are nurse researchers, practitioners and academicians, have suggested innovative strategies based on evidence for the prevention and control of common NCDs. Authors have tried to blend different realities into a unique perspective of how people can be motivated to take action to avoid falling into the traps of chronic illnesses.

The members of the NRSI understand their role and responsibility in the promotive, preventive and restorative activities contributing to health, and this has led to the creation of this book.

I commend the authors for bringing out this volume with its many features which provide very useful supplementary reading material for undergraduate and graduate students in nursing. The volume will also serve as a reference book for post graduate students, nursing faculty and other health care professionals.

– **Dr. Usha Ukande**

President, NRSI
Principal, Choithram College of Nursing
Indore (M.P.)

Preface

Nursing Research Society of India (NRSI) believes that the nursing fraternity in India is poised for a great leap forward. It has been over 10 years since the idea of a manual on Non-Communicable Disease (NCDs) germinated in the minds of NRSI executives. Who could have foreseen how that seed would grow into a flower and take the shape of a book?

As various studies and research evidenced, the prevalence of NCDs in the late 90's, which was around 29% of overall diseases prevailing in India during that time has presently increased to around 59%. Literature and research about NCDs can now be found literally around the world; almost everybody is talking about it. Technology has not only made a huge impact on delivery of nursing care but also facilitated access to knowledge about various health problems including NCDs.

The first edition of **NRSI book on "Preventive Strategies for Non-Communicable Diseases"** focuses on prevention and control of various NCDs. This volume is being brought out especially for the health professionals with extensive matter on various preventive aspects for Cardiovascular disease, Cancer, Chronic respiratory diseases, Diabetes, Osteoporosis and Alzheimer's disease, with a comprehensive approach to the subject.

NRSI is very grateful to those who helped us directly or indirectly in preparing this volume. The growth of our profession depends on its members being active producers and consumers of research. We firmly believe that there is always scope for improvement and accordingly we shall look forward to receiving suggestions for further enriching the quality of this book.

– **Dr. Anil Sharma**
Jt. Secretary, NRSI

Chapter I
Overview of Non-Communicable Diseases (NCDs)

Janarthanan B

Non-Communicable Disease (NCD) is a medical condition or disease that is non-infectious and non-transmissible among people. NCDs can refer to chronic disorders which last for long periods of time and progress slowly. Sometimes, NCDs result in sudden deaths such as seen in certain types of disorders such as Cardiovascular disorders, Cancers, Chronic respiratory illnesses and Diabetes Mellitus, which are usually considered to be the 4 common types of non-communicable diseases. (WHO Report, 2009)

NCDs are to some extent synonymous with "chronic diseases." NCDs however, are distinguished by their non-infectious nature and not necessarily by the duration of the illness. Chronic diseases with longer duration, such as HIV/AIDS, are caused by infections that can be easily transmitted. Disorders of longer duration require long-term management, as do all diseases that are slow to develop and last for long duration.

Risk Factors

NCDs usually affect people in the older age groups, but evidence shows that nearly 16 million deaths which are attributed to non-communicable diseases (NCDs) occur before 70 years of age. Among the premature deaths, 82% occurred in low and middle-income countries. Children, adults and the elderly are affected by risk factors such as improper balanced diet, improper activities, smoking and alcohol intake.

Aging, rapid unplanned urbanization, and the unhealthy lifestyles provoke the incidences of these diseases. For example, unhealthy lifestyles like improper diets can cause raised blood pressure, increased blood glucose, elevated blood lipids, and obesity. These are called 'intermediate risk factors' that can lead to cardiovascular diseases. An individual's family background, lifestyle practices and environment are known to increase the likelihood of certain non-communicable diseases. Improper lifestyle practices can result in hypertension and obesity, in turn leading to increased risk of many NCDs.

The WHO's *World Health Report 2002* identified 5 important risk factors for non-communicable diseases in the top 10 leading risks factors to health. These are raised blood pressure, raised cholesterol, tobacco use, alcohol consumption, and overweight. The other factors associated with higher risk of NCDs include a person's economic and social conditions, also known as the "social determinants of health."

It has been estimated that if the primary risk factors are eliminated, 80% of the cases of heart disease, stroke and type 2 diabetes, and 40% of cancers could be prevented. Interventions targeting the major risk factors could have a significant impact on reducing the disease burden worldwide. Efforts focused on better diet and increased physical activity have been shown to control the prevalence of NCDs. These risk factors are categorized as modifiable behavioral risk factors and Metabolic/physiological risk factors. **(WHO Report on Global Health Risks, 2009)**

Modifiable Behavioral Risk Factors
(i) Tobacco

Tobacco use and exposure come in both smokeless and smoking forms. Smokeless tobacco is consumed in unburnt forms through chewing or sniffing and contains several carcinogenic, or cancer causing, compounds. Smokeless tobacco has been associated with oral cancer, hypertension, heart disease and other conditions. Smoking tobacco, by far the most commonly used form globally, contains over 4000 chemicals, of which 50 are known to be carcinogenic. There are currently about 1 billion smokers in the world. Manufactured cigarettes represent the major form of smoked tobacco. Current smokers are estimated to consume about 6 trillion cigarettes annually. In India alone, about 700 billion 'bidis' (a type of filter-less hand-rolled cigarette) are consumed annually. Risks to health from tobacco use result not only from direct consumption of tobacco but also from exposure to secondhand smoke. **(WHO Report, 2002)**

Almost 6 million people die from tobacco use and exposure each year, accounting for 6% of all female and 12% of all male deaths in the world. Of these deaths, just over 600000 are attributable to secondhand smoke exposure among nonsmokers and more than 5 million to direct tobacco use (both smoking and smokeless). By 2020, annual tobacco-related deaths are projected to increase to 7.5 million, accounting for 10% of all deaths in that year, and the deaths are projected to increase to 8 million by 2030. Smoking is estimated to cause about 71% of all lung cancer deaths, 42% of chronic respiratory disease and nearly 10% of cardiovascular disease. Smoking is also an important risk factor for communicable diseases such as tuberculosis and lower respiratory infections. Among men, the highest prevalence of smoking was in lower middle-income countries. Smoking then declines as country income rises. Among women, relatively high rates (around 15%) are reported in upper middle and high-income countries, and about 5 times lower (between 2% and 4%) in low and lower middle-income countries. **(Shafey O et al., 2009)**

(ii) Insufficient Physical Activity

Insufficient physical activity is the fourth leading risk factor for mortality. Approximately 3.2 million deaths and 32.1 million Disability Adjusted Life Years (DALYs) (representing about 2.1% of global DALYs) each year are attributable to insufficient physical activity. People who are insufficiently physically active have a 20–30% increased risk of all-cause mortality compared to those who engage in at least 30 minutes of moderate intensity physical activity on most days of the week. It is postulated that participation in 150 minutes of moderate physical activity each week (or equivalent) is estimated to reduce the risk of ischemic heart disease by approximately 30%, the risk of diabetes by 27%, and the risk of breast and colon cancer by 21–25%. Additionally, physical activity lowers the risk of stroke, hypertension and depression. It is a key determinant of energy expenditure and thus fundamental to energy balance and weight control. Globally, 31% of adults aged 15 years or older were insufficiently active (men 28% and women 34%) in 2008. **(McMurray RG et al., 2000)**

The prevalence of insufficient physical activity rose according to the level of country income. High-income countries had more than double the prevalence compared to low-income countries for both men and women, with 41% of men and 48% of women being insufficiently physically active in high-income countries as compared to 18% of men and 21% of women in low-income countries. In other words nearly every second woman in high-income countries was insufficiently physically active. These data may be explained by increased work and transport-related physical activity for both men and women in the low and lower middle-income countries. The increased automation of work and other aspects of life in higher-income countries is a likely determinant of insufficient physical activity. **(WHO Report, 2002)**

(iii) Harmful Use of Alcohol

The harmful use of alcohol is a major risk factor for premature deaths and disabilities in the world. Hazardous and harmful drinking was responsible for 2.3 million deaths worldwide in 2004. That amounts to 3.8% of all deaths in the world. More than half of these deaths occurred as a result of NCDs, including cancers, cardiovascular disease and liver cirrhosis. An estimated 4.5% of the global burden of disease—as measured in DALYs—is caused by the harmful use of alcohol. Cancers, cardiovascular disease and liver cirrhosis are responsible for a quarter of this burden. There is a direct relationship between higher levels of alcohol consumption and rising risk of some cancers, liver diseases and cardiovascular diseases. The relationship between alcohol consumption and ischemic heart and cerebrovascular diseases is complex. It depends on both the amount and the pattern of alcohol consumption. **(Mukamal KJ et al., 2010)**

Some epidemiological data, generated mainly in high-income countries, suggest that low-risk patterns of alcohol consumption may have a beneficial effect on selected disease outcomes and in some segments of populations, but these effects tend to disappear if the patterns of drinking are characterized by heavy episodic drinking. Although alcohol consumption is deeply embedded in the cultures of many societies, an estimated 45% of the global adult population has never consumed alcoholic beverages in their lives. An estimated 55% of women have never consumed alcohol. There is a high level of variation in alcohol consumption around the world. On an average, global adult per capita consumption was estimated at 6.0 liters of pure alcohol in 2008. Adult per capita consumption was highest in the European Region (12.2 liters) and lowest in the Eastern Mediterranean Region (0.6 liters). In general, abstention rates are lower and per capita consumption is higher in the countries with higher income. The adult per capita consumption in upper middle and high-income countries (around 10 liters) was more than double the level of low and lower-middle-income countries (around 3 to 4 liters). **(Ronksley PE et al., 2011)**

(iv) Unhealthy Diet

Approximately 16 million (1.0%) DALYs and 1.7 million (2.8%) of deaths worldwide are attributable to low fruit and vegetable consumption. Adequate consumption of fruits and vegetables reduces the risk of cardiovascular diseases, stomach cancer and colorectal cancer. There is convincing evidence that the consumption of high levels of high-energy foods, such as processed foods that are high in fats and sugars, promotes obesity as compared to low energy foods such as fruits and vegetables. The amount of dietary salt consumed is an important determinant of blood pressure levels and overall cardiovascular risk. A population salt intake of less than 5 grams per person per day is recommended by WHO for the prevention of cardiovascular disease. However, data from various countries indicate that most populations are consuming much more salt than this. It is estimated that decreasing dietary salt intake from the current global levels of 9–12 grams per day to the recommended level of 5 grams per day, would have a major impact on reducing blood pressure and cardiovascular disease. **(Report of a joint WHO/FAO expert consultation, 2003)**

There is convincing evidence that saturated fat and trans-fat increase the risk of coronary heart disease and that replacement with monosaturated and polyunsaturated fat reduces the risk. There is also evidence that the risk of type 2 diabetes is directly associated with consumption of saturated fat and trans-fat and is inversely associated with polyunsaturated fat from vegetable sources. In the absence of comparable data on individual dietary intakes around the world, the availability of food for human consumption derived from national *Food balance sheets* has been used. However, these may not accurately reflect actual consumption and should be treated as indicative only. The availability of total fat increases with country income level, while the availability of saturated fats clusters around the value of 8% in low and lower middle-income countries and 10% in upper middle-income and high-income countries. In relation to cancer, dietary contaminants—as well as dietary constituents—are a significant problem in some regions. One example is widespread naturally occurring aflatoxins, which contaminate cereals and nuts and cause liver cancer when eaten. Aflatoxin was estimated to have a causative role in 5–28% of all hepatocellular cancers. **(Liu Y & Wu F, 2010)**

Metabolic/Physiological Risk Factors

There are 3 key metabolic/physiological changes that increase the risk of NCDs: raised blood pressure, overweight/obesity, and raised cholesterol level (hyperlipidemia, i.e., high levels of fat in the blood). The effects of these changes are discussed in detail below:

(i) Raised Blood Pressure

Worldwide, raised blood pressure is estimated to cause 7.5 million deaths, about 12.8% of the total of all annual deaths. This accounts for 57 million DALYs or 3.7% of total DALYs. Raised blood pressure is a major risk factor for coronary heart disease and ischemic as well as hemorrhagic stroke. Blood pressure levels have been shown to be positively and progressively related to the risk of stroke and coronary heart disease. In some age groups, the risk of cardiovascular disease doubles for each incremental increase of 20/10 mmHg of blood pressure, starting as low as 115/75 mmHg. In addition to coronary heart diseases and stroke, complications of raised blood pressure include heart failure, peripheral vascular disease, renal impairment, retinal hemorrhage and visual impairment. Treating systolic blood pressure and diastolic blood pressure so they are below 140/90 mmHg is associated with a reduction in cardiovascular complications. Globally, the overall prevalence of raised blood pressure in adults aged 25 and over was around 40% in 2008. The proportion of the world's population with high blood pressure, or uncontrolled hypertension, fell modestly between 1980 and 2008. However, because of population growth and aging, the number of people with hypertension rose from 600 million in 1980 to nearly 1 billion in 2008. Across the income groups of countries, the prevalence of raised blood pressure was consistently high, with low, lower middle and upper middle-income countries, all having rates of around 40% for both sexes. The prevalence in high-income countries was lower, at 35% for both sexes. **(Chobanian A V et al., 2003)**

(ii) Overweight and Obesity

Worldwide, 2.8 million people die each year as a result of being overweight (including obesity) and an estimated 35.8 million (2.3%) of global DALYs are caused by overweight or obesity. Overweight and obesity lead to adverse metabolic effects on blood pressure, cholesterol, triglycerides and insulin resistance. Risks of coronary heart disease, ischemic stroke and type 2 diabetes mellitus increase steadily with increasing body mass index (BMI), which is a measure of weight relative to height. Raised BMI also increases the risk of cancer of the breast, colon/rectum, endometrium, kidney, esophagus (adenocarcinoma) and pancreas. Mortality rates increase with increasing degrees of overweight, as measured by BMI. To achieve optimal health, the median BMI for adult populations should be in the range of 21 to 23 kg/m^2, while the goal for individuals should be to maintain a BMI in the range 18.5 to 24.9 kg/m^2. There is increased risk of co-morbidities for BMIs in the range of 25.0 to 29.9 kg/m^2, and moderate to severe risk of co-morbidities for a BMI greater than 30 kg/m^2. In 2008, 35% of adults aged 20 years and older were overweight (BMI ≥ 25 kg/m^2)—(34% men and 35% of women). The worldwide prevalence of obesity has nearly doubled between 1980 and 2008. **(Martinez JA et al., 1999)**

In 2008, 10% of men and 14% of women in the world were obese (BMI ≥30 kg/m^2), compared with 5% for men and 8% for women in 1980. An estimated 205 million men and 297 million women over the age of 20 were obese in 2008—a total of more than half a billion adults worldwide. The prevalence of raised BMI increases with income levels of countries, up to upper middle-income levels. The prevalence of overweight in high-income and upper middle-income countries was more than double that of low and lower middle-income countries. For obesity, the difference more than triples from 7% obesity in both sexes in lower middle-income countries to 24% in upper middle-income countries. Women's obesity was significantly higher than men's, with the exception of high-income countries where it was of similar prevalence. In low and lower middle-income countries, obesity among women was approximately double that among men. The prevalence of obesity varies across socio-economic groups within individual countries. In high-income countries, an inverse relationship has been identified between socio-economic status and obesity in women for several decades. In medium and low-income countries a positive relationship between socio-economic status and obesity in men, women and children has instead been observed. **(Sobal J & Stunkard AJ, 1989)**

(iii) Elevated Cholesterol

Elevated cholesterol levels increase the risks of heart disease and stroke. Globally, a third of ischemic heart disease is attributable to high cholesterol. Overall, raised cholesterol is estimated to cause 2.6 million deaths (4.5% of total) and 29.7 million DALYs, or 2.0% of total DALYs. Raised total cholesterol is a major cause of disease burden in both the developed and developing world as a risk factor for ischemic heart disease and stroke. For example, a 10% reduction in serum cholesterol in men aged 40 has been reported to result in a 50% reduction in heart disease within 5 years; the same serum cholesterol reduction for men aged 70 years can result in an average 20% reduction in heart disease occurrence in the next 5 years. **(Law MR, Wald NJ & Thompson SG, 1994)**

In 2008, the global prevalence of raised total cholesterol among adults was 39% (37% for males and 40% for females). Globally, mean total cholesterol changed little between 1980 and 2008, falling by less than 0.1 m mol/L per decade in men and women. The prevalence of raised total cholesterol increased noticeably according to the income level of the country. In low-income countries, around a quarter of adults had raised total cholesterol, while in lower middle-income countries this rose to around a third of the population for both sexes. In high-income countries, over 50% of adults had raised total cholesterol, more than double the level of the low-income countries. **(Farzadfar F et al., 2011)**

Socio-Economic Impacts of NCDs

Non-communicable diseases have potentially serious socio-economic consequences, through increasing individual and household impoverishment and hindering social and economic development. The incidence and impact of NCDs and their risk factors is highly inequitable and imposes a disproportionately large burden on low and middle-income countries where nearly three quarters of NCD deaths—28 million—occur. NCDs threaten progress towards the UN Millennium Development Goals and post-2015 development agenda. Poverty is closely linked with NCDs. The rapid rise in NCDs is predicted to impede poverty reduction initiatives in low-income countries, particularly by increasing household costs associated with health care. Vulnerable and socially disadvantaged people get sicker and die sooner than people of higher social positions, especially because they are at greater risk of being exposed to harmful products, such as tobacco or unhealthy food. Besides, they also have limited access to health services. **(Van Lenthe FJ et al., 2004)**

Once thought of as diseases of the rich, NCDs are now the leading causes of death in low and middle-income countries. As mentioned previously, nearly 30% of NCD-related deaths in low-income countries occur under the age of 60, whereas in high-income countries the proportion is only 13%. In low-resource settings, healthcare costs for cardiovascular diseases, cancers, diabetes or chronic lung diseases can quickly drain household resources, driving families into poverty. The exorbitant costs of NCDs, including often lengthy and expensive treatment and loss of breadwinners, are forcing millions of people into poverty annually, stifling development. In many countries, harmful drinking and unhealthy diet and lifestyles occur both in higher and lower-income groups. However, high-income groups can access services and products that protect them from the greatest risks while lower-income groups can often not afford such products and services. Without targeted and sustained interventions, these health inequities are likely to widen, causing even greater individual, social and economic consequences. NCDs can pose socio-economic, wellness and developmental threat to both rich and poor. **(Ezzati M et al., 2002)**

(i) Social Determinants of NCDs

Structural determinants and the conditions of daily life constitute the social determinants of health and are crucial to explaining and addressing health inequities. As with other priority health issues, prevailing social and economic conditions influence people's exposure and vulnerability to NCDs, as well as related healthcare outcomes and consequences. People in developing countries eat foods with higher levels of total energy. **(Van Lenthe FJ et al., 2004)**

Increasing NCD levels are being influenced by many factors including tobacco use and availability, cost and marketing of foods high in salt, fat and sugar. A considerable proportion of global marketing targets children and adolescents as well as women in developing countries to promote tobacco smoking and consumption of 'junk' food and alcohol. Rapid, unplanned urbanization also changes people's way of living through more exposure to the shared risk factors. NCDs are exacerbated in urban areas by changes in diet and physical activity, exposure to air pollutants (including tobacco smoke) and harmful use of alcohol. Overwhelmed by the speed of growth, many governments are not keeping pace with ever-expanding needs for infrastructure and services and people are less likely to be protected by interventions like smoke free laws, regulations to phase out trans-fats, protections against harmful use of alcohol, and urban planning to promote physical activity. **(WHO Global Status Report, 2010)**

As a consequence, vulnerable and socially disadvantaged people get sicker and die sooner than people of higher social positions; the factors determining social positions include education, occupation, income, gender and ethnicity. There is strong evidence on the links between poverty and lower life expectancy, and on the associations between a host of social determinants, especially education, and prevalent levels of NCDs: people of lower social and economic positions fare far worse in countries at all levels of development. Evidence now shows that the poor may begin life with increased vulnerability to NCDs and are then exposed to additional risks throughout life. Under-nutrition in-utero and low birth weight, particularly prevalent among low-income populations, increases the subsequent risk of cardiovascular disease and diabetes. There is evidence that childhood low socio-economic status is associated with type 2 diabetes and obesity in later life. As a consequence, the poor are more likely to die prematurely from NCDs. The WHO Commission on Social Determinants of Health made an initiative for closing the health gap in a generation. To ensure that the call is fulfilled, focused research, coherent policies and multi-sectoral partnerships for action are required to expand the evidence base and implement interventions that show evidence of effectiveness in combating NCDs and their risk factors. **(WHO Report on Global Health Risks, 2009)**

(ii) Economic Impacts of NCDs

Measuring the economic impacts of NCDs remains a relatively complex and under-developed discipline. However, they invariably affect low and middle-income countries and households more severely because they have the least financial cushion to withstand the economic consequences of NCDs. The World Health Report 2010 states that each year, 100 million people are pushed into poverty because they have to pay directly for health services; in some countries, this may represent 5% of the population forced into poverty each year. Financial hardship is not restricted to low and middle-income countries. At the household level, unhealthy behaviors, poor physical status, and the high cost of NCD-related health care, lead to loss of household income. People often become trapped in a dangerous cycle where poverty and NCDs continually reinforce one another. In low-resource settings, treatment for cardiovascular disease, cancer, diabetes or chronic lung disease can quickly drain household resources, driving families into impoverishment. NCDs exacerbate social inequity because most payments for health care in low and middle-income countries are private and out-of-pocket; such costs weigh more heavily on those least able to afford them, increasing the risk of impoverishment. **(WHO Global Status Report, 2010)**

If those who become sick or die are the main income earners, NCDs can force a drastic cut in spending on food and education, causing the liquidation of family assets and a loss of care and investment in children. Where males are the primary income earners, widowhood or the burden of caring for a permanently disabled partner are routes to poverty. The high rate of disability due to NCDs is a particular burden on women and children. This may result in children losing opportunities for schooling, women losing the main sustenance for their families, and families losing their stability. Studies from India show that the contribution to poverty of high out-of-pocket expenditure for health care and NCDs is significant. An estimated 1.4 million to 2 million Indians experienced catastrophic spending in 2004 and 600000 to 800000 people were impoverished by the costs of caring for cardiovascular disease and cancer. The findings of another study also reveal that 1 of every 4 families living in the world's poorest countries borrows money or sells assets to pay for health care. **(Sharma K, 2013)**

NCDs and Global Health

Referred to as "lifestyle" diseases, because the majority of these diseases are preventable illnesses, the most common causes for non-communicable diseases (NCD) include tobacco use (smoking), alcohol abuse, poor diets (high consumption of sugar, salt, saturated fats, and trans-fatty acids) and physical inactivity. Currently, NCDs kill 36 million people a year, a number that by some estimates is expected to rise by 17–24% within the next decade.

General Burden of NCDs

All countries, irrespective of their stage of economic development or demographic and epidemiological transition, face an increasing burden of non-communicable diseases. In 2000, around 60% of all deaths and 43% of the global burden of disease were due to coronary heart disease, stroke, cancers, and type 2 diabetes mellitus. Among developing countries, around 50% of deaths and 40% of burden are due to non-communicable conditions. Heart disease, stroke, cancer, diabetes, and respiratory disease are responsible for an increasing proportion of disease burden in many developing countries undergoing an epidemiological transition. Based on current trends, these diseases are predicted to account for 73% of global deaths and 60% of the global burden of disease by the year 2020. **(Mathers CD & Loncar D, 2006)**

The emergence of epidemics of NCDs is the result of demographic and epidemiological transitions, along with increase in levels of risk factors resulting from social and economic changes. Now NCDs are recognized as a major public health threat in the developing world. For example, over the next 30 years, the burden of disease from NCDs in developing and newly industrialized countries is expected to rise by more than 60%. In comparison, the increase in developed countries is expected to be less than 10%. The increasing burden of NCDs threatens to overwhelm already stretched health services. The factors underlying the major NCDs (heart disease, osteoporosis, Alzhiemer's disease, diabetes, cancer, and respiratory disease) are well documented. Primary prevention based on comprehensive population-based programs is the most cost-effective approach to containing the emerging epidemic of NCDs. **(Alwan et al., 2010)**

An example of cardiovascular disease (CVD), which contributes a substantive part of both mortality and morbidity, illustrates the problem. There is strong evidence that smoking, blood pressure and cholesterol are the cause of at least two-thirds of heart attacks and strokes. It has also been shown that major changes in the rates of CVD are explained by changes in levels of risk factors in populations. CVD (mainly heart disease and stroke) is responsible for approximately half of all NCD deaths and one-fourth of the worldwide NCD burden. Low and middle-income countries suffer the major impact of the CVD epidemic, with two-thirds of the global CVD deaths and three quarters of the global CVD disability occurring in these countries. Furthermore, CVD is more likely to affect people at younger ages in low and middle-income countries. 47% of CVD deaths in developing countries occur in people below the age of 70 years, in comparison with 23% in established market economies. **(Ronksley PE et al., 2011)**

Burden Related to Mortality

The World Health Organization (WHO) reports NCDs to be by far the leading cause of death in the world, representing over 60% of all deaths, and by some estimates expected to rise by 17–24% within the next decade. Out of the 36 million people who died from NCDs in 2005, half were under age 70 and half were women. Of the 57 million global deaths in 2008, 36 million were due to NCDs. That is approximately 63% of total deaths worldwide. Every year, at least 5 million people die because of tobacco use and about 2.8 million die from being overweight. High cholesterol accounts for roughly 2.6 million deaths and 7.5 million die because of high blood pressure. With two-thirds of people who are affected by diabetes now residing in developing nations, NCD can no longer be considered just a problem affecting affluent countries. Deaths from non-communicable diseases are on the rise, with the developing world hit hardest. As previously stated, in 2008 alone, NCDs were the cause of 63% of deaths worldwide, a number that is expected to rise considerably in the near future if effective measures are not taken. NCDs account for 53% of deaths in India. Based on available evidence, cardiovascular diseases (24%), chronic respiratory diseases (11%), cancer (6%) and diabetes (2%) are the leading causes of mortality in India. Treatment cost in India is almost double for NCDs as compared to other conditions and illnesses. **(WHO Global Status Report, 2010)**

If the present growth trends are maintained, by 2020, 7 out of every 10 deaths in developing countries, killing 52 million people annually worldwide by 2030, will be attributed to NCDs. With statistics such as these, it comes as no surprise that international entities such as the World Health Organization and World Bank Human Development Network have identified the prevention and control of NCDs as an increasingly important discussion item on the global health agenda.

In addition to information about NCD-related deaths, morbidity data are important for the management of healthcare systems and for planning and evaluation of health service delivery. However, reliable data on NCD morbidity are unavailable in many countries. The most comprehensive morbidity data available relate to cancer and are available from population or hospital based cancer registries. Such data are important since information on the incidence and types of cancer is required for planning cancer control programs. Only population-based cancer registries can provide an unbiased description of the cancer profile in a given population. Although disease registries for diabetes, hypertension (raised blood pressure) and renal insufficiency exist in some countries, these are generally only available for well-resourced settings, rather than for entire populations. Data on the prevalence of diabetes and raised blood glucose are available from population-based surveys. **(WHO report on Global Health Risks, 2009)**

Key Points

Non-communicable diseases are the biggest global killers today.

- Non-communicable diseases (NCDs) kill 38 million people each year.

- Almost three quarters of NCD deaths—28 million—occur in low and middle-income countries.

- Sixteen million NCD deaths occur before the age of 70; 82% of these "premature" deaths occurred in low and middle-income countries.

- Cardiovascular diseases account for most NCD deaths, or 17.5 million people annually, followed by cancers (8.2 million), respiratory diseases (4 million), and diabetes (1.5 million). These 4 groups of diseases account for 82% of all NCD deaths.

- 63% of all deaths in 2008—36 million people—were caused by NCDs. Nearly 80% of these deaths occurred in low and middle-income countries, where the highest proportion of deaths under the age of 70 from NCDs occur.

- Tobacco use, physical inactivity, the harmful use of alcohol and unhealthy diets all increase the risk of dying from an NCD.

- The prevalence of NCDs, and the resulting number of related deaths, are expected to increase substantially in the future, particularly in low and middle-income countries, due to population growth and aging, in conjunction with economic transition and resulting changes in behavioral, occupational and environmental risk factors.

References

1. "New network to combat non-communicable diseases." World Health Organization report, July 2009.

2. Sharma, K. (2013). Burden of Non-communicable diseases in India: Setting priority for Action. International Journal of Medical Science and Public Health. 2(1); 7–11.

3. World Health Organization. Global Status Report on non-communicable diseases 2010.

4. World Health Organization. Non-communicable Diseases Country Profile 2011.

5. Global health risks: Mortality and burden of disease attributable to selected major risks. World Health Organization report, 2009.

6. Global estimate of the burden of disease from secondhand smoke. Geneva, World Health Organization, 2009.

7. Mathers CD, Loncar D. Projections of global mortality and burden of disease from 2002 to 2030. PLoS Medicine, 2006, 3: e442.

8. Ronksley PE et al. Association of alcohol consumption with selected cardiovascular disease outcomes: a systematic review and meta-analysis. BMJ, 2011, 342: d671.

9. Bazzano LA, Serdula MK, Liu S. Dietary intake of fruits and vegetables and risk of cardiovascular disease. Current Atherosclerosis Reports, 2003, 5: 492–499.

10. The world health report 2002: Reducing risks, promoting healthy life. Geneva, World Health Organization, 2002.

11. Chobanian AV et al. The seventh report of the Joint National Committee on Prevention, Detection, Evaluation, and Treatment of High Blood Pressure: the JNC 7 report. *JAMA*, 2003, 289: 2560–2572.

12. Alwan A et al. Monitoring and surveillance of chronic non-communicable diseases: progress and capacity in high-burden countries. The Lancet, 2010, 376: 1861–1868.

13. Shafey O et al. The Tobacco Atlas, 3rd ed. Atlanta, GA, American Cancer Society, 2009.

14. Mathers CD, Loncar D Projections of global mortality and burden of disease from 2002 to 2030. PLoS Medicine, 2006, 3: e442.

15. Mukamal KJ et al. Alcohol consumption and cardiovascular mortality among US adults, 1987 to 2020. Journal of the American College of Cardiology, 2010, 55: 1328–1335.

16. Rehm J et al. The relation between different dimensions of alcohol consumption and burden of disease: an overview. Addiction, 2010, 105: 817–843.

17. Ronksley PE et al. Association of alcohol consumption with selected cardiovascular disease outcomes: a systematic review and meta-analysis. *BMJ*, 2011, 342: d671.

18. Sobal J, Stunkard AJ. Socioeconomic status and obesity: a review of the literature. Psychological Bulletin, 1989, 105: 260–275.

19. Martinez JA et al. Variables independently associated with self-reported obesity in the European Union. Public Health Nutrition, 1999, 2: 125–133.

20. Farzadfar F et al. National, regional, and global trends in serum total cholesterol since 1980: systematic analysis of health examination surveys and epidemiological studies with 321 country-years and 3.0million participants. The Lancet, 2011, 337(9765): 578–586.

21. McMurray RG et al. The influence of physical activity, socio-economic status, and ethnicity on the weight status of adolescents. Obesity Research, 2000, 8: 130–139.

22. Ezzati M et al. Selected major risk factors and global and regional burden of disease. The Lancet, 2002, 360: 1347–1360.

23. Diet, nutrition and the prevention of chronic diseases: report of a joint WHO/FAO expert consultation. Geneva, World Health Organization, 2003.

24. Liu Y, Wu F. Global burden of aflatoxin-induced hepatocellular carcinoma: a risk assessment. Environmental Health Perspectives, 2010, 118: 818–824.

25. Law MR, Wald NJ, Thompson SG. By how much and how quickly does reduction in serum cholesterol concentration lower risk of ischemic heart disease? British Medical Journal, 1994, 308: 367–372.

26. Van Lenthe FJ et al. Investigating explanations of socioeconomic inequalities in health: the Dutch GLOBE study. European Journal of Public Health, 2004, 14: 63–70.

Chapter II

Monitoring and Surveillance of the Risk Factors of Non-Communicable Diseases

Janarthanan B

Introduction

Non-communicable Diseases (NCDs) are contributing towards the increasing burden of diseases at present. It is quite evident that there are a lot of risk factors contributing to this. Monitoring and surveillance of these risk factors has really become the need of the hour. The WHO report of the year 2000 had already stressed upon the importance of introducing a well-structured monitoring and surveillance system of the various risk factors associated with the occurrence of non-communicable diseases. The underlying cause of this NCD epidemic is the increase in lifestyle related risk factors resulting from social and economic changes. In many countries the increasing impact of globalization has given momentum to this process.

Importance of Identifying the Risk Factors

A "risk factor" refers to any attribute, characteristic, or exposure of an individual which increases the likelihood of developing a non-communicable disease. In the context of public health, population measurements of these risk factors are used to describe the distribution of future diseases in a population, rather than predicting the health of a specific individual. Knowledge of risk factors can then be applied to shift population distributions of these factors in a positive direction.

Emphasis in surveillance should be given to risk factors that are amenable to intervention. Some factors not suitable for intervention, such as sex and age, are also important for estimating trends in NCDs. Intervention strategies can often be delivered cost effectively by community-wide activities, including information and education campaigns, and legislative reform or structural changes that encourage health-preserving behavior.

Monitoring and Surveillance for NCDs should cover monitoring of risk factors, health outcomes (mortality and morbidity) and system capacity. Based on the survey, more than 80% of countries reported NCD mortality as part of their national health information systems. Although the data reported suggest improvements over the past decade, they do not provide information on completeness and quality of mortality data, since fewer countries currently report reliable cause-specific mortality data on a regular basis to WHO. Regardless of the completeness and reliability of data, 16% of countries still have no mortality or morbidity surveillance at all. Significantly, far fewer countries reported that they had population-based mortality data for NCDs.

Written reporting on NCD mortality in national health information systems is another specific challenge: only 61% of countries said they had produced a report on these data in the last 3 years (2007 or later). Overall, the gaps in reporting these data were much greater in lower-income countries. High-income countries were 16 times more likely to have population-based NCD mortality data in their national health information system than low-income countries. The same pattern was observed for population-based morbidity monitoring, with high-income countries 3 times more likely to have morbidity data in their reporting system.

Significant progress has been made over the past 10 years on risk factor surveillance, including surrounding population-based data and in lower-income countries. Tobacco use surveillance in Member States has increased from 61% to 92%, physical inactivity from 38% to 73%, blood glucose from 53% to 76%, diet from 59% to 78%, blood pressure from 49% to 81%, and overweight/obesity from 62% to 80%. Analysis suggests that lower-income countries are catching up with higher-income groups in risk factor surveillance—and in some cases surpassing high-income countries. Nevertheless, despite this progress, data on NCD risk factors are still less likely to be included in a country's national health information system than mortality and morbidity data. **(Rockhill B, 2001)**

Characteristics of a NCD surveillance system

The critical components in the definition of a surveillance system include the ongoing collection, analysis, and use of health data. Demographic or health information systems (for example, registration of births and deaths, routine abstraction of hospital records, health surveys in a population) that are not linked to specific prevention and control programs, do not constitute a surveillance system. However, data collected from ongoing health information systems may be useful for surveillance when systematically analyzed and applied to policy on a timely basis. In this regard the link between information collected and its use to influence both the national and global health policies characterizes a surveillance system. The reverse situation is also a characteristic of the integration of surveillance into a system: surveillance can also be used as a tool to evaluate health policies and preventive interventions.

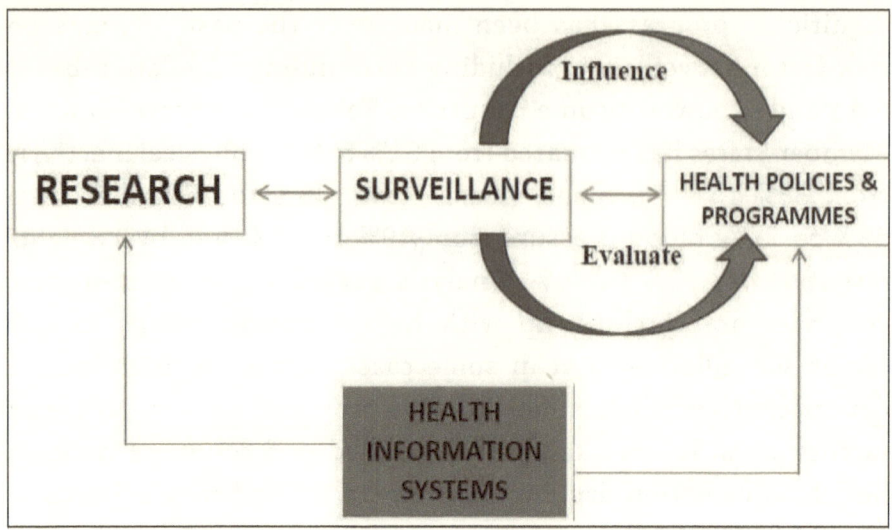

Fig. 2.1: *"characteristics of a surveillance system"*
(Source: WHO Action Plan Report on the Prevention & Control of NCD, 2008)

A well-functioning NCD surveillance system is an integral part of public health surveillance and the wider health information system. It provides information for planning, implementation, monitoring and evaluation of public health intervention programs. The use of the information determines the data collected and the speed necessary for the information flow within the system. Surveillance needs to be grounded in evidence-based approaches. This document stresses that NCD surveillance is an essential national public health function. Multiple sources of information can contribute to an ongoing surveillance system as indicated below.

Table No. 2.1: Information Sources from Surveillance Purposes

Source	Information
Surveys	Population-based data
Disease registries	Incidence and case fatality
Hospital activity data	Morbidity and health service use indicators

Administrative data	Births, deaths, insurance claims, medication use
Aggregate consumption data	Per capita consumption
Economic activity data	Economic indicators

Transition from Disease Surveillance to Risk Factor Surveillance

(Courtesy: WHO Report on Global Health Risks, 2009)

The key to the control of the global epidemics of NCDs is primary prevention. The aim is to avert epidemics wherever possible and to reverse them where they have begun. The basis of prevention of NCDs is identification of the major risk factors and their prevention and control. Where resources are available it is recommended to include data on diseases (for example, heart disease, stroke, and cancer) in the surveillance process. This information is important in assisting health services in planning, determining public health priorities and monitoring the long-term effectiveness of disease prevention campaigns. However, from a primary prevention perspective, surveillance of those major risk factors which are known to predict disease has a high priority.

Research has identified a number of "independent" risk factors common to many NCDs. The conventional approach often focuses on the isolated contribution each of them makes to causality rather than on the totality of risk. In the context of public health, risk factors are a probabilistic concept that applies to an aggregate of individuals and not to a specific individual.

Knowledge about risk factors should be applied to shift population distributions of these factors, and for achieving that, to understand their social, economic, and political determinants. At the individual level, however, such risk factors might be quite poor screening tools. In addition, results from community-intervention trials aimed at the reduction of individual risk factors have been disappointing and this has led to a more comprehensive look at the fundamental determinants of disease and the need to integrate prevention efforts across several factors.

A multidimensional view of disease determinants includes grouping of risk factors along a causal scale from more distant to closer to the actual disease process. A number of these determinants are common to several NCDs. Socio-economic status is a key determinant of health status and many indicators have been developed to describe the social structure for public health purposes. This view illustrates also that some of the risk factors (for example, obesity) are themselves often the outcome of other factors (for example, physical inactivity), a distinction that should be used for guiding interventions to reduce the risk to health.

The multidimensional understanding of the determinants of disease requires targeting of various preventive actions to different levels of causation. For instance, at the physiological level, clinical (pharmacological) interventions may be appropriate, whereas at the level of social structure, the intervention might be directed at alleviation of poverty. Community interventions aimed at changing the pattern of behaviors that predict the occurrence of disease—for example, physical inactivity or smoking—are midway in the scale.

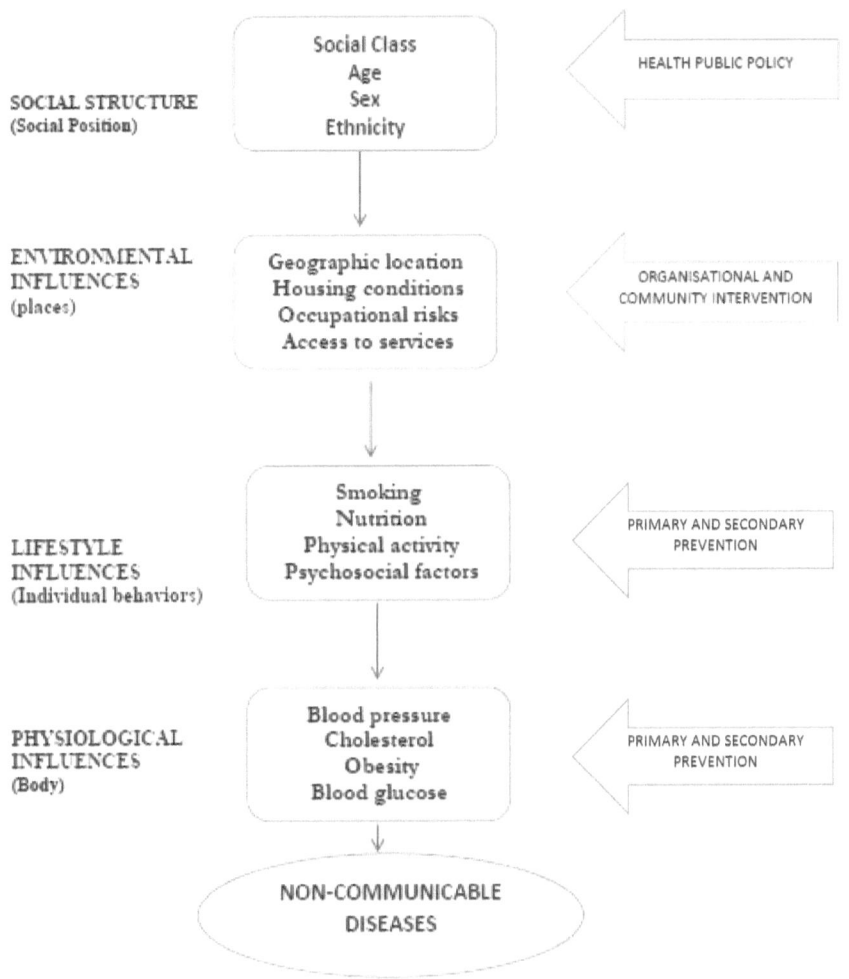

Fig. 2.2: *Levels of Causation and the Related Intervention*
Source: *WHO STEPS Surveillance Manual, 2005*

Role of WHO in Responding to the Increasing NCD Epidemics

In 2000, the Fifty-third World Health Assembly of WHO passed a resolution on the "Prevention and Control of Non-Communicable Diseases" with the goal to support Member States in their efforts to reduce the toll of morbidity, disability and premature mortality related to NCDs. This global strategy has 3 main objectives:

- ❖ To map the emerging epidemics of NCDs and to analyze their social, economic, behavioral and political determinants to provide guidance for policy, legislation and finance;
- ❖ To reduce the level of exposure of individuals and populations to the common risk factors for NCDs;
- ❖ To strengthen health care for people with NCDs.

Risk factor surveillance contributes to the implementation of this resolution by providing data on critical and modifiable risk factors associated with the leading causes of NCD mortality and morbidity. Information on risk factors also helps to guide the development and implementation of disease prevention and health promotion policies and programs and to measure their impact. The overall goal of the WHO global NCD surveillance strategy is to enable countries to build and strengthen their capacity to conduct risk factor surveillance within the framework of an integrated, systematic approach aimed at sustainable national collection of data on NCDs. This process enables countries to use the data collected for decision making and also contributes to the collection of standardized information for global comparisons. **(McKinlay J & Marceau L, 2000)**

The WHO NCD global surveillance strategy includes:

- ❖ Identification of the key risk factors to be addressed together with recommended WHO standardized definitions;
- ❖ A coordinated approach for conducting surveillance of risk factors that upholds scientific principles and is sufficiently flexible to meet local and regional needs and allows international comparisons;
- ❖ Technical materials and tools, including training, to support the implementation of the surveillance tools;

- ❖ Effective communication strategies for providing data to planners of policy and intervention programs, decision-makers, potential funding sources, as well as to the general public; and

- ❖ Use affordable and accessible technology to share information within and between countries.

STEP Wise Approach: Surveillance of NCD Risk Factors

(Courtesy: WHO STEPS Surveillance Manual, 2005)

The WHO STEP wise approach to surveillance (STEPS) is the WHO recommended NCD surveillance tool. This framework unifies all WHO approaches to defining core variables for population-based surveys, surveillance and monitoring instruments. The goal is to achieve data comparability over time and between countries. STEPS offers an entry point for low and middle – income countries to get started in NCD activities. STEPS for NCD risk factors is based on the concept that surveillance systems require standardized data collection as well as sufficient flexibility to be appropriate in a variety of country situations and settings. The STEP wise approach, therefore, allows for the development of an increasingly comprehensive and complex surveillance system depending on local needs and resources.

For surveillance to be sustainable, the STEP wise approach advocates that small amounts of good quality data are more valuable than large amounts of poor quality data. A strong argument can also be made for the benefits of monitoring a few modifiable NCD risk factors since they reflect both a large part of future NCD burden as well as indicating the success of interventions considered to be beneficial to a wide range of NCDs.

In the STEPS approach, the recommended surveillance measures are categorized according to the degree of complexity and cost in obtaining the data. The degree of difficulty equates to whether instruments alone are used, physical measures are collected in the field, or laboratory measurements needing external expertise are required.

The key feature of the STEPS framework is the distinction between the different levels of risk factor assessment:

- self – report information by questionnaire **(Step 1)**,
- objective information by physical measurements **(Step 2),** or
- objective information by blood samples for biochemical analyzes **(Step 3)**.

  The 3 modules involved in describing each risk factor

  - core
  - expanded core
  - optional

The STEPS approach moves along a sequential process. The key premise is that, by using the same standardized questions and protocols, all countries can use the information not only for informing within-country trends, but also for between-country comparisons. The questionnaires and methods recommended must therefore be relatively simple. Because they have been selected on the basis of their ability to provide trends in summary measures of population health, they may not necessarily give a complete picture of each risk factor.

A good illustration in the form of conceptual framework underlying STEPS is given in the following Table, where the different levels of risk factor data assessment (self-report, physical or biochemical measurement) are related to the 3 categories of comprehensiveness involved in describing each risk factor: core, expanded core and optional modules.

Table No. 2.2: Levels of Risk Factor as per STEPS Approach

Measures	Step 1 (Self-Report)	Step 2 (Physical)	Step 3 (Biochemical)
Core	Socio-economic and demographic variables, years of education, tobacco and alcohol use, physical inactivity, intake of fruit and vegetables	Measured weight and height, waist circumference, blood pressure	Fasting blood sugar, total cholesterol
Expanded Core	Ethnicity, income, education, household indicators, dietary patterns	Hip circumference, pulse rate	HDL cholesterol, Triglycerides
Optional (Examples)	Other health related behaviors, mental health, disability, injury	Timed walk, pedometer, skinfold thickness	Oral glucose tolerance test; urine examination

The STEPS approach encourages a focus on obtaining core data at each level on the established risk factors that determine the major disease burden. It is sufficiently flexible to allow each country to expand on the core variables and risk factors, and to incorporate optional modules related to local or regional interests. By including optional modules, the surveillance system can provide more in-depth information but the balance between quantity of data and quality of data must always be considered.

An important feature of the STEP wise approach is that it allows expansion of the key variables by the addition of optional modules if there is strong (local) interest in them. However the focus of WHO STEPS is to propose at each level, a minimum of core standardized variables and methods that will not only be useful at the country level, but will also allow comparability of the collected information for more countries participating in the global surveillance network. This does not apply to the extensions chosen and developed locally. The STEP wise approach is also designed so that, independent of any additions made, data sets should always be 'downwards compatible' by using exactly the same methods such as an agreed common denominator for surveillance.

In countries where health promotion activities, such as campaigns to promote use of seat belt are in place, data on the use of seat belts would be appropriate. A system for monitoring a range of factors related to intentional and unintentional injury is under preparation. In some settings, the teams responsible for the surveillance process may also wish to add more sophisticated laboratory measures to the STEP wise protocols recommended.

Monitoring Outcomes: Mortality and Morbidity

An accurate measure of adult mortality is one of the most informative ways to measure the extent of the NCD epidemic and to plan and target effective programs for NCD control. All-cause and cause-specific death rates, particularly premature deaths before age 60 or 70, are key NCD indicators. High quality mortality data can only be generated by long-term investment in civil registration systems.

Registering every death is a key first step. Accurate reporting of the cause of death on the death certificate is a challenge, even in high-income countries. Death registration by cause is neither accurate nor complete in a large proportion of countries. From a global perspective, there has been only limited improvement in the registration of births and deaths over the past 50 years.

Ascertaining all deaths and their cause on a country level is a critical requirement. Only about two-thirds of countries have vital registration systems that capture the total number of deaths reasonably well. **(Mathers D et al., 2005)**

Although total all-cause mortality may be reported, significant accuracy problems exist in many countries with cause-specific certification and coding. National initiatives to strengthen vital registration systems, and cause-specific mortality statistics, are a key priority. In the meantime, where cause-specific mortality data are not available or inadequate from a coverage and/or quality perspective, countries should establish interim measures such as verbal autopsy for cause of death, pending improvements in their vital registration systems. **(Stamler J, Stamler R, Neaton JD, Wentworth D, Daviglus ML, Garside D et al., 1999)**

Monitoring Health System Response and Country's Capacity

(Ref: WHO, Global strategy for prevention and control of NCD, 2000)

Assessing individual country capacity and health system responses to address NCD prevention and control in a comprehensive manner, and measuring their progress over time, are some of the major components of the Global Action Strategy Plan. To monitor country capacity to respond to NCDs, periodic assessments of the major components of national capacity in all the countries was carried out in 2000–2001, following the endorsement of the Global Strategy for the Prevention and Control of Non-communicable Diseases, and again in 2009–2010.

The capacity assessments examined the public health infrastructure available to deal with NCDs, the status of NCD-relevant policies, strategies, action plans and programs, the existence of health information systems, surveillance activities and surveys, access to essential healthcare services including early detection, treatment and care for NCDs, and the existence of partnerships and collaborations related to NCD prevention and control.

A number of countries also monitor activities in tackling risk factors such as tobacco, harmful alcohol use and obesity. WHO supports this process, for example by conducting regular reviews of tobacco demand reduction policy measures, and the status of policies and programs to address harmful use of alcohol.

Opportunities for Enhancement

The significance of reliable information and capacity, which includes important gaps in surveillance data, is a major challenge to NCD prevention and control in many countries. Tracking NCDs and their risk factors and determinants is one of the 3 key components of the prevention and control of Non-communicable Diseases. Strengthening surveillance is a priority for every country. There is an urgent and pressing need for concerted efforts to improve the coverage and quality of mortality data, to conduct regular risk factors surveys at a national scale with standardized methods, and to regularly assess national capacity to prevent and control NCDs. Technical, human, and fiscal resource constraints are major impediments in some countries. With judicious use of scarce resources and capacity building, the surveillance framework can be implemented in all countries. Such a framework is essential for policy development and assessment and for monitoring of trends in population behaviors and diseases. The adoption and use of a standardized core set of indicators is of crucial importance for national and global monitoring of NCD trends.

Numerous recommendations have been made to improve country capacity for the development and maintenance of health information systems, and many are clearly applicable to NCDs. A permanent infrastructure for surveillance activities is required. Data collection can be organized in several ways, but an institution or a network with the relevant expertise is needed to guarantee the sustainability and quality of surveillance over time. However, knowing what to do is not the only obstacle; lack of experience in establishing health information systems, and obtaining the necessary resources, also remain. key challenges.

Common Issues in Monitoring and Surveillance of NCDs

(Courtesy: WHO Action Plan, 2008: Document A61/8)

1. The target population

The risk factors and determinants chosen for population surveillance in the present framework are primarily related to habits that are potentially amenable to intervention. Several aspects should be taken into account when considering risk factor surveillance. Chronic disease generally occurs following prolonged exposure, usually of several years if not decades, to certain behaviors. For this reason, surveillance of risk factors is generally recommended in the population aged 25 to 64 years.

In countries with high life expectancies, such as most developed countries, extension of the age range of the target population to 74 years would be appropriate. As a standard, 10-year age groups (25–34, 35–44, 45–54, 55–64) are recommended. Monitoring the current levels for risk factors at both older ages (65–74 or 75–84 years) as well as younger ages (15–25 years) presents additional challenges with respect to recruitment and response fractions. Surveillance of the entire target population is neither feasible nor desirable. Surveys in random samples of the target population provide the most cost-effective method for risk factor surveillance needs. Provided the appropriate sampling method is used, the results of the survey can be generalized to provide estimates for the entire target population.

2. Health indicators

Health Indicators for populations are summary measures of the health of individuals and if related to some aspect of a health system, they are measures of the status of its performance, or outcomes. As such the definition and selection of health indicators is closely linked with their intended use as markers of performance.

Health indicators have the potential to increase the impact of public health programs by establishing a small number of key health areas that can be brought to the attention of policy makers. They can motivate actions to promote positive changes in these areas, and provide ongoing feedback about progress towards achieving the desired changes. Such a set of health indicators can focus national attention on a limited number of measures that have relevance to, and can be acted upon by, the general public, public and private policy makers, and health and science professionals.

As health interventions will differ regionally and nationally, the most appropriate health indicators chosen will be specific to the setting. Therefore, universally accepted health indicators are few and often do not meet the specific purpose. Nevertheless, definitions and methods of data assessment can be standardized on a global level together with recommendations on how to derive appropriate health indicators from the data.

Health indicators have a focus on either primary, secondary, and tertiary prevention issues or environmental and sociocultural determinants of health, with the goal of eliminating health disparities and improving the number and quality of years of healthy life. They are characterized by an ability to promote positive changes in behaviors by encouraging and supporting the general public and policymakers to develop interventions that will result in significant and sustained changes in the status of that indicator. Selected health indicators should have a level of credibility with support from individuals, groups, organizations, health professionals, and others involved in the delivery of healthcare, education and services to the general population.

3. Population means as statistical measures

The optimal statistical indicator for a given risk factor varies with the nature of the risk factor and how it is measured. With smoking, for example, the population fits into one of 3 mutually exclusive categories for smoking (current smoker, ex-smoker and never smoker).

The key indicator for such a categorical variable is the prevalence, the proportion of the population that is in a given category at a given point in time. Judging whether prevalence changes or whether differences are statistically significant must take into account the level of statistical uncertainty surrounding each measurement and this is to a large extent related to the size of the sample on which it is based. Large samples yield more precise estimates of the true population mean and will allow smaller differences or trends to be detected. From the perspective of the health of the whole population, measures of central tendency and dispersion provide important information. The proportion of the population exceeding any given level of a continuous variable is directly related to the average level and the spread of the distribution in that population.

4. Quality control

To be able to trust surveillance results, it is crucial that surveillance systems include quality control measures for all key surveillance functions. These functions include:

- ensuring that common questions are used by all participating locations
- standard data collection procedures are adhered to so that results will be valid
- data are analyzed consistently across all participating locations
- participation in a global or regional network such as WHO STEPS, which includes guidelines and training materials, which will enhance standardized data collection.

5. Surveillance infrastructure

The design of surveillance systems requires ongoing commitment and resources including personnel and technology for communication and data use. Efficiencies are gained by building infrastructure for surveillance, rather than conducting a series of repeat surveys, in which new staff and new administrative and procedural guidelines must be developed.

As the team begins planning to conduct surveillance across more locations and on a more ongoing basis, a central or lead agency should be identified to coordinate the surveillance activities and to ensure quality control so as to ensure that data collected is used for public health action and interventions influenced by health policy. Using a partnership approach that includes receiving input from all participating agencies and locations to help develop, maintain, and expand the surveillance system, will result in a participatory system. These participants, whether at national or local level, will share ownership of the system and the surveillance information produced.

Key Points

- Current capacities for NCD surveillance are inadequate in many countries and urgently require strengthening.
- High quality NCD risk factor surveillance is possible even in low-resource countries and settings.
- A surveillance framework that monitors exposures (risk factors and determinants), outcomes (morbidity and mortality) and health system responses (interventions and capacity) is essential.
- A common set of core indicators is needed for each component of the framework.
- Cancer morbidity data are essential for planning and monitoring cancer control initiatives.
- Population-based cancer registries play a central role in cancer control programs because they provide the means to plan,

monitor and evaluate the impact of specific interventions in targeted populations.

o Sustainable NCD surveillance systems need to be integrated into national health information systems and have to be supported with adequate resources.

References

1. Last J. The dictionary of epidemiology. 4 ed. Oxford: Oxford University Press; 2000.

2. McQueen DV. A world behaving badly: the global challenge for behavioral surveillance. American Journal of Public Health. 1999; 89: 1312–14.

3. World Health Organization. International Guide for Monitoring Alcohol Consumption and Related Harm. Geneva: WHO, 2000.

4. Action plan for the global strategy for the prevention and control of non-communicable diseases. Geneva, World Health Organization, 2008 (document A61/8).

5. McKinlay J, Marceau L. US public health and the 21st century: diabetes mellitus. Lancet 2000; 356: 757–61.

6. Rockhill B. The privatization of risk. Am J Public Health. 2001; 91: 365–68.

7. Regidor E, Gutierrez-Fisac JL, Rodriguez C. Increased socio-economic differences in mortality in eight Spanish provinces. SocSci Med. 1995; 41: 801–7.

8. World Health Organization. World Health Report 2000. Health Systems: Improving Health Performance. Geneva: WHO, 2000.

9. Labarthe DR. Prevention of cardiovascular risk factors in the first place. Prev Med. 1999; 29: S72-S78.

10. Stamler J, Stamler R, Neaton JD, Wentworth D, Daviglus ML, Garside D et al. Low risk-factor profile and long-term cardiovascular and non-cardiovascular mortality and life expectancy: findings for 5 large cohorts of young adult and middle-aged men and women. JAMA 1999; 282: 2012–18.

11. Mathers D et al. Counting the dead and what they died from: an assessment of the global status of cause of death data. Bulletin of the World Health Organization, 2005, 83: 171–177.

12. Global strategy for the prevention and control of non-communicable diseases (WHAA53/14). Geneva, World Health Organization, 2000.

13. WHO STEPS surveillance manual: the WHO STEP-wise approach to chronic disease risk factor surveillance. Geneva, World Health Organization, 2005.

14. Global health risks: mortality and burden of disease attributable to selected major risks. World Health Organization report, 2009.

Chapter III

Risk Reduction Strategies for Non-Communicable Diseases

Dr. Assuma Beevi

Behavioral risk factors, including tobacco use, physical inactivity, unhealthy diet and the harmful use of alcohol are estimated to be responsible for about 80% of coronary heart disease and cerebrovascular diseases in India.[1] According to ICMR findings the prevalence of risk factors for non-communicable diseases (NCD) in India is as follows[1]:

- Tobacco use (40% men, 4% women)
- Low fruit and vegetable intake (69% men, 75% women)
- Obesity (19% men, 28% women)
- High cholesterol (33% men, 35% women)
- Hypertension (20% men, 22% women)
- Underweight (21% men, 18% women)

This statistics shows that it is crucial to initiate risk reduction strategies to prevent the development of non-communicable diseases in all populations. Risk reduction strategies as a whole consists of primordial prevention and primary prevention strategies.

Primordial prevention is prevention of the emergence or development of risk factors among population groups in which they have not yet appeared. Primordial prevention consists of actions to minimize future hazards to health and resultantly inhibit the establishment of risk factors (environmental, economic, social, behavioral and cultural) known to increase the risk of disease.

The major interventions are through individual and mass education to avoid the development of risk factors in the first place itself.

Primary prevention can be defined as "action taken prior to the onset of diseases which removes the possibility that a diseases will ever occur." It signifies intervention in the pre-pathogenesis phase of diseases or health problem. The WHO has recommended the following approaches for the primary prevention of chronic NCDs where the risk factors are established[2]. Primary prevention consists of actions to prevent the onset of specific diseases via risk reduction. This will be done by altering behaviors or exposures that can lead to disease, or by enhancing resistance of the body to diminish the effects of exposure to the disease agent.

- Population-based strategies for preventing NCDs in whole population.
- High risk strategies for target people with identified risk factors.

Population-based strategies are lifestyle linked community programs that address most of the NCDs. This strategy needs both 'bottom–up' (community health education and empowerment of people) and 'top down' (legislation and regulation from government agencies) approaches. For example, if it is food, then the strategy starts from the production, pricing and labeling to control price and making available free insecticide and healthy food materials to people. If it is tobacco, a control is exerted on production, sale and advertisement to curtail the use for preventing cancer. In the same way, for physical activity, it would be putting in place a conducive transport system that caters to the needs of people but curbs vehicular transport, as well as providing facilities for leisure time exercise in community play grounds. Active health policies are required for implementing population-based strategies. An effective policy and an empowered community can work together to control the epidemics of NCDs in India.

High risk strategies for target people include:

a. Creating awareness and empowering people for adopting healthy living habits;

b. Early identification of persons with risk factors and providing cost-effective interventions for reducing the risks;

c. Cost-effective care to people with clinical disease to prevent complications; and

d. Acute care, utilizing low-cost, high yield technologies.

In this chapter, the interventions for risk reductions are dealt with under the following headings.

1. Interventions to promote mental health.

2. Avoiding harmful habits and promoting good behavioral attributes (avoiding tobacco and alcohol consumption).

3. Healthy dietary practices, and

4. Promoting physical activities.

These strategies are intended to prevent development of NCDs, increase productivity and promote better quality of life for people belonging to all walks of life and avert premature deaths.

1.0 Interventions to Promote Mental Health

The modern world is moving at a great pace and every individual is faced with multiple stressors in daily life. Better adaptation towards stress is important to maintain a healthy life. To keep healthy, individuals should maintain mental health. If an individual wants to be mentally healthy he should be able to cope with the stressors in a positive manner. A positive living requires mental health.

A sound mind in a sound healthy body makes a person happier. At present there is an increasing focus on powerful 'mind-body connection' through which emotional, mental, spiritual, social and behavioral factors can directly affect our health. Mental health denotes how a person thinks, feels and acts in order to face life situations, handles stress, how a person relates to others, and how decisions are made.[3]

Ways to maintain Mental Health

The following are simple rules of happy and contented life which form the basis for sound mental health suggested by Dr. C R Chandrasekhar, Professor of Psychiatry, NIMHANS.[4]

The acronym of MENTAL HEALTH stated below will be of use for understanding a mentally healthy living.

M – Money management. Be wise in spending money according to earning. Be realistic. Lead a simple and contented life.

E – Expectations about others: Nobody is perfect. It is difficult to change others. So try to adapt with people by making them understand you.

N – Negative thinking: Remove negativity with positive aspects of the situations.

T – Today is important, neither the past, nor the future. Remember nobody is inevitable. The world will move on even if people, property or products which we usually think are essential are nonexistent.

A – Accept reality: Adapt yourself to it. Appreciate yourself and others.

L – Loneliness to be avoided. Get the support of others. Develop religious and spiritual activities. Join social organizations.

H – Hobbies to divert your attention, to relax: Music, reading, creative activities, sports, yoga and meditation are some of the hobbies that can be added to life to enrich the feeling of wellness.

E – Express your feelings with someone you like. Write a diary, keep good environment.

A – Be Active. Enjoy the work you do. Keep yourself busy.

L – Learn skills; improve your knowledge to manage your problems. Prepare for and manage life events.

T – Take things as they come. Tackle one problem at a time. Have realistic targets.

H – Healthy lifestyle—Regular Food—Exercise (walking), Good living Environment, Treatment for health problems from family doctor.

Mental well-being is an integral part of an individual's capacity to lead a fulfilling life, including the ability to form relationships, study, work or pursue leisure interests, education, employment and housing as well as to make day-to-day decisions and choices.

According to WHO, 2008, mental health problems contribute to an estimated 1.1% of the total DALY's. Mental disorders contribute to 12% of the global burden of disease and will rise to roughly 15% by the year 2020. It has been seen that neurotic illnesses, including depression, anxiety and severe mental illnesses such as bipolar disorder and schizophrenia are some of the mental health challenges[3].

1.1 Mental Health and NCDs

Increased morbidity and mortality are associated with factors related to living with mental illness. Lifestyle behaviors such as smoking, lack of physical activity and the effects of psychotropic medication cause increased weight gain and are 2 to 3 times more prevalent in people with serious mental illness than in the general population.

People suffering from other illnesses like cancer also have increased risk of depression and they also suffer from heart diseases. So sound mental health is very important for preventing NCDs; and therefore, strategies for improving mental health should be part of everyday life.

1.2 Effects of Stress on Mental Health

There are lots of ups and downs in life. When an individual is unable to maintain equilibrium between these ups and downs effectively, stress develops. Everyone experiences stress differently and it influences the health in different ways. Stress is an inevitable and necessary evil. Stress in small amount is productive while too much stress is counterproductive. So for healthy living one has to develop effective coping strategies to resolve stress. Unhealthy ways of coping up, leads to various forms of risk behaviors such as[3]:

- smoking
- alcoholism
- over eating or under eating
- spending more time with computer
- excessive use of mobile
- withdrawing from friends, family and society
- use of excessive sleeping pills
- sleeping too much, and
- projective behaviors (putting stress on others through angry outbursts, physical violence, etc.).

Unmanaged or mismanaged stress activates the neuroendocrine system causing physical and physiological changes in the body systems. The impact of such bodily changes for a long period will be renamed as non-communicable diseases like Diabetes Mellitus, Myocardial Infarction, Hypertension, Dyslipidemia, Arthritis, Asthma and so forth.

1.3 Stress Reduction Strategies

Every individual is unique and has enormous potential to adapt to situations. Human beings are bestowed with adaptability and one good example is Eskimos living in Arctic and Antarctic regions. They adjust their lifestyle according to climatic conditions. It is the individual who has to find a suitable adaptation strategy. So there is no single mantra for resolving stress. Everyone can deal with stress either through changing the stress producing situations or changing their reaction to stressful situations. Experts in the field of stress management suggest 4 strategies to deal with stress. Techniques that empower the mind are:

- Avoid stressors
- Alter stressors
- Accept stressors
- Adapt stressors

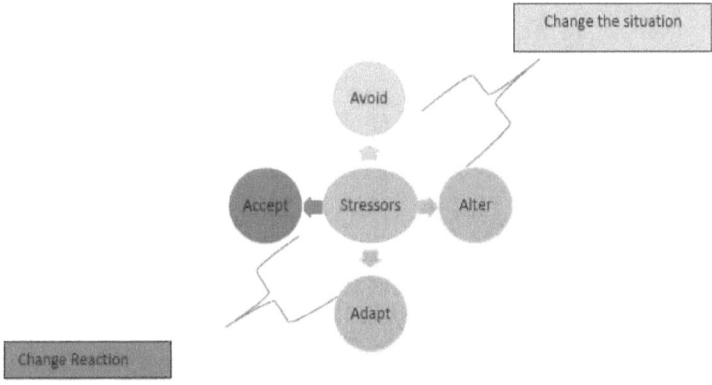

Fig. No. 3.1: *Stress Management Strategies*

These strategies help to cope with neurotic, psychotic, and psychopathic disorders like depression, anxiety disorders, stress syndromes and eating disorders, and mold individual to be strong enough to resist against non-communicable diseases. These are elaborated below.[5]

1.3.1 Avoid the stressors

It is not always easy to avoid stress. But there are many unnecessary situations or moments that cause discomfort in an individual's life and deteriorate his health as well as mental wellness.

It's better to avoid relationships that cause extreme tension either by simple negligence or saying 'NO' to them. People should commit themselves to those tasks that are within their capacity to fulfill. Otherwise unachievable commitments can increase stressors and eventually cause physical and mental ill health. In addition, it is better to avoid sensitive talks, unpleasant TV programs, busy roads, and busy shopping areas; instead one can find out better alternatives. Prioritize daily activities, and plan accordingly.

1.3.2 Alter the stressors

Changing the stressful situations through certain behavioral tactics in communications and changing the mode of operation in daily life will help to alter stress. Best methods of changing stressors are through speaking directly to annoying persons in an open and respectful way, rather than keeping frustrations in one's mind. Certain behaviors such as poor time management, inability to compromise on certain things, lack of flexibility, perfectionism, and lack of assertiveness can act as stressors.

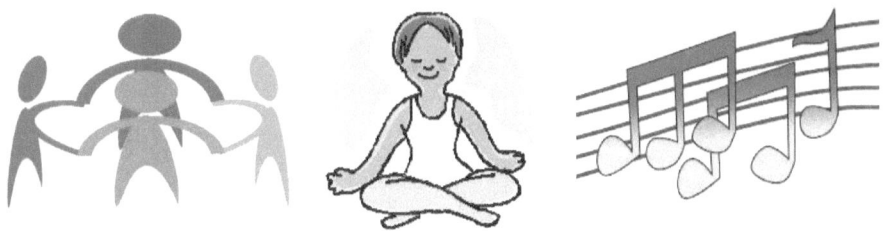

Fig.No. 3.2: *Methods to alter the stressors*

1.3.3 Accept the stressors

There are certain stressors that are unavoidable such as death of loved ones, chronic illness, and natural calamities. These inescapable stresses are to be accepted as the facts of life. Challenges can be taken as opportunities, as business people see in SWOT (strength, weakness, opportunities and threats) analysis.

1.3.4 Adapt to the stressors

One has to find out measures to cope up with unavoidable stressful situations. Be realistic in setting goals and divert your mind to pleasurable events. It doesn't mean having inappropriate behavior for enjoyments. Learn to accept things if they are good enough. It is important not to expect excellence everywhere. An individual who focuses on positives in every situation and tolerates some sort of discomforts gets something good in future or changes his perspectives. Such individuals can adapt to stress very well. If 8 out of 10 decisions or activities of an individual are successful, that person is great. We need not be adamant to have 10 out of 10 successes.

There are various strategies to reduce stress and improve mental health. These strategies guard against mental disorders and other preventable non-communicable diseases namely diabetes, hypertension, depression and asthma. Daily practice of such strategies acts as a great wall in preventing these disorders. These strategies are:

- Breathing exercises
- Yoga
- Progressive relaxation technique
- Humor/laughter
- Laughter therapy
- Mindful awareness
- Meditation
- Journaling
- Social events
- Music
- Assertive behaviors
- Time management, etc.

These activities will not take much time. Remember there are 24 hours in a day. Every individual is entitled to take 30–40 minutes for himself.

1.3.5 ABC strategy for stress control

- **A** = Awareness (What causes you stress and how do you react?)
- **B** = Balance (There is a delicate balance between positive and negative stress and how much you can cope with before it becomes negative)
- **C** = Control (What can you do to help yourself combat the negative effects of stress)

So it is the individual who has to decide how to handle stress and live positively in this beautiful world which is full of diversity.

2.0 Avoiding Harmful Habits and Promoting Good Behavioral Attributes

Mental health is connected to many factors. Behavioral attributes are proximal determinants for mental health. Harmful behaviors like use of alcohol and substance abuse have direct link to mental health. Mentally healthy individuals have the mental ability and strength to adapt their lifestyles.

Set a **powerful mind** against alcoholism, drug abuse and smoking. Powerful mind against addictions is key to successful life and healthy body. Individuals who have determination to stay away from dangerous behaviors such as alcoholism, smoking and drug dependency, will be far away from non-communicable diseases. There are some ground rules that help a person to be away from dangerous behaviors that lead to non-communicable diseases[6].

1. Don't be afraid to say 'NO': if somebody pressurizes you to drink, just say 'NO' to them assertively and don't spend time to describe the several reasons behind your refusal.

2. Avoid negative peer pressure: it is better to avoid a friends' circle that can't live without addictive behaviors.

3. Find ways to make life enjoyable without smoking, alcohol or drugs: certain social, personal and moral values will in the long run give long-term pleasure rather than what can be had from smoking, alcohol or drugs.

4. Adopt stress reduction strategies: emotional instability is the commonest reason behind alcoholic and smoking behavior among most people. Stress reduction strategies in daily life play a pivotal role in living away from substance dependence.

5. Strong bond with family: Open communication in family helps to ventilate frustrating feelings and makes one mentally healthy.

6. Avoid all sorts of addictive beverages: there are many beverages which tend to be addictive in the future. These drinks are primary teaching for future alcoholic behaviors. Say goodbye to those liquids and rely on natural homemade drinks.

7. Internalize the harmful effects of alcoholism, smoking and drugs: collect adequate information of negative effects of these behaviors to teach oneself to abstain from addictive behaviors. A determined and self-motivated mind is needed to fight against cravings for substances and provocations from peers. Knowledge is a powerful force to defend against substance abuse.

8. Be courageous to declare non-alcoholic status in public places: this will help one to be a role model in society and take responsibility to emphasize safe health care practices in public gatherings.

9. Plan ahead for get together or journey: Plan ahead in mind that, "I will not be a victim of somebody else's alcohol or drug abuse."

Get support: It is better to get counseling support when an individual feels vulnerable to be influenced. Chemicals such as central nervous system depressants and alcohol increase desires but decrease performances. There are many counseling centers throughout the world to help people from depressive feelings along with the family members and good friends. Seek help and be strong. Many research studies show that a stress-free mind relaxes our organs and maintains our cells positive and productive. Let us fight against non-communicable disease with beautiful cum solid mind.

So far the discussions concentrated on avoiding stressors and staying away from dangerous behaviors as risk reduction strategies for preventing NCDs. The next important aspect is healthy dietary practices.[11]

3.0 Healthy Dietary Practices

A healthy diet should include all essential nutrients needed for the body but it should not be leading to either overweight or obesity or to under nourishing. Balanced nutrition enables us to maintain good health. Unhealthy diet can lead to intermediate risk factors such as high blood pressure, impaired glucose tolerance and ultimately causes non-communicable disease like diabetes, cardiovascular disease, obstructive pulmonary disease, etc.

It is important to remember that eating habits are established early in life. So it is desirable to inculcate healthy food habits from an early age itself. Introduction of free sugars and salts in weaning food in early childhood are found to produce high blood pressure in adult life. The quality of food is based on composition, periodicity and amount of energy derived along with microelements and vitamins and with bulk of foods.[6]

3.1 Nutrition and Non-Communicable Disease

A healthy diet prevents non-communicable disease to a certain extent. Here are some tips for maintaining a healthy diet that may reduce the risk of non-communicable disease:

- Avoid fatty diet because that increases cholesterol and the chance of developing NCDs like Coronary Artery Disease, DM, stroke, etc.

- Avoid foods containing Trans-fatty acid such as fried and baked foods.

- Take food rich in poly unsaturated fatty acid instead of saturated fat. Example: soybean, sunflower oil, fish like mackerel and salmon, nuts and green leafy vegetables. Healthy living program in Mauritius, which combined health education of people along with policy changes leading to the substitution of palm oil with soya bean oil as ration oil, resulted in the reduction of multiple NCD risk factors within a 5-year period.

- Avoid eating too much sweets and drinks rich in free sugar.
- Limit the salt intake to not more than 4–6 gm per day.
- Avoid soft drinks and carbonated beverages.
- Drink plenty of water, at least 2 liters/8 glasses per day.
- Take 2–3 servings of variety of fruits and vegetables per day.

According to WHO recommendation, total intake of fat is 15–30% of total caloric intake, and WHO recommends restricting free sugar to 10% of total caloric intake, because free sugar increases the total caloric intake. WHO also recommends intake of 400 gm of fruits and vegetables per day because they have minerals and vitamins essential to health. Given below is a list of nutrients generally available.[7]

3.2 Nutrients Present in Fruits and Vegetables Are

- Minerals like iron and calcium.
- Vitamins: Vitamin C, B complex, carotenoids (a precursor of vitamin A), folic acid.
- Phytochemicals.
- Carbohydrate and fiber.

3.3 Role of Fruits and Vegetables in Prevention of NCDs

- Fruits and vegetables are rich sources of fiber. Dietary fibers block the absorption of fat and thereby reduce the plasma cholesterol level. Thus it reduces the risk of diseases like Coronary Artery Disease and diabetes. Dietary fibers which are abundant in fruits and vegetables have protective effect against colon cancer.

- Consumption of a variety of fruits and vegetables reduces caloric intake except tuberous vegetables like yam, tapioca, potato and colacasia, and fruits like banana which provide more than 100Kcl/gm.

- Fruits and vegetables are rich sources of antioxidants that play a protective role against the harmful effect of oxygen free radicals in body.

- Plenty of Vitamin C and carotenoid (precursor of vitamin A) are present in fruits and vegetables. They are powerful antioxidants that help to reduce the risk of NCDs like DM, atherosclerosis, and cancer.

- Folic acid deficiency increases the Homocysteine level thereby increasing the risk of heart disease. Green leafy vegetables are rich sources of folate, and thus help to reduce the risk of heart disease.

- Fruits and vegetables are rich sources of potassium, which plays a role in maintaining blood pressure.

3.4 Methods to Preserve Nutrients in Fruits and Vegetables

- Wash fruits and vegetables before cutting.

- Never soak the cut vegetables in water for a long time, because it causes loss of water soluble minerals and vitamins.

- Cut vegetables just before cooking rather than refrigerating.

- Avoid cutting fruits and vegetables into small pieces, because it causes exposure of greater surface area of food stuff to atmospheric air, resulting in loss of vitamin due to oxidation.

- Boiling is the most common method of cooking, during which heat labile and water soluble vitamins like vitamin B complex and vitamin C are lost.

- Steaming and microwaving are best methods of cooking, because they minimize cooking time, temperature and water needed and preserve the nutrients in food stuff.

- Cooking food in vessel covered with lid helps to hold heat and steam and also reduces cooking time.

- Do not discard the excess water after cooking and use as vegetable stocks to prepare gravy.

- Try to consume fruits as a whole rather than drinking fruit juice, because juices reduce the fiber content of fruits.

3.5 Methods to Remove Pesticides from Fruits and Vegetables

Even though fruits and vegetables are beneficial to health, pesticides used during cultivation and preservation can have a deleterious effect on the body. They are found to be the number one cause of various types of cancers. Measures to remove pesticides from fruits and vegetables are:

- Wash in running water.
- Washing with 2% salt water is also helpful to remove pesticides.
- Steam or wash in hot water, after pre-washing.
- Always purchase locally available fruits and vegetables.
- Encourage people to cultivate fruits and vegetables at home.
- Distribute fruits and vegetable seeds at village level through gram panchayat.

- Encourage local farmers to use biological methods like composting to cultivate vegetables and fruits and educate them about harmful effect of pesticides on our body.

3.6. Health Benefits of Locally Available Fruits and Vegetables

Name of fruits and vegetable	Nutrients and Health benefits
Red and pink fruits and vegetables Papaya Tomato Pomegranate Guava Watermelon Beetroot Red apple Kidney bean	Lycopene and Anthocyanin Lycopene, Ellagic acid, Quercetin, Hesperidin Reduces risk of prostate cancer Helps to lower blood pressure Reduces cholesterol Reduces harmful effect of free radicals
Blue or purple fruits and vegetables Black Currants Brinjal Raisins	**Lutein, Zeaxanthin, Resveratrol, vitamin c, fiber, flavonoids, Ellagic acid, Quercetin** Good for eye health Decrease LDL cholesterol Improve immune system Increase calcium and other mineral absorption Decrease tumor growth Act as anticarcinogen in GI tract

Name of fruits and vegetable	Nutrients and Health benefits
Green vegetables Green leafy vegetables Green peas Beans Cucumber Green pepper Spinach Ladies finger	**Contains Lutein and Zeaxanthin, chlorophyll, fiber, folate, vitamin C, Beta carotene** Reduce risk of cancer Lower blood pressure Reduce LDL cholesterol level Boost immune system Reduce harmful effect of free radicals
Yellow/orange Carrot Mango Pineapple Orange Lemon Sweet potato	**Beta carotene, Zeaxanthin, flavonoids, Lycopene, Potassium, vitamin C** **Beta Carotene:** Powerful antioxidant which reduces the risk of cancer, heart disease, boosts immune system, slows aging and helps in maintaining good eyesight. **Bioflavonoids**: Work with vitamin C to strengthen bones and teeth, heal wounds, keep skin healthy.
	These orange foods also give us the right amount of potassium and vitamin A, which keep our eyes and skin healthy, and protect against infections. They are also known to boost the immune system because of the vitamin C content in them.

Name of fruits and vegetable	Nutrients and Health benefits
White vegetables	
Garlic	**Allicin, beta-glucan, lignans**
Onion	Allicin helps to lower cholesterol and blood pressure and increases the ability to fight against infections
Mushrooms	Beta-glucan and lignans activate B and T cells, reduce the risk of colon cancer, breast cancer and prostate cancer. The selenium in mushrooms helps prevent cancer.

3.7 Overweight and Obesity

Impact of overweight and obesity are costing a lot in the national economy. There are 43 million children who are estimated to be overweight (WHO, 2009).[7] It attributes to 44% of DM burden, 23% of ischemic heart disease burden and 7–41% of certain cancer burdens.

Baby friendly initiatives had created an impact on complementary feeding practices. The provision of Amrut through aganwadies for infants and adolescent girls and lactating and pregnant mothers along with health education had made people aware of healthy dietary practices. Curtailing of advertisement on junk food needs to be implemented properly along with other measures mentioned above for promoting good dietary practices. Increasing tax on fast foods may be required as education itself is not enough. The best chance for success is to increase tax per ounce on sugar-sweetened beverages.[10]

4.0 Promoting Physical Activities

Physical activity is an innate characteristic of human beings. Human history reveals that physical demands were typical of daily life and were an expected part of everyday life. The characteristics of movement made mankind have progress. Human beings not only survived but flourished for several thousand generations prior to the advent of the automobile, television, video games and the Internet. The technological advancements in the modern era made people have an easy life with machines and robots. Many of the non-communicable diseases of today are associated fundamentally with the pervasive sedentariness of modern life. Physical activity has a biological basis with central control and there is an inherent need to be exercised. Physical inactivity disturbs normal functions and contributes to chronic energy imbalance.[8, 9, 10]

4.1 Simple Steps to Promote Physical Activities

American Heart association proposes certain tips to promote physical activities as follows:

4.1.1 At home

- Carry out all household work yourself instead of hiring someone else to do it.
- Do some garden work and feel the happiness.
- Go out for a short walk before breakfast, after dinner or both! Start with 5–10 minutes and work up to 30 minutes.
- Walk to the nearby shops instead of driving.
- When walking, pick up the pace from leisurely to brisk. Choose a hilly route.
- While watching TV, sit up instead of lying on the sofa. While watching TV pedal on your stationary bicycle. Try not to use remote controls. Get your drinks by yourself rather than asking someone to bring it.
- Stand up while talking on the telephone.

- Park farther away at the shopping mall and walk the extra distance.
- Stretch and get items in high places and squat or bend to look at items at floor level.
- Keep exercise equipment always in working condition and use it!

4.1.2 At work place

- Use stairs whenever possible.
- Park your vehicle far and walk to the office.
- Engage in walk meetings.
- Participate in sponsored walks and fun run as a team from your institution.
- Formulate a sports team in office.
- Walk around the building in break time, if possible.

4.2 Harmful Effects of Physical Inactivity

The fourth leading risk factor for NCDs is physical inactivity. It is an independent risk factor for cardiorespiratory health, metabolic health, musculoskeletal health, cancer and mental health[8]. Moderate to vigorous activity should be planned and performed by individuals to promote health. Domains of activity can be recreation and sports, transportation as far as possible by walk or cycling, household chores, work at school and work place.

Results from laboratory studies, clinical trials and epidemiological investigations provide convincing evidence that increasing one's level of physical activity—especially for those who are sedentary—has multiple beneficial health effects. These include reducing the risk of prematurely dying from coronary heart disease (CHD), type 2 diabetes and colon cancer. Endurance-type exercise can improve mental health, and reduce the risk of developing obesity and osteoporosis. Regular physical activity also preserves functional independence in older adults. Among adults and older adults, physical activity can lower the risk of:

- Early death
- Coronary heart disease
- Stroke
- High blood pressure
- Type 2 diabetes
- Breast and colon cancer
- Falls
- Depression[8, 9, 10]

4.3 Benefits of Physical Activity

- Physical activity relaxes and lowers cholesterol (LDL) and triglycerides in the blood.
- It is the best way to increase HDL cholesterol (good cholesterol) in the blood.
- It lowers blood pressure.
- It prevents diabetes by improving glucose control in diabetes by increasing insulin sensitivity and bringing the glucose level close to normal.
- It promotes weight control.
- It reduces risk for developing myocardial infarction, stroke, diabetes, colon and breast cancers.

- It is one of the best ways to reduce stress.

Among children and adolescents, physical activity can:

- Improve bone health.
- Improve cardiorespiratory and muscular fitness.
- Decrease levels of body fat.
- Reduce symptoms of depression.

4.4 Recommended Schedule of Physical Activities for Different Age Groups[8, 13]

There will be questions on what type of activities, how often and for how long and how much in total?

4.4.1 Children and youth

Children and youth are advised to do at least 60 minutes of moderate to vigorous intensity physical activity daily. Physical activity for more than 60 minutes has additional health benefits. Most of the activity can be aerobic. Vigorous intensity activities increase muscle strength and bone strength. Such activities must be done at least 3 times per week.

4.4.2 Adults aged 18-64 years

Adults aged 18–64 should do at least 150 minutes of moderate intensity aerobic physical activity. This can be spread throughout the week or at least 75 minutes of vigorous intensity aerobic physical activity should be done biweekly. Aerobic activities should be performed in bouts of at least 10 minutes. Increasing the time and type of activity has added health benefits. It is better to do muscle strengthening activities involving major muscle groups on 2 or more days a week.

4.4.3 Older people of 65 years and above

Older adults with poor mobility should perform physical activity 3 or more days in a week to enhance balance and prevent falls. Muscle strengthening exercises should be done involving the major muscles. If they have health problems that do not permit them to have such activities, they should be active according to their permissive limits as their abilities permit.

People should change their lifestyle of using more automotive for short distance travel. Use walking as a means of travel for short distance. As far as possible, curtail the use of lifts when it is possible to climb stairs. Use bicycle for short distance travel. It saves fuel and promotes health. Create social network groups for physical activities in the local area. Make local facilities for play activities. Ensure that the working population has facilities for their physical activities in the work place and also at their local area. Find space for local recreation facilities.[13]

4.5 Supportive Policies in Promoting Physical Activity

- Ensure that walking, cycling and other forms of physical activity are accessible and safe.

- Provide local play facilities for children (e.g., building walking trails and panchayat grounds or other public places for play activities).

- Facilitate transport to work (e.g., cycling and walking and other physical activity strategies) for the sedentary working population.

- Ensure that schools provide physical education classes and play grounds to support the provision of opportunities and programs for physical activity.

- Provide schools with safe and appropriate spaces and facilities so that students can be physically active.

- Provide advice or counsel in primary care.
- Create social networks that encourage physical activity.

5.0 Public Health Intervention to Tackle Some Risk Factors That Contribute to Non-Communicable Disease and Health Promotion

5.1 Health Promotion

Health promotion is very relevant today. There are various approaches to health promotion. They are **setting based approach, population-based approach, and issue based approach**. **Setting based approach** acknowledges the interrelationship between the environment and humans. E.g., healthy cities, villages, schools, markets, etc. The setting based approach builds on the principles of community participation, partnership, empowerment and equity and replaces an over reliance on individual methods with a more holistic and multidisciplinary approach to integrate action across risk factors. Healthy cities program launched by WHO in 1986 was followed by all similar initiatives like health promoting schools and healthy work places.[9]

5.1.1. Population-based approaches

Address needs of diverse population groups like children, women, lactating mothers, adolescent girls, elderly or workers.

Up-scaled population interventions are health promoting interventions to reduce the risk factors that contribute to non-communicable disease in the whole community. Traditional preventive measures are not effective in low and middle-income countries. Up-scaled population intervention addresses many factors and it could influence a larger population.[14]

Approaches to implement the up-scaled population interventions are health education, social marketing, community mobilization, structural environmental change and social change, policies and legislative initiatives.

5.2 Approaches

5.2.1 To reduce tobacco use:

- In order to reduce the tobacco use, increase the tax on tobacco products. It has been seen that taxation is a means to change behavior.
- Restrict smoking in public places.
- Mass health education on health impact of smoking and dependence on tobacco.
- Prohibition of advertisement on tobacco use.
- Health warning on tobacco package reduces the demand.
- Creative mass media campaigns against tobacco use.

It is also important to inform the public and use behavioral change communication model to include 6 policies by WHO to reverse the tobacco epidemic **(MPOWER)**.[11]

- **M**onitor tobacco use and prevention policies.
- **P**rotect people from tobacco smoke.
- **O**ffer help to quit tobacco use.
- **W**arn about the dangers of tobacco.
- **E**nforce bans on tobacco advertising, promotion and sponsorship.
- **R**aise taxes on tobacco.

The tobacco experience proved that education is not enough: regulation, litigation and legislature are important too. The best example for this is the verdict given by the Honorable High Court of Kerala prohibiting smoking in places and levying high penalty on those who do so.

5.2.2 To reduce harmful use of alcohol:

- Increase the excise tax on alcoholic beverages
- Regulate availability of alcoholic beverages by
  - ✓ Limiting minimum legal purchase age.
  - ✓ Dispensing of alcohol only for the person who produces the identity which proves age.
  - ✓ Limit outlet density and time of sale.
  - ✓ Observing dry day.
  - ✓ Limit the quantity of alcohol that a person can keep in hand.
  - ✓ Strict regulation on licensing outlets.
- Drink-driving counter measures
  - ✓ Random check points, breath test and Blood alcohol concentration (blood alcohol concentration limit is 0.03% or 30µl alcohol in 100 ml blood).
  - ✓ Penalties for drunk driving.
- Prohibit advertisement of alcohol.
- Health warning label shall be mandatory on bottles of alcoholic beverage.
- Compulsory health warning labels in TV shows where scenes are related to alcohol or tobacco use.
- Public education and mass media campaign on harmful effect of alcohol and alcohol dependence.
- Restrict illicit production and use of alcohol.
- Conduct school health programs and involve teachers to teach the ill effects of alcohol consumption.

5.2.3 To promote physical activity:

- Make physical fitness mandatory for all jobs.
- Include physical fitness as a component in recruitment policy.
- Include physical training in school curriculum and provide time for physical training in each day.
- Renovate unused public spaces for recreational purposes.
- Provide street gyms and fixed exercise equipment in local parks.
- Introduce sports interest groups in workplaces.
- Establish walking clubs in local communities.
- Stick posters that encourage use of stairs near elevators and escalators.

5.2.4 To promote healthy diet:

- Display posters of healthy dietary choices in workplace canteens, community centers and local recreational areas.
- Encourage local restaurants, hospitals and workplace canteens to add less salt and oil in food preparation and to use healthier cooking methods.
- Encourage local farmers to cultivate fruits and vegetables and establish markets to provide healthy food.
- Encourage health professionals to screen and support dietary change.
- Encourage farmers to use organic methods to cultivate fruits and vegetables rather than using chemicals and pesticides.

6.0 Legal Movement by Government of India against Use of Tobacco and Alcohol Consumption

6.1 Tobacco Control Measures

- The Government enacted the Cigarettes and Other Tobacco Products Act (COTPA), in 2002. The provisions under the act include:

  ✓ Prohibition of public place smoking

  ✓ Prohibition of advertisements of tobacco products, prohibition on sale of tobacco products to and by minors (persons below 18 years)

  ✓ Ban on sale of tobacco products within 100 yards of all educational institutions

  ✓ Mandatory display of pictorial health warnings on tobacco products packages

  ✓ Testing all tobacco products for their tar and nicotine content

- The Cable Television Networks (Amendment) Act in 2000 prohibited tobacco advertisement in state controlled electronic media and publications including cable television.

- In 2004, the Government approved the WHO Framework Convention on Tobacco Control (WHO FCTC), which gives strategies to reduce demand and supply of tobacco.

6.1.1 Demand reduction strategies include price and tax measures and non-price measures

Price and tax measures include increasing the prices of such commodities that are categorized as high risks factors and increase their sale taxes so that it will not be easily available to everyone.

Non-price measures are

- ✓ statutory warnings,
- ✓ comprehensive ban on advertisements,
- ✓ Tobacco product regulation.

6.1.2 The supply reduction strategies

- ✓ Combating illicit trade.
- ✓ Providing alternative livelihood to tobacco farmers and workers.
- ✓ Regulating sale to and by minors.

6.2 Measures to Reduce Alcohol Consumption

- The laws which regulate the sale and consumption of alcohol vary significantly from state to state in India; consumption of alcohol is prohibited in the states of Gujarat, Manipur, Mizoram and Nagaland.
- The Blood Alcohol Content (BAC) legal limit is 0.03% or 30 µl alcohol in 100 ml blood.
- According to motor vehicle act higher penalties were introduced, including fines from 2,000 to 10,000 and imprisonment from 6 months to 4 years.
- Dry Days are specific days when the sale of alcohol is not permitted. Most of the Indian states observe these days on major national festivals/occasions such as Republic Day (January 26), Independence Day (August 15) and Gandhi Jayanti (October 2). Dry days are also observed on and around voting days.
- According to cable television amendment bill advertising alcoholic beverages is prohibited in India.

7.0 Issue Based Approach

Targets a wide range of determinants of health or risk factors (diet, smoking, unsafe sex, road safety, patient safety, etc.)

Community-Based Initiatives for the Prevention of Non-Communicable Diseases

Chronic non-communicable diseases (NCDs) such as Cardiovascular diseases, Cancer, Chronic lung diseases and Diabetes are the leading cause of death in the world. In the South-East Asia Region of WHO, they accounted for 54% of deaths in 2005. On the basis of available data, by 2020, NCDs are estimated to account for 73% of deaths and 60% of the disease burden (WHO, 2005). A combination of a population or community-based approach and an individual-focused intervention is important in preventing NCDs. Health workers can use behavior change communication model in planning community-based programs. Along with bringing in behavioral changes, the community action includes strengthening the community, encouraging it to act as change agent and helping it to use its own resources for action.

Awareness level of the community has to be raised so as to change risk perceptions. By providing simple tools, technologies and lifestyle choices the community can be motivated towards adoption of the actions appropriate to them, which will lead to preventing NCDs. Since early 1970s, a number of community-based health intervention projects have started in developed countries. WHOs regional office for the Eastern Mediterranean introduced the following Community-Based Initiatives:

– Basic development needs approach (BDN)

– Health villages programs (HVP)

- Healthy neighborhood programs (HNP)
- Healthy cities programs (HCP)
- Healthy lifestyle programs
- Women in Health and development

These community-based initiatives provided a new stimulus for health and human developments and have initiated a transformation process whereby communities are playing an active role. Multi-sectoral government functionaries are providing support for sustainable local development in order to improve the quality of life and health of the people.

7.1 How Community-Based Initiatives Bring about Changes

Changes take place through the following actions:

- Encouraging change in self and society.
- Introducing intersectoral coordination and partnership.
- Breaking the vicious cycle of dependency through active community participation.
- Developing awareness among the masses concerning coping with problems, practicing healthy lifestyles and health care measures.
- Encouraging decentralization and local empowerment for bottom-up planning and self-management.
- Mobilizing local and public resources.
- Transforming the attitude of government functionaries to be more supportive of the community.
- Improving health status through increased family income and self-care.
- Reducing poverty and improving quality of life and health.

Community-based initiatives can successfully solve all the issues related with NCDs, if done in a well-organized manner. All traditional medicines and practices contribute to health and wellness of the people. WHO urge people across the globe to practice yoga in their daily lives. Such practices will reduce the risk of non-communicable diseases including heart diseases, diabetes and respiratory diseases.

Yoga can be practiced anywhere by people of all age groups, irrespective of their socio-economic status. It fits in very well with the healthy lifestyle that WHO has been strongly advocating, throughout the lifecycle, from childhood to healthy aging. Yoga is mostly viewed as a helpful form of exercise that focuses on easing the body into several postures which are intended to increase flexibility, balance and strength and enhance one's sense of well-being.

There are different styles of yoga including Hatha, Ashtanga, Iyengar and many more which help to prevent various diseases. People who practice yoga report a deep sense of relaxation, substantially increased flexibility and blood and oxygen supply after regular classes.

The practice of **yoga** helps in preventing all non-communicable diseases which are often caused by hectic lifestyle and internal stress. Including yoga in daily regimen can help to maintain the level of sugar in blood, along with a normal BP rate and body weight.[13]

Just as in yoga, practicing meditation regularly for a few minutes acts as an excellent stress-buster for the mind and body. It also helps in restoring one's confidence level to fight any condition including Cancer, COPD, Hypertension and Diabetes Mellitus.

8.0 Public Health Laws and NCDs

The public health laws can help much in preventing the occurrence of non-communicable diseases. Some of those laws are:

1. Protecting people from tobacco smoke and banning tobacco in public places.
2. Warning about the dangers of tobacco use.
3. Enforcing bans on tobacco advertising, promotion and sponsorship.
4. Raising taxes on tobacco.
5. Restricting access to retailed alcohol.
6. Enforcing bans on alcohol advertising.
7. Raising taxes on alcohol.
8. Reducing salt intake and salt content of food.
9. Replacing Trans-fats in food with polysaturated fat.
10. Promoting public awareness about diet and physical activity through mass media.

When thinking about risk reduction strategies, one needs to think on best buys and good buys as far as the public laws are concerned.

9.0 Grass Root Level Prevention

Grass root level prevention is aimed at preventing NCDs by teaching children healthy lifestyle habits during their early developmental period itself. Children are the future of a nation. Health of children is the actual wealth of a nation. But today due to demographic changes, globalization and lifestyle transitions, there has been a significant increase in the risk of non-communicable diseases even among children. Grass root level risk reduction strategies should start from childhood onwards. A recent study conducted in one of the affluent schools in Kerala had found that type 2 diabetes exists in children as young as 9 years of age. The other NCDs that have an impact, especially on school-age children, include injuries, oral diseases, stress and mental illnesses, which result in a reduced quality of life and poor academic performance of children. Habits are developed in childhood and school children and adolescents are more receptive to behavioral changes. It is wise to start strategies for primordial prevention among school children to curtail risk factors early in life and promote healthy living to prevent development of NCDs. It is also important because many NCDs have their roots in exposure to risk factors and unhealthy habits established during childhood and adolescence. So it is essential to empower school teachers, school children, their parents and community on aspects of healthy living throughout the life span.

School children should be taught on topics like healthy nutrition, benefits of physical activity, harmful effects of tobacco and alcohol, importance of mental health and risk of bad behaviors. Behavioral change communication strategies must be utilized in empowering the young and youth to risks mainly related to exposure to 4 key risk factors: unhealthy diet, physical inactivity, tobacco use and the harmful use of alcohol.

Key Points

NCDs take a heavy toll on human life and productivity prematurely. If individuals follow risk reduction strategies by modifying the life style by curtailing the distal determinants and proximal determinants as causes of risk factors, NCDs can be prevented. Health care professionals should concentrate on best buys and good buys that are advocated by WHO as risk reduction strategies. A **best buy** is an intervention that is highly cost-effective and cheap. It is feasible and culturally acceptable to implement. **Good buys** are interventions that may cost more than best buys or generate less health gain but still provide good value for money.

The most common best buys and good buys suggested by WHO are:

For tobacco use

Best buys are protecting people from tobacco smoke, warning about the dangers of tobacco, enforcing ban on tobacco advertising, and raising tax on tobacco and its products. The good buy is to offer counseling to smokers.

For alcohol use

Best buys are restricting access to retailed alcohol, enforcing bans on alcohol advertising, and raising tax on alcohol. The good buys are enforcing drink-driving laws (breath testing) and offering brief advice on hazards of drinking.

For unhealthy diet

The best buys are restricting marketing of fast and junk foods and alcoholic beverages to children, replacing saturated fat with unsaturated fat, managing food taxes and subsidies, offering counseling in primary care, providing health education in work sites and promoting healthy eating in schools.

For physical inactivity

The best buys are promoting physical activity through mass media, promoting physical activity in communities, supporting active transport strategies, and promoting physical activity in schools and colleges. Another best buy to prevent liver cancer is to provide hepatitis B vaccination.

References

1. Reddy, SK (July 2003) "Prevention and control of non-communicable diseases: status and strategies" Indian council for research on international economic relations,

Core-6A, 4ᵗʰ Floor, India Habitat Center, Lodi Road, New Delhi-110 003.

2. Anand K. Report on Assessment of Burden of Major Non-communicable disease in India. World Health Organization, New Delhi, March 2000.

3. Allison DB and Casey DE "Antipsychotic-induced weight gain: a review of literature" J Clin. Psychiatry, 2001: 62 Suppl. 7: 22–31.

4. CR Chandrasekhar's presentation, Jan 9, 2012 uploaded by Napsonic.

5. www.clipart.com.

6. Simopoulos AP "Nutrition and Fitness, Cultural, Genetic and Metabolic aspects" World Review on Nutrition and Dietetics. Vol. 98. 2006.

7. Indian Council of Medical Research. Nutrient Requirements and Recommended.

8. Dietary Allowances for Indians, National Institute of Nutrition, Hyderabad (2010), retrieved on July 2015 from icmr.nic.in (Preventing non-communicable diseases, Promoting fruit and vegetable consumption, World Health Organization 2010).

9. WHO (2010) Global Status report on non-communicable disease, Reprint, 2011. 20 Avenue Appia, 1211 Geneva 27, Switzerland.

10. Global Action Plan for the prevention and control of Non-communicable diseases, 2013–2020, Printed by the WHO, 2008 Document Production Services, Geneva, Switzerland.

11. Rose G (1992) The strategy of preventive medicine. Oxford: Oxford University Press.

12. Cherian Varghese: Health Promotion for NCD Prevention, Jan 25, 2011 WHO, Western Pacific Region, 201. Vol.1.

13. Dietary Allowances for Indians, National Institute of Nutrition, Hyderabad (2010), retrieved on July 2015 fromicmr.nic.in.

14. www.healthbridge.ca. Physical Activity and NCD prevention: A development Agenda for research.

15. Dyson PA, Anthony D, Fenton B, Stevens DE, Champagne B, Li LM, et al. (2015) Successful Up-scaled Population Interventions to Reduce Risk Factors for Non-Communicable Disease in Adults: Results from the International Community Interventions for Health (CIH) Project in China, India and Mexico. PLoS ONE 10(4).

16. Action plan for global strategy for prevention and control of non-communicable disease. Geneva, World Health Organization, 2008. Retrieved on July 2015 from Action plan for global strategy for prevention and control of no communicable disease. Geneva, World Health Organization, 2008.

Chapter IV

Strengthening Health System Infrastructure for Combating Non-Communicable Diseases

Dr. Jogindra Vati

Cardiovascular diseases, Diabetes, Cancers and Chronic Respiratory Diseases are common Non-Communicable Diseases (NCDs), also known as chronic diseases which are of slow progression and of long duration. These are preventable diseases as they are linked with lifestyle factors such as intake of unhealthy diets, physical inactivity, tobacco use, and consumption of excessive alcohol. Various steps and strategies have been taken and initiated to prevent and control NCDs. Strengthening health system infrastructure is one of the important strategies to combat these NCDs.

Cardiovascular Diseases

Cardiovascular diseases (CVDs) are the leading cause of death globally and account for most NCD deaths. An estimated 17.5 million people died due to CVDs in 2012, which means 3 in every 10 deaths, representing 31% of all global deaths. Of these, 7.4 million people died of ischemic heart disease and 6.7 million from stroke. The incidences of CVDs have gone up significantly for people between the ages of 25 and 69 to 24.8%, thus losing more productive people to these diseases. (WHO, 2014 May)

In India, there has been an alarming increase in the prevalence of CVDs over the past 2 decades. According to government data, the prevalence of heart failure in India due to coronary heart disease, hypertension, obesity, diabetes and rheumatic heart disease ranges from anywhere between 1.3 to 4.6 million, with an annual incidence of 491,600 to 1.8 million (Singh, 2015).

According to WHO (2014 May), Cardiovascular diseases (CVDs) are a group of disorders of the heart and blood vessels which include: coronary heart disease (disease of the blood vessels supplying the heart muscle); cerebrovascular disease (disease of the blood vessels supplying the brain); peripheral arterial disease (disease of blood vessels supplying the arms and legs); rheumatic heart disease (damage to the heart muscle and heart valves from rheumatic fever, caused by streptococcal bacteria); congenital heart disease (malformations of heart structure existing at birth); deep vein thrombosis and pulmonary embolism (blood clots in the leg veins, which can dislodge and move to the heart and lungs). Coronary heart disease, hypertension, dyslipidemia and stroke are discussed below.

Coronary Heart Disease

Coronary heart disease (CHD) is the most common type of cardiovascular disease. It is caused due to narrowing and damage of coronary arteries supplying to the heart, mainly due to deposition of cholesterol, calcium and formation of plaques or atherosclerosis (hardening of the arteries due to lipids deposition) resulting in its blockage and reduced blood flow to heart.

This disease is gradual and progressive in nature and goes unnoticed, and may take many years to develop clinical manifestations. The person experiences chest pain (angina) and breathlessness due to reduced blood flow and oxygenation to heart; and complete blockage of the artery may lead to heart attack or myocardial infarction.

Coronary heart disease is the major cause of mortality and morbidity globally. Out of total deaths due to CVDs, an estimated 7.4 million died due to coronary heart disease. In India, approximate

45 million people, out of the estimated population of 1.27 billion suffer from CAD; 7–13% in urban and 2–7% in rural India. A conservative estimate indicates that there could be 30 million CHD patients in India, of whom 14 million are in urban and 16 million in rural areas. If the current trend continues, by the year 2020 the burden of this disease in India will surpass other regions of the world. (Kaul & Bhatia, 2010)

Manifestation of Coronary Heart Disease

The manifestations of CAD are chronic stable angina, acute coronary syndrome or sudden cardiac death, heart failure. Ischemic heart disease was the leading cause of death globally, killing 7.4 million people (13.2%) in the world as compared to 6 million deaths in 2000. In India also, it was the leading cause of death, killing 1215.4 thousand people (12.4%) in 2012. (WHO, 2015, Global Health Observatory (GHO) data)

Factors contributing to Coronary Heart Diseases

In India, many risk factors seem to accelerate coronary heart disease in recent time. These factors are i) non-modifiable risk factors such as men ≥45 years and women ≥55 years of age are having risk of CADs, persons having family history of early heart diseases, and familial hypercholesterolemia are at risk for CADs; ii) modifiable (behavioral) risk factors include persons taking unhealthy diet, diet rich in saturated fats and cholesterol, fast food, food rich in salt, increased salt intake, lack of adequate physical exercise, sedentary lifestyle, physical inactivity, tobacco usage, mental stress and depression and harmful use of alcohol which lead to metabolic/physiological changes including raised blood pressure, raised blood glucose, elevated serum lipids, overweight and obesity. An elevated serum lipid level indicates increased risk of developing *atherosclerosis*. The primary reason for insufficient blood flow to heart is the narrowing of coronary arteries by atherosclerosis. When the artery is 75% or more obstructed, it leads to *ischemia* (decreased supply of oxygen to heart or increased demand for oxygen) secondary to atherosclerosis, which is a major cause of CAD. Social, economic and cultural driving forces, globalization, population aging, and urbanization have changed the behavioral patterns or the life style of people at large resulting in increased prevalence of CADs. (WHO, 2014, Global status of report on non-communicable diseases) (Figure 4.1)

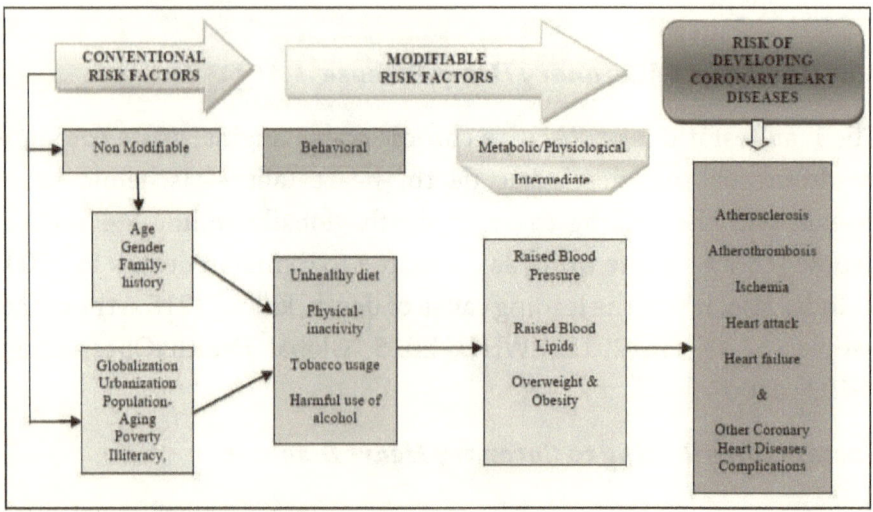

Fig. 4.1: *Factors contributing to Coronary Heart Diseases and other complications*

Hypertension

Hypertension is defined as a persistent systolic blood pressure ≥140 mmHg and/or diastolic blood pressure ≥90 mmHg, or individuals on antihypertensive medications (self-reported). (US Department of Health and Human Services, 2004 Aug)

It is also referred to as high blood pressure or raised blood pressure. Blood is carried from the heart to all parts of the body through blood vessels. Blood pressure is the force exerted by blood against the walls of the blood vessels (arteries). The normal adult blood pressure is 120 and diastolic blood pressure is 80 mm Hg. In raised blood pressure the heart has to pump blood harder. Raised blood pressure is one of the leading risk factors of cardiovascular disease. If uncontrolled it can lead to heart attack, enlargement of heart and heart failure, stroke, kidney failure or blindness.

The global prevalence of raised blood pressure can be gauged from the fact that 40% of adults aged 25 years and over had raised blood pressure in 2008. Out of approximately 17 million deaths due to CVDs, it contributes for 9.4 million deaths worldwide every year and is responsible for at least 45% of deaths due to heart disease and 51% of deaths due to stroke. Hypertensive heart disease is a major risk factor for CADs. Globally hypertensive heart disease caused 1.1 million (13.2%) deaths in 2012 as compared to 0.8 million deaths in 2000. (WHO, 2013 — A global brief on Hypertension: Silent killer, global public health crisis)

Prevalence of hypertension in India is 25% in urban and 10% in rural inhabitants. According to NCD Country profiles, 2014, raised blood pressure is the most prevalent risk factor of all in India (32.5%). A study of men and women aged 35–69 years in Mumbai showed that on average 20% had a medical history of hypertension, rising to 26% based on measurement of blood pressure (Pandey, 2010). It has been estimated that even 7–10% of schoolchildren in India suffer from hypertension and 15–16% have high cholesterol levels (Daniel et al., 2011). In terms of numbers, estimates suggest the number of people in India with hypertension will almost double, from 118.2 million in 2000 to 213.5 million by 2025 (Shokeen & Aeri, 2015).

Hypertension is a silent, invisible killer and is a global public health concern. It rarely causes symptoms in the early stages and sometimes hypertension causes symptoms like headache, dizziness, shortness of breath, chest pain, and palpitation of heart and nose bleed. If these symptoms are ignored, the consequences to heart and other organs will be higher, resulting in hypertensive heart disease, cardiovascular diseases, peripheral vascular diseases, nephron-sclerosis, or retinal damage.

Dyslipidemia

According to National Cholesterol Education Program (NCEP) guidelines, Dyslipidemia is defined as a person having hypercholesterolemia (serum cholesterol levels ≥200 mg/dl (≥5.2 m mol/l; hypertriglyceridemia (serum triglyceride levels ≥150 mg/dl (≥1.7 m mol/l); low HDL cholesterol (HDL cholesterol levels <40 mg/dl (<1.04 m mol/l) for men and <50 mg/dl (<1.3 m mol/l) for women); high LDL cholesterol (LDL cholesterol levels ≥130 mg/dl (≥3.4 m mol/l) calculated using the Friedewald equation); high total cholesterol to HDL-C ratio (a total cholesterol to HDL-C ratio of ≥4.5); isolated hypercholesterolemia (Serum cholesterol ≥200 mg/dl and triglycerides <150 mg/dl; isolated hypertriglyceridemia (Serum triglycerides ≥150 mg/dl and cholesterol <200 mg/dl); isolated low HDL-C (HDL-C ≤40 mg/dl (male) and ≤50 mg/dl (female) without hypertriglyceridemia or hypercholesterolemia) (Expert Panel on Detection, Evaluation, and Treatment of High Blood Cholesterol in Adults, 2001).

Prevalence of dyslipidemia is about 37.5% among adults of 15 to 64 years of age. Dyslipidemia has been closely linked to the pathophysiology of CVD and is a key independent modifiable risk factor for cardiovascular disease. People having unhealthy dietary habits (diet rich in saturated fat and cholesterol, lacking in complex carbohydrate, e.g. whole grains, fruits, and vegetables), lack of adequate physical exercise on a regular basis, use of tobacco, and obesity, have higher risk for Coronary Artery Disease.

Low Density Lipoproteins (LDLs) have more cholesterols and have an affinity for arterial walls. Both cholesterol and triglycerides are thought to be deposits in arterial walls. Elevated LDLs is closely correlated with an increased risk of developing atherosclerosis and CAD. Life style factors such as high alcohol consumption, high intake of refined carbohydrates and simple sugars, and physical inactivity can also contribute to elevated triglycerides. Diseases like type 2 diabetes and chronic renal failure are also associated with increased triglycerides. Increased risk for CAD is proportional to the degree of obesity. Obese persons are thought to produce higher level of LDLs and triglycerides than normal weight persons; moreover obesity is often associated with hypertension and having higher incidence of CAD **(Berra & Klieman, 2003).**

Stroke

A stroke or brain attack occurs due to inadequate or interruptions in the blood supply to brain, usually because of blockage (ischemic stroke) or rupture of blood vessels (hemorrhagic stroke). The most common symptom of a stroke is sudden weakness or numbness of the face, arm, or leg, usually on one side of the body. Other symptoms include: confusion, difficulty in speaking or understanding speech, difficulty in seeing with one or both eyes, dizziness, loss of balance or coordination, severe headache with no known cause, fainting or unconsciousness. Stroke can even cause a sudden death.

Stroke is a major public health concern. It is the second leading cause of death after CADs. It was reported that, in 2013, globally, there were nearly 25.7 million stroke survivors, 6.5 million deaths due to stroke, 113 million DALYs lost because of stroke, and 10.3 million new cases of strokes[1]. A majority of the stroke burden was observed in developing countries, accounting for 75.2% of all stroke-related deaths and 81.0% of the associated DALYs lost. **(N. Venkatasubramaniam, 2016)**

Stroke burden is projected to increase from around 38 million DALYs globally in 1990 to 61 million DALYs in 2020, along with the numbers of disabled stroke survivors and deaths related to stroke. It is estimated that, if current trends continue, by 2030 there will be 20 million annual stroke deaths and 70 million stroke survivors worldwide (Krishnamurthi et al., 2013). In India it caused 881.7 thousand (9%) deaths in 2012 and the estimated age-adjusted prevalence rate for stroke ranges between 84/100,000 and 262/100,000 in rural and between 334/100,000 and 424/100,000 in urban areas **(Stroke fact sheet India, Taylor & Kumar, 2012)**.

Certain racial, ethnic and socio-economic groups are also at greater risk of stroke. The most important modifiable cause of stroke is high blood pressure; for every 10 people who die of stroke, 4 could have been saved if their blood pressure had been regulated. Among those aged under 65, two-fifths of deaths from stroke are linked to smoking. Other modifiable risk factors include unhealthy diet, high salt intake, underlying heart disease, diabetes and high blood lipids (WHO, 2015, Global burden of stroke). It has been estimated that hypertension causes 54% of stroke in low-income and middle-income countries, followed by hypercholesterolemia (15%) and tobacco smoking (12%) **(Preventing stroke: saving lives around the world, Strong, Mathers, & Bonita, 2007)**.

Diabetes

Diabetes is a chronic multisystem disease, primarily a disorder of glucose metabolism in which either the pancreas does not produce sufficient insulin, or there is ineffective utilization of insulin produced by the body, or both, thus resulting in increased concentration of glucose level in the blood termed as hyperglycemia. Diabetes mellitus is described as a metabolic disorder of multiple etiologies characterized by chronic hyperglycemia with disturbances of carbohydrate, fat and protein metabolism resulting from defects in insulin secretion, insulin action, or both. The effects of diabetes mellitus include long-term damage, dysfunction and failure of various organs (WHO, 1999), especially the eyes, kidneys, nerves, heart, and blood vessels. The normal glucose range is approximately 70 to 120 mg/dl.

The classical symptoms due to hyperglycemia are increased thirst (polydipsia), increased urination (polyuria), increased hunger (polyphagia), and unexplained weight loss. The patient may feel weakness and fatigue, have blurred vision, become anemic, develop recurrent infections, prolonged wound healing and in the long-term if untreated, it will cause micro vascular and macro vascular complications. *Micro vascular complications* are due to damage to small blood vessels such as damage to eyes (retinopathy) leading to blindness and visual disability, to kidneys (nephropathy) leading to renal failure, and to nerves (neuropathy) leading to sensory loss, damage to limbs, impotence and foot disorders, possibly leading even to amputation due to severe infections. *Macro vascular complications* are the diseases of the large and medium sized blood vessels such as cardiovascular, cerebro-vascular and peripheral vascular diseases. Persons with diabetes have higher risk for developing macro vascular complication. The data revealed that 50% of people with diabetes die of cardiovascular disease **(Morrish et al., 2001).**

According to an International Expert Report 1997, diabetes is classified into 2 major forms of diabetes, insulin-dependent diabetes mellitus (IDDM, type 1 diabetes) and non-insulin-dependent diabetes mellitus (NIDDM, type 2 diabetes) **(The Expert Committee on the Diagnosis and Classification of Diabetes Mellitus, 1997).**

Type 1 Diabetes (T1D): It is also known as 'juvenile onset' or 'insulin-dependent' Diabetes Mellitus (IDDM). It usually develops in childhood and in adolescents, or people under 30 years of age, with a peak onset between ages 11 and 13, but can occur in any age. In this type of diabetes, T cells of its own body attack and destroy pancreatic beta (β) cells (insulin producing cells). It is of 2 types, autoimmune (Type 1A) and idiopathic (Type 1B). In autoimmune type of diabetes, genetic factors are predisposing to disease, while Type 1B diabetes is caused by non-immune factors of unknown origin. The patients with this type of diabetes require lifelong insulin therapy for survival.

The onset of T1D is rapid and initially clinical manifestations are acute and severe. Apart from classical symptoms, the patient experiences numbness in extremities, pain in feet (dysesthesias), fatigue and blurred vision. Loss of consciousness, severe nausea and vomiting due to ketoacidosis is more common in this type of diabetes. The patients may develop micro vascular and macro vascular complications.

The diagnosis is made by (i) the presence of classical symptoms of hyperglycemia, and (ii) a plasma glucose concentration >=7 m mol/L (or 126 mg/dL) or >= 11.1m mol/L (or 200 mg/dL) 2 hours after a 75g glucose drink, or without presence of classical symptoms with 2 abnormal blood tests done on separate days. Glycated hemoglobin (HbA1c) of 6.5% is recommended as the cut point for diagnosing diabetes. A value of less than 6.5% does not exclude diabetes diagnosed using glucose tests. **(WHO, 2015, About Diabetes)**

Type 2 Diabetes (T2D): This is the most prevalent type of diabetes, representing 90% cases worldwide. Earlier this type of diabetes was known as non-insulin-dependent diabetes mellitus (NIDDM). It usually occurs in adulthood but is on the rise in children and adolescents. It is related to obesity, lack of physical activity, and unhealthy diets and involves insulin resistance. It is associated with hypertension, Dyslipidemia, and central obesity. It may be caused due to genetic and environmental factors. The treatment may involve lifestyle changes and weight loss alone, or in combination with oral medications or with addition of insulin injections. Those who are affected by T2D are at higher risk of getting micro vascular and macro vascular complications.

The onset of Type 2 diabetes is gradual; initially the patient may have no symptoms at all or minimal symptoms for years before being diagnosed. The patients have similar symptoms as in Type 1 diabetes. Loss of consciousness is less common. Diagnosis is made similar to T1D.

Other Categories of Diabetes Are

i. **Pre-diabetes:** Pre-diabetes is condition in which there is impaired glucose tolerance (IGT) which is higher than normal plasma glucose concentration 2 hours after 75 gram oral glucose load, but less than the diagnostic cut-off for diabetes; and impaired fasting glucose (IFG), i.e., blood glucose level higher than normal (>100 mg/dl but <126 mg/dl). Such patients are not diagnosed as diabetic. The patients with pre-diabetes have high risk for developing type 2 Diabetes.

ii. **Gestational diabetes mellitus (GDM):** This type of diabetes develops during pregnancy. According to American Diabetes Association it is defined as glucose intolerance of varying degree with onset or first recognition during pregnancy. Depending on the population studied and criteria used for diagnosis, the prevalence may range from 2.4 to 21% of all pregnancies (Schmidt et al., 2001). This is related to increasing urbanization, physical inactivity, changes in dietary patterns and increasing prevalence of obesity. The women with gestational diabetes and their children are at risk of developing diabetes in future, and risks during pregnancy itself such as congenital malformations, increased birth weight and perinatal mortality.

Polydipsia and polyuria are the most common symptoms; other symptoms may also present. During prenatal checkup, the larger baby than normal may indicate GDM. Glucose tolerance test is done at 24–28 weeks of pregnancy after an overnight fasting for fasting plasma glucose level and a plasma glucose 2 hours after 75g glucose drink (postprandial). A 2 hour level >=7.8 m mol/L (or 140 mg/dL) is diagnostic of gestational diabetes. If fasting and postprandial blood sugars are elevated in the first trimester, this may indicate pre-existing diabetes mellitus and may not be GDM.

iii. **Secondary diabetes:** Secondary diabetes occurs because of other medical conditions or due to treatment of a medical condition that causes increased blood glucose levels. These conditions include pancreatic diseases, metabolic diseases, endocrinopathies, drugs and chemical induced (e.g., corticosteroids, thiazides, atypical antipsychotics), infections, immune mediated, and genetic syndrome. This type of diabetes can result from damage or injury to pancreas and usually resolves when underlying condition is treated.

Magnitude of Diabetes

According to WHO, globally 347 million people worldwide have diabetes. The global prevalence was estimated to be 9% among adults 18 years and older (WHO, 2014, Global status report on non-communicable diseases). In 2012, an estimated 1.5 million (2.7%) deaths were caused due to diabetes, up from 1.0 million (2.0%) deaths in 2000, and it is projected that it will be double between 2005 and 2030, and will be the 7th leading cause of death. More than 80% of people with diabetes deaths occur in low and middle-income countries **(Mathers & Loncar, 2005; WHO, 2015, Global Health Estimates).**

The International Diabetes Federation reported that 387 million people worldwide have diabetes as on 2014, and it will increase to 592 million by 2035. It caused 4.9 million deaths and 179 million people with diabetes are undiagnosed. In 2013, more than 79,000 children developed type-1 diabetes, type-2 diabetes is increasing and more than 21 million live births were affected by diabetes during pregnancy. 77% of people with diabetes live in low and middle-income countries **(International Diabetes Federation, 2014).**

Factors associated with increased risk of developing type-1 diabetes are people having family history; and certain environmental factors and viral infections have been linked with the pathogenesis of immune-related type1 diabetes. Multiple modifiable and non-modifiable factors are associated with increased risk for developing type 2 diabetes. The main associated modifiable factor is obesity (specifically abdominal and visceral adiposity) which is associated with rising living standards, steady urban migration and life style changes, consuming unhealthy diet, excessive calorie intake, higher dietary glycemic load and trans-fat (vegetable and animal ghee used for cooking), higher consumption of sugar-sweetened beverages and food items, consumption of grains changed from coarse grains to policed rice and refined wheat, physical inactivity, lack of regular exercise and changing dietary habits. High blood pressure, elevated cholesterol level, family history of diabetes, history of gestational diabetes, poor nutrition during pregnancy, increased age and smoking also contribute towards the development of type 2 diabetes **(International Diabetes Federation, 2015; Frank, 2011).**

Cancer or Neoplasm

Cancer or neoplasm is an uncontrolled and unregulated growth and spread of cells. It is a large group of more than 200 diseases of multiple causes, characterized by defective proliferation and defective differentiation of any cell of the body and capable of invading adjoining parts of the body and spreading to other organ/s termed as metastasis.

Cancer is a major public health problem and leading cause of morbidity and mortality worldwide, accounting for 14 million new cases and 8.2 million deaths in 2012. It is expected that annual cancer cases will be 22 million (about 70%) within the next 2 decades. The most common sites of cancer cases diagnosed were breast, colorectum, lung, cervix, and stomach. The most common causes of cancer death are cancers of lung (1.6 million or 2.9% deaths), liver (745 000 deaths), stomach (723 000 deaths), colorectal (694 000 deaths), breast (521 000 deaths), and esophageal cancer (400 000 deaths). Lung cancer was the 5th leading cause of death **(Bernard & Christopher, 2014).**

An estimated 683,500 deaths (357,000 males and 326,300 females) in India were caused by cancer. Among women, 21.5% deaths occurred due to breast cancer, followed by cervix uterus cancer (20.7%) and among males, 18.3% deaths occurred due to mouth and oropharynx cancer (WHO, 2014, Cancer Country Profiles-2014). The incidence of cancer is low in India as compared to high-income countries, but incidence is projected to rise to 1.7 million individuals in 2035. Breast cancer (145 000 cases per year), tobacco-related head and neck cancers (141 000), cervical cancer (123 000), lung cancer (70 000), large bowel cancer (64 000), and stomach cancer (63 000) accounted for more than half of the burden in 2012 **(IARC, WHO, 2015, GLOBOCAN – 2012).**

Cancer is a genetic complex disease caused primarily by environmental or *external factors*. The external factors include i) physical carcinogen such as ultraviolet and ionizing radiation; ii) chemical carcinogens such as component of tobacco smoke, asbestos, aflatoxin (a food contaminant) and arsenic (a drinking water contaminant) and; iii) biological carcinogens such as infections from certain viruses, bacteria or parasites. Carcinogen agents are present in polluted air, water, food, chemicals, sunlight, and indoor smoke that the people are exposed to it.

Cancer is developed in 3 stages: initiation, promotion and progression stage. In the *initiation stage*, due to inherited mutation, or following exposure to physical, chemical, biological carcinogen agents, there is a mutation in the cell's genetic structure and the cell develops into a clone or a group of identical cells of neoplastic cells. This stage is usually irreversible and additive, but not all these cells go on to establish a tumor. Altered cell has dysfunction in differentiation and proliferation which turns into a cancer or neoplastic cell. The second stage in the development of cancer is *promotion stage*. This stage is characterized by reversible proliferation of altered cells with increased additional mutation. The behavior and dietary risk factors such as obesity, smoking, dietary fat, alcohol consumption, etc. exert activity against specific types of body tissues or organs. Lifestyle modification can reduce the chance of cancer development. During *progressive* or metastasis stage, the tumor grows in large scale, increased invasiveness and spreads to adjoining and distant sites. Metastasis process involves many steps. The tumor cells detach from primary tumor and travel to distant sites through lymphatic and hematogenous routes and create conducive environment to grow in the distant site.

The most common sites for metastasis are lungs, brain, bone, liver, and adrenal glands. Lung cancers (along with trachea and bronchus cancers) went up to become the 5th leading cause of death in 2012, causing 1.6 million (2.9%) deaths, killing 1.1 million men and 0.5 million women in 2012. These figures are up from 1.2 million (2.2%) deaths in 2000 **(WHO, 2015, Global Health Observatory (GHO) data).**

Behavioral and dietary risks factors such as high BMI (obesity), low fruit and vegetable intake (unhealthy diet), lack of physical activity, tobacco usage, and alcohol use are also responsible for deaths accounting for around one-third of cancer deaths. Cancer causing *viral infections* such as Hepatitis B (HBV), Hepatitis C (HCV) and sexually transmitted Human Papilloma Virus (HPV) infections are responsible for up to 20% of cancer deaths in low and middle-income countries. Tobacco use is the most important risk factor for cancer, causing around 20% of global cancer deaths and around 70% of global lung cancer deaths **(de Martel et al., 2012).**

Factors associated with increased prevalence of cancers in India are consumption of unhealthy and improper diet, a low intake of fresh fruits and high cooking temperatures, improper life style, poor dietary habits, consumption of tobacco (unrefined form), smoking (cigarette, hookah), consumption of Pan Masala, Dohra and Zarda, betel nut, opium and bhang, alcohol consumption, radiation exposure (both ionizing and non-ionizing), and other environmental pollutants (indoor and outdoor). **(Ali, Wani, & Saleem, 2011)** (Figure 4.2)

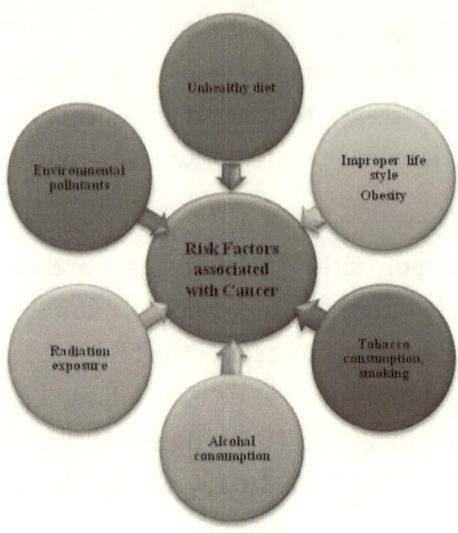

Fig. 4.2: *Risk factors associated with Cancer in India*

Chronic Respiratory Diseases

Chronic respiratory diseases are the group of chronic diseases that affect airways and other structures of lungs. The common chronic respiratory diseases are asthma, Bronchiectasis, Chronic obstructive pulmonary disease, Chronic rhinosinusitis, Hypersensitivity pneumonitis, Lung cancer and neoplasms of respiratory and intrathoracic organs, Lung fibrosis, Chronic pleural diseases, Pneumoconiosis, Pulmonary eosinophilia, Pulmonary heart disease and diseases of pulmonary circulation, Rhinitis, Sarcoidosis, and Sleep apnea syndrome. The most common preventable respiratory diseases are asthma, COPD, Occupational lung diseases, Sleep apnea syndrome, and pulmonary hypertension.

Respiratory diseases are one of the leading causes of death. Hundreds of millions of people of all ages (from infancy to old age) suffer from preventable chronic respiratory diseases and respiratory allergies in all countries of the world (WHO, 2015 Jun, Chronic respiratory diseases). Lung infections, mostly pneumonia and tuberculosis, lung cancer and chronic obstructive disease accounted for 9.5 million deaths worldwide (one-sixth of the global total) during 2008. World Health Organization estimated for these 4 diseases one tenth of DALYs lost worldwide in 2008, and for India made an estimation of 53% of all deaths due to NCDs. (WHO, 2008, The global burden of disease-2004 Update). 7% deaths were accounted for chronic respiratory disease in 2005 as reported by ICMR in 2009 **(ICMR-MRC Workshop, 2009)**.

Asthma

Asthma is one of the non-communicable diseases and is common among children. According to World Health Organization estimates, 235 million people currently suffer from asthma. Most asthma-related deaths occur in low and lower-middle-income countries **(WHO, 2015, Asthma)**.

It is a chronic inflammatory disorder of the airways characterized by recurrent episodes of wheezing, breathlessness, chest tightness, cough, particularly at night or in the early morning. It is associated with airway hyper-responsiveness and variable airflow obstruction, that is often reversible spontaneously or with treatment **(Global Initiative for Asthma, 2015)**.

Asthma is caused due to combination of multi-factors which are non-modifiable, modifiable, certain demographic, environmental and other inciting factors. *Non-modifiable factors* include family history of asthma (especially parent or sibling), genetic factor, premature birth, and low birth weight baby, bronchiolitis during childhood; *modifiable factors* are such as obesity, exposure to tobacco smoke, particularly if the mother smokes during pregnancy; *environmental factors* are such as allergens inhalation such as animal dander, house dust mite, pollens, molds etc., air pollutants, viral upper respiratory infection; *socio demographic factors* are such as urbanization and changing life style; *other inciting factors* are such as exercise, stress, laughing, crying, drugs, occupational exposure, food additives, psychological factors, changes in temperature, etc. It varies in severity and frequency from person to person. The strongest risk factors for developing asthma are allergens' inhalation that may trigger allergic reactions or irritate the airways.

On exposure of allergen, allergen-specific IgE antibodies are formed that attach to the surface of mast cells and basophiles in the bronchial wall. The mast cells release chemical mediators of inflammation such as histamine, bradykinin, prostaglandin and slow reacting substance of anaphylaxis. The chronic inflammatory process produces mucosal edema, mucus secretion, and airway inflammation or bronchospasm. During bronchospasm, the patient has symptoms of shortness of breath, chest tightness, and wheezing and peak flow variability. The initial clinical manifestation is known as early-phase reaction or response. This phase is developed immediately or 30–60 minutes after exposure to allergens or irritants and lasts about an hour.

The patient may develop similar symptoms within 4 to 10 hours after the initial attack due to eosinophil and lymphocyte activation and further release more chemical mediators of inflammation. This delayed response is termed as delayed or late phase reaction. During recurrent attacks, the chemical mediators create self-sustaining cycle of obstruction and inflammation. Asthma may be classified as mild intermittent, mild persistent, moderate persistent or severe persistent.

Severe acute bronchospasm can result in complications such as status asthmaticus which is severe and life-threatening. During this, the patient may develop acute cor pulmonale, the right sided heart failure resulting from lung disease.

Chronic Obstructive Pulmonary Disease

Chronic obstructive pulmonary disease (COPD) is a progressive, multi-component disorder associated with abnormal inflammatory response of the lungs characterized by chronic bronchitis, airway thickening and emphysema. It is a combination of chronic obstructive bronchitis, emphysema, and asthma. It affects lungs and also systemic consequences develop. The major systemic co-morbid conditions associated with COPD are cardiovascular diseases.

Chronic obstructive bronchitis resulting from inflammation of bronchi is characterized by chronic productive cough for 3 months in each 2 consecutive years. There is increase in size and number of subcutaneous and goblet glands in the large bronchi, thus increasing the mucus production, and impaired ciliary function which reduces mucus clearance, and increased susceptibility to infection. During infection mucus production is more, initially affecting the bronchi only but eventually involving all the airways.

Emphysema is an abnormal permanent enlargement of the air spaces distal to the terminal bronchioles, and with the destruction of their walls, and without obvious fibrosis. The most common type of emphysema, Centriacinar or Centrilobular emphysema causes destruction of bronchioles usually in the upper lung region; Panacinar emphysema destroys the entire alveolus usually involving lower portion of the lungs; and paraseptal or distal Acinar emphysema involves the distal airway structures, alveolar ducts and alveolar sacs, around the septa of lungs.

Asthma, we have discussed in previous section.

According to WHO estimates, 65 million people have moderate to severe chronic obstructive pulmonary disease (COPD). More than 3 million people died of COPD in 2005, which corresponds to 5% of all deaths globally; almost 90% of COPD deaths occur in low and middle-income countries and affects men and women almost equally. It was the fifth leading cause of death in 2002 and was estimated that it will be the third leading cause of death worldwide in 2030 (WHO, 2015, Chronic obstructive pulmonary disease). COPD was ranked 4th in 1990 and 3rd in 2010 for death, and ranked 6th in 1990 and 5th in 2010 for years lived with disability, while comparing the contribution of major diseases to deaths and disability worldwide for 1990 and 2010 in a study conducted on The Global Burden of Disease (GBD, 2012).

India contributes a significant and growing percentage of COPD mortality which is estimated to be among the highest in the world; i.e., more than 64.7 estimated age standardized death rate per 100,000 among both sexes. This would translate to about 556,000 in case of India (>20%) out of a world total of 2,748,000 annually (Lopez et al., 2006). Crude estimates suggest there are 30 million COPD patients in India (Salvi & Agrawal, 2012). COPD was responsible for killing 3.1 million people in the world in 2012 and in India 1061.9 thousand people (10.8%) died due to COPD **(WHO, 2015, Burden of COPD).**

The risk factors are genes, exposure to particles such as tobacco smoking, indoor air pollution from heating and biomass fuel in poorly ventilated houses, prolonged exposure to occupational dusts, organic and inorganic, outdoor air pollution, poor lung growth and development, previous tuberculosis, early childhood recurrent lower respiratory infections, poor nutrition, female gender, old age and low socio-economic status.

The primary cause of COPD is *smoking*; 5.4 million people died due to tobacco use. Tobacco-related deaths are projected to increase to 8.3 million deaths per year by 2030. In high and middle-income countries tobacco smoke is the biggest risk factor, while in low-income countries exposure to *indoor air pollution*, such as the use of biomass fuels (including from the burning of wood) for cooking and heating, is estimated to kill 2 million women and children each year. Occupational dusts and chemicals (such as vapors, irritants, and fumes) and frequent lower respiratory infections during childhood are other causes of COPD. **(WHO, 2015, Burden of COPD)**

Strenthening Health System Infrastructure
Health system

Heath system is the ensemble of all the activities whose primary purpose is to promote, restore and/or maintain health. It comprises of people, institutions and resources, arranged together in accordance with established policies, to improve the health of the population they serve, while responding to people's legitimate expectations and protecting them against the cost of ill health through a variety of activities whose primary intent is to improve health. **(Arlington, 2015; World Health Organization, 2000)**

Health system is comprised of all those people and actions whose primary purpose is to provide health services to improve and maintain health. It includes not only the government hospitals and dispensaries, the doctors, nurses and other professionals working in these organizations, but also the philosophy of health care, management of health professionals both formal and informal and all the health professionals' activities which people carry out to remain healthy (Vati, 2015). Each health system is responsible for improving health and also to protect people against financial risk for medical care and for providing care to them with dignity.

Health System in India

India has a three-tier system of health care with 3 main links: Center, State, and local or peripheral level. Center makes policies, plans and guidelines and assists and coordinates activities of State Health Ministries. Each state has developed its own system of health care machinery, independent of the central government. At regional district level, people at large receive health care services through public sector, private sectors, indigenous system of medicines, voluntary health agencies and vertical health program. At Taluka (Tehsil) level, hospitals/Community Health Centers (CHCs) provide basic and comprehensive emergency obstetric and neonatal services.

Health Systems Strengthening

According to USAID, health systems strengthening is 'a process that concentrates on ensuring that people and institutions, both public and private, undertake core functions of the health system (governance, financing, service delivery, health workforce, information, and medicines/vaccines/other technologies) in a mutually enhancing way, to improve health outcomes, protect citizens from catastrophic financial loss and impoverishment due to illness, and ensure consumer satisfaction, in an equitable, efficient and sustainable manner.' It encompasses many subsystems, such as human resources, information systems, health finance, and health governance, all of which can be weakened by different types of constraints **(USAID: https://www.hfgproject.org/about-hfg/about-health-systems-strengthening).**

National Health Programs and NCDs

At the national level efforts have been made to combat the burden of NCDs especially cardiovascular diseases, diabetes mellitus, cancer, strokes and chronic respiratory diseases which have emerged as major public health problems and contribute to a substantial burden of diseases. Various health programs and strategies at the national level are being implemented in phase-wise manner to address 4 main modifiable behavioral risk factors that contribute to NCDs and which are totally preventable, including tobacco use in all forms, physical inactivity, unhealthy diets (increased intake of salt, fats) and harmful use of alcohol. These programs are:

- National Programme for Prevention and Control of Cancer, Diabetes, Cardiovascular Diseases & Stroke (NPCDCS)
- National Tobacco Control Programme (NTCP)
- National Mental Health Programme (NMHP)
- National Programme for Health Care of the Elderly (NPHCE)
- National Injury Prevention Framework

Ministry of Health and Family Welfare (MOHFW) integrated cancer control (NCCP) with the national program for prevention and control of diabetes, cardiovascular disease, and stroke (NPCDS) as NPCDCS, as a National Program which was launched on 8th July 2010. It was implemented in 100 districts under the Umbrella of National Health Mission with the following objectives.

- To prevent and control common NCDs through behavior and life style changes.

- To provide early diagnosis and management of common NCDs.

- To build capacity at various levels of health care for prevention, diagnosis and treatment of common NCDs.

- To train human resources within the public health setup via doctors, paramedics and nursing staff to cope with the increasing burden of NCDs.

- To establish and develop capacity for palliative and rehabilitative care.

Health System Infrastructure Building Blocks

Health system infrastructure includes all resources including men, money, material, methods (technologies) and machines (equipment, laboratory support, etc.) required to deliver quality and equitable health services to all people, when and where they are needed. It needs to respond in a balanced way to the needs and expectations of the community at large to improve their health status, defend them against health threats and provide equitable access to people or community centered care.

Adequate resources include physical infrastructure, laboratory support and essential drugs against NCDs, sufficient number and type of human resources, e.g., generalists, specialists, nurses, paramedical staff, etc. according to service requirements and burden of disease, their production, training curricula relevant to population needs, and skill development at each level, through continuing education, regulatory measures, etc.

Evidence shows that improving health is impossible without intersectoral actions addressing the social determinants of health and other contributing factors plus a mix of services targeted at individuals (personal health services) and populations at large (non-personal health services).

Health care in India is provided at primary, secondary and tertiary level through public health sector, private sector, indigenous system of medicine, voluntary health agencies and through national health programs.

Strengthening Health System Infrastructure at Various Levels

In order to meet the objectives of the national health program to combat NCDs, infrastructure of health system at different levels needs to be strengthened. Health system infrastructure building blocks needing special focus to combat NCDs at different levels are explained below (Figure 4.3).

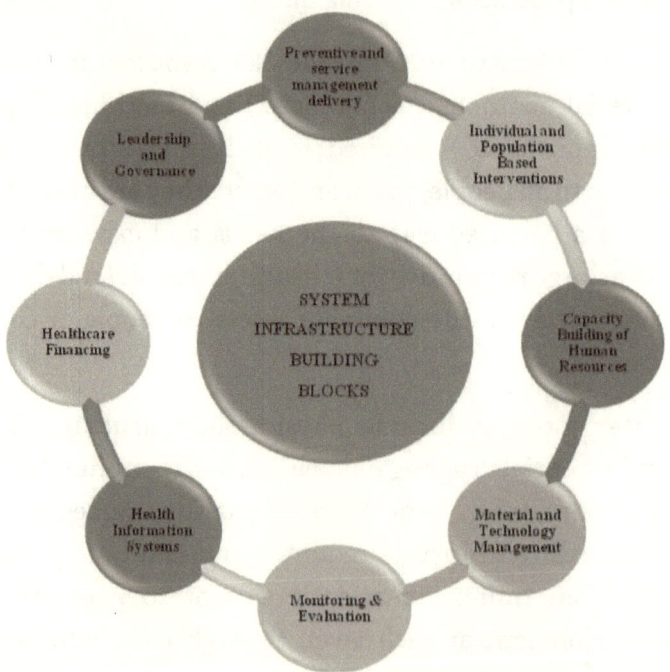

Fig. 4.3: *System infrastructure building blocks*

Strengthening Preventive and Service Management Delivery

A safe, effective and high quality service delivery with optimum cost efficacy is one of the building blocks needed to be strengthened to tackle NCDs effectively. There is a need to provide comprehensive preventive, curative, palliative and rehabilitative services and also health promotion activities. These services should be financially, culturally and geographically accessible to all, especially for the population at risk for NCDs. Services provided should be utilized by people with minimum waste and improved health outcomes.

At the PHC & sub-center level: Strengthening of health system at the PHC level is important, since most cost-effective interventions for the prevention and treatment of NCDs can be delivered at this level. Primary prevention is targeted to reduce risk factors like physical inactivity (life style), unhealthy diet (low fruit and vegetable consumption, excessive intake of saturated fats, refined sugars, trans-fatty acids), and tobacco use, smoking or exposure to second hand smoke, alcohol consumption and high stress levels which are modifiable but precipitate the development of physiological risk factors such as obesity.

It is provided through primary health centers, its sub-centers, at village level by suitably trained workforce like multipurpose health workers, health worker (female), health assistant male, village guides, and trained Dais. Village Health Guides, under *village health guide scheme* (October, 1977 &May, 1986) who provide the primary health care, are the first contact with the people. ASHA (Accredited Social Health Activist) who is trained community-based to provide the health services to Tribal and Non-tribal population is a link worker and acts as bridge between the Government functionaries and Tribal and Non-tribal population. Following services are provided by these workforces:

i. Promotion of health for behavior change through:

- Use of various approaches, e.g. mass media, community education and interpersonal communication to focus on: i) increased intake of healthy food; ii) Increased physical activity through sports, exercise, etc.; iii) Avoidance of tobacco and alcohol; iv) Stress management; and v) Warning signs of cancer, etc.

- Interpersonal communication through ASHAs/AWWs/SHGs/Youth clubs, Panchayat members, etc.

- Social mobilization for diagnostic camps through ASHAs/AWWs/SHGs/Youth clubs, Panchayat members, etc.

- Opportunistic screening of persons <30 years of age by doing simple clinical examination comprising of asking relevant questions (such as taking history of tobacco or alcohol consumption), taking blood pressure measurement, blood glucose estimation by strip method, etc.

- Referring suspected cases to community health center.

Various models/approaches can be exercised to strengthen health system to improve the primary health care response to NCDs, such as: i) integration of the management of chronic NCDs with that of chronic communicable diseases; ii) adapting DOTS (Directly Observed Therapy, Short-Course) framework for NCDs; and iii) Integration of NCDs with other health programs.

At the CHC level: At this level usually the target is to provide secondary prevention for the people diagnosed for NCDs. Secondary prevention aims to prevent or reduce the physiological risk factors such as increased BMI, raised blood pressure, deranged blood glucose and Dyslipidemia. Services provided at this level by health care workers needing to be strengthened are:

- Opportunistic screening of persons <30 years of age at the point of primary contact
- Identifying individuals who are at a high risk of developing diabetes and CVD, warranting further investigation/action
- Early diagnosis through clinical and laboratory investigations such as blood sugar, lipid profile, ECG, Ultrasound, X-ray, etc.
- Providing counseling (including diet counseling, lifestyle management)
- Management of common CVD, diabetes and stroke cases in outpatient and inpatient departments
- Providing home based care for bed ridden chronic cases through 'NCD clinic' at Community Health Center and District Hospital
- Referring difficult cases to District Hospital, higher health care facility to be provided

At District hospitals and tertiary level: At district hospital level, the main focus is on tertiary prevention that aims to prevent and treat diseases like heart diseases, stroke, diabetes, cancers, and COPD, etc. At tertiary level comprehensive cancer care including prevention, early detection, diagnosis, treatment, minimal access surgery after care, palliative care and rehabilitation like services are to be provided. NCDs services are to be provided through NCD clinics, having cardiac care unit and cancer care facility. All services as mentioned above are to be provided at first contact of person having risk for NCD or with diagnosed NCD or referred from CHC. The services provided at different levels needing special attention to achieve the targets are depicted in Figure 4.4.

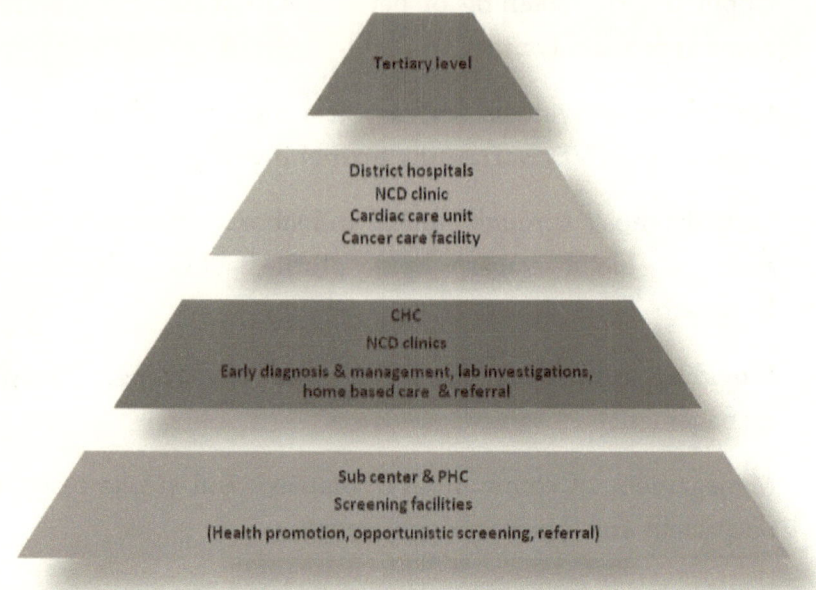

Fig. 4.4: *Services at different level under NPCDCS*

Strengthening Cost-Effective Interventions

NCDs can be prevented and life of many can be saved through cost-effective interventions. Thus priority needs to be given for individual and population-based interventions at different levels of prevention. These are:

- *'Best Buys' interventions,* e.g., protecting people from tobacco smoke and banning smoking in public places; warning about the dangers of tobacco use; restricting access to retailed alcohol; enforcing bans on alcohol advertising; reducing salt intake and salt content of food; replacing trans-fat in food with polyunsaturated fat; and promoting public awareness about diet and physical activity through mass media.

- *Low-cost population-wide interventions* include Nicotine dependence treatment; promoting adequate breastfeeding and complementary feeding; restrictions on marketing of foods and beverages high in salt, fats and sugar, especially to children; subsidies to promote healthy diets, etc.

- *Evidence-based interventions* such as healthy nutrition environments in schools; nutrition information and counseling in health care; school-based physical activity programs for children; workplace programs for physical activity and healthy diets; community programs for physical activity, exercises and healthy diets.

- *Interventions focused on cancer prevention* include vaccination against Hepatitis B, HPV, protection against environmental or occupational risk factors for cancer, screening for breast and cervical cancer.

- *Individual based interventions*: Healthcare systems should undertake interventions for individuals who either already have NCDs or who are at high risk of developing them.

Strengthening Capacity Building of Human Resources

Human resources for health are crucial in any of the health care systems. It is important to ensure right health care workers, at right place, at the right time with the right skills. At each level appropriate numbers of skilled health care workers are required to deliver various NCDs interventions.

Planning quality and quantity of staff such as professionals, technicians, and auxiliaries required under NCPDCS at different levels, and managing them in a cost-effective manner is one of the challenges to fight against NCDs. Health workforce should be well performing, competent, and responsive at all the levels. Training and continuing education for NCD health personnel at various levels regarding health promotion, prevention, early detection and management of NCDs should be planned and imparted by a team of trainers at identified Training Institutes/Centers. There should be emphasis on self-management education. The educational curricula need revision for NCD health personnel at different levels to include necessary knowledge and skills for them. There should be coordination among various functionaries for NCD prevention and control.

Strengthening Material and Technology Management

In health sector, material management deals with providing drugs, supplies and equipment needed by the staff to deliver health services. It is concerned with the flow, conservation and utilization of the materials as well as quality and cost of the materials. Medical products, vaccines and technologies need to be safe, and cost-effective. There should be proper utilization of medical drugs, equipment and supplies to achieve the objectives of national health programs to combat NCDs.

The National Monitoring Framework has targeted 80% availability of the affordable basic technologies and essential NCD medicines, including generics, and basic technology in both public and private facilities to prevent and control NCD by 2025. It is also planned that at least 50% eligible people will receive drug therapy and counseling (including glycemic control) to prevent heart attacks and strokes by 2025. Emphasis should be given on quality and safety of medicines and medical devices and should be monitored through national regulatory authorities **(GOI, 2013).**

Strengthening Monitoring and Evaluation at Different Level

To fight against NCDs, monitoring and evaluation system should be improved at District, State and Central level. There is initiative from the Health and Family Welfare Department, Government of India, New Delhi to improve monitoring of NCDs by launching 'New Delhi calls for Action on combating NCDs in India' focusing on related risk factors such as obesity, junk food, and tobacco consumption and co-morbidities. This venture includes 26 'mini interventions' to combat NCDs in 2011 (Sinha, 2011). These need to be disseminated to the community at large.

India is also committed to implement an appropriate action plan based on consultative approach with relevant stakeholders to meet the objectives and targets within time frame to combat NCDs. The Government of India is taking immediate action and targeting the greatest risk factors contributing to NCDs—unhealthy diets, physical inactivity, tobacco and alcohol use, and air pollution—by means of multi-sectoral collaboration and cooperation at national, regional and global levels (WHO, 2015, India: first to adapt the Global Monitoring Framework on non-communicable diseases). The National Monitoring Framework has 10 targets and 21 indicators to monitor progress of actions planned to prevent and control NCD by 2025.

Strengthening health information systems

National health information systems (including registries) for monitoring and evaluation of NCDs and risk factors, as well as morbidity/mortality statistics by cause should be strengthened. The production, analysis, dissemination and use of timely information from individual to population level should be a part of information management.

Strengthening healthcare financing

A strong and effective health system is to ensure sustainable financing system, stable availability of sufficient funds in a way maximizing health results and providing financial risk protection to the population. There is a need to prioritize NCDs and to develop health financing models/schemes and financing mechanisms that can reduce out-of-pocket expenditure and catastrophic spending related to NCDs. Since a major portion of health treatment for NCD is paid out-of-pocket in India, 70% expenditure is incurred by households, mostly at the point of service use. The hospital expenditure due to cancer is higher as compared to hospitalization due to communicable diseases **(Duran & Knot, 2011).**

Strengthening leadership and governance

Leadership and governance are important managerial functions to implement the system effectively. It is concerned with inspiring and encouraging health workforce working at different levels, and creating understanding among them. Supervision, communication, exhibiting leadership and motivating workforce are important ingredients for combating NCDs and for achieving the objectives of national health programs. It is also important to ensure policy frameworks with effective oversight, coalition building, regulation, attention to system design and accountability to tackle NCDs effectively.

Key Points

- Non-communicable diseases (NCDs) are chronic, having slow progression and being of long duration, but can be prevented.
- NCDs are number one leading cause of mortality and morbidity globally.
- Cardiovascular diseases, cancers, chronic respiratory diseases and diabetes fall under this category.
- The common risk factors are grouped under non-modifiable risk factors and modifiable behavioral risk factors.
- Cardiovascular diseases (CVDs) are a group of disorders of the heart and blood vessels including Coronary heart disease, hypertension and Dyslipidemia and Stroke.
- Coronary heart disease is caused due to narrowing and damage of coronary arteries supplying to the heart, resulting in chest pain (angina) and breathlessness or even leading to heart attack.

- Hypertension is a persistent systolic blood pressure ≥140 mmHg and/or diastolic blood pressure ≥90 mmHg. Individuals on self-reported antihypertensive medications are to be included in the numbers of afflicted persons.

- Dyslipidemia (abnormal lipid profile) closely linked to the pathophysiology of CVD, is a key independent modifiable risk factor for cardiovascular disease.

- A stroke, the second leading cause of death occurs due to inadequate or interruptions to the blood supply to brain, either because of blockage (ischemic stroke) or rupture of blood vessel (hemorrhagic stroke).

- Diabetes mellitus is multi-system, a disorder of glucose metabolism of multiple etiologies, either with insufficient insulin production by pancreas, or due to ineffective utilization of insulin produced by the body, or both, characterized by chronic hyperglycemia.

- Cancer, an uncontrolled and unregulated growth and spread of cells is a large group of more than 200 diseases of multiple causes and is a leading cause of morbidity and mortality worldwide.

- Chronic respiratory diseases are the group of chronic diseases that affect airways and other structures of the lungs.

- Lung infections (pneumonia and tuberculosis), lung cancer and chronic obstructive disease, asthma are the most common chronic respiratory diseases.

- India has a three-tier system of health care with 3 main links: Center, State, and local or peripheral level.

- Heath system comprises all the activities whose primary purpose is to promote, restore and/or maintain health.

- The main function of a health system strengthening is to ensure that people and institutions, both public and private, undertake core functions of the health system.

- Various health programs and strategies at the national level are working to address 4 main modifiable behavioral risk factors such as tobacco use in all forms, physical inactivity, unhealthy diets (increased intake of salt, fats) and harmful use of alcohol.

- Health system infrastructure includes all resources required to deliver quality and equitable health services to all people at the right time.

- System infrastructure building blocks such as preventive and service management delivery, cost-effective interventions, human resources, material and technology management, surveillance, monitoring and evaluation, health information systems, healthcare financing and leadership and governance need to be strengthened at various level to tackle the burden of NCDs.

References

1. Ali, I, Wani, AW, & Saleem, K (2011). Cancer scenario in India with future perspectives. *Cancer Therapy*, 8, 56–70.

2. Arlington, VA (2015). *Management Sciences for Health*. Available from:

    http://www.healthsystems2020.org/content/resource/detail/528/

3. Bernard, WS, & Christopher, PW (Ed.) (2014). *World Cancer Report 2014*. WHO: IARC Publication. Available from:

    http://www.iarc.fr/en/publications/books/wcr/wcr-order.php

4. Berra, K, Klieman, L (2003). National Cholesterol Education Program: Adult Treatment Panel III-new recommendations for lifestyle and medical management of dyslipidemia. *J Cardiovasc Nurs*, 18, 85.

5. Daniel, CR, Prabhakaran, D, Kapur, K, Graubard, BI, Devasenapathy, N, et al. (2011 Jan 28). A cross-sectional investigation of regional patterns of diet and cardio-metabolic risk in India. *Nutr J*, 10, 12. doi: 10.1186/1475–2891–10–12.

6. de Martel, C, Ferlay, J, Franceschi, S, Vigna, J, Bray, F, Forman, D, Plummer, M (2012). Global burden of cancers attributable to infections in 2008: a review and synthetic analysis. *The Lancet Oncology*, 13(6), 607–15.

7. Duran, A, & Knot, A (2011 Dec). Strengthening the Health System to Better Confront Non-communicable Diseases in India. *Indian J Community Med*, 36 (Supp. 11), S32–S37. doi: 10.4103/0970–0218.94706 PMCID: PMC3354901.

8. Expert Panel on Detection, Evaluation, and Treatment of High Blood Cholesterol in Adults. (2001). Executive summary of the third report of the National Cholesterol Education Program (NCEP) expert panel on detection, evaluation, and treatment of high blood cholesterol in adults (Adult Treatment Panel III) *JAMA*, 285, 2486–97. doi: 10.1001/jama.285.19.2486.

9. Frank, B, Hu. (2011 Jun). Globalization of diabetes: the role of diet, lifestyle, and genes. *Diabetes Care*, 34 (6), 1249–57. doi: 10.2337/dc11–0442.

10. GBD. (2012 Dec 13). The Global Burden of Disease study 2010. *Lancet*, 380 (9859), 2053–60.

11. Global Initiative for Asthma. (2015 Apr.) *Pocket guide for Asthma management and prevention*. Available from:

http://www.ginasthma.org/documents/1

12. GOI (2013) *National action plan and monitoring framework for prevention and control of non–communicable diseases in India 2012–13*. Available from:

    http://www.searo.who.int/india/topics/cardiovascular_diseases/National_Action_Plan_and_Monitoring_Framework_Prevention_NCDs.pdf

13. IARC, WHO (2015). *GLOBOCAN 2012: Estimated cancer incidence, mortality and prevalence worldwide in 2012*. Available from:

    http://globocan.iarc.fr/Pages/fact_sheets_cancer.aspx

14. ICMR-MRC Workshop (2009). *Building Indo-UK Collaboration in chronic diseases*. Available from:

    http://www.icmr.nic.in/final/chronic/Chronic_Diseases_Report.pdf

15. International Diabetes Federation (2014). *IDF Diabetes Atlas*. 6th ed. Brussels, Belgium. Available from:

    http://www.idf.org/diabetesatlas/update-2014

16. International Diabetes Federation (2015). Risk factors. Available from:

    https://www.idf.org/about-diabetes/risk-factors

17. Kaul, U, & Bhatia, V (2010 Nov). Perspective on coronary interventions & cardiac surgeries in India. *Indian J Med Res*, 132, 543–8.

18. Krishnamurthi, RV, Feigin, VL, Forouzanfar, MH, Mensah, GA, Connor, M, Bennett, DA, et al. (2013). Global and regional burden of first-ever ischemic and hemorrhagic stroke during 1990–2010: findings from the Global Burden of Disease Study 2010. *Lancet Glob Health*, 1, 259–81.

19. Lopez, AD, Shibuya, K, Rao, C, Mathers, CD, Hansell, AL, Held, LS, Schmid, V, Buist, S (2006 Feb). Chronic obstructive pulmonary disease: current burden and future projections. *Eur Respir J*, 27(2), 397–412.

20. Mathers, CD, & Loncar, D (2005 Oct). *Updated projections of global mortality and burden of disease, 2002–2030: data sources, methods and results*. Available from:

    http://www.who.int/healthinfo/statistics/bodprojectionspaper.pdf

21. Morrish, NJ, Wang, SL, Stevens, LK, Fuller, JH, Keen, H (2001). Mortality and causes of death in the WHO multinational study of vascular disease in diabetes. *Diabetologia*, 44 (Suppl 2), S14–S21.

22. Pandey, V (2010 Nov 13). *Mumbai Number 2 on Child obesity list: study. Daily News & Analysis (DNA)*. Available from:

    http://www.dnaindia.com/mumbai/report-mumbai-number-two-on-child-obesity-list-study-1465897

23. Salvi, S, & Agrawal, A (2012 Feb). India needs a national COPD prevention and control program. *J Assoc Physicians India*, 60 (Suppl), 5–7.

24. Schmidt, MI, Ducan, BB, Reichelt, AJ, Branchtein, L, Matos, MC, et al. (2001). For the Brazilian Gestational Diabetes Study Group. Gestational diabetes mellitus diagnosed with a 2-h 75 gm oral glucose tolerance test and adverse pregnancy outcomes. *Diabetes Care*, 24, 1151–5.

25. Shokeen, D, & Aeri, BT (2015) Risk Factors Associated with the increasing cardiovascular diseases prevalence in India: a review. *J Nutr Food Sci*, 5, 331. doi: 10.4172/2155-9600.1000331.

26. Singh, PK (2015 Jan). *India: first to adapt the Global Monitoring Framework on non – communicable diseases (NCDs)*. Available from

    http://www.who.int/features/2015/ncd-india/en/

27. Sinha, K (2011 Oct 3). India will roll out world's largest drive against NCDs. *The Times of India*. Available from:

    http://timesofindia.indiatimes.com/india/India-will-roll-out-worlds-largest-drive-against-NCDs/articleshow/10212828.cms?

28. Strong, K, Mathers, C, Bonita, R (2007 Feb). Preventing stroke: saving lives around the world. *Lancet Neurol*, 6(2), 182–7.

29. Taylor, FC, & Kumar, SK (2012). *Stroke in India fact sheet (updated 2012)*. Available from:

    http://www.sancd.org/Updated%20Stroke%20Fact%20sheet%202012.pdf

30. The Expert Committee on the Diagnosis and Classification of Diabetes Mellitus (1997 Jul). Report of the expert committee on the diagnosis and classification of diabetes mellitus. *Diabetes Care*, 20 (7), 1183–97. Available from:

    http://care.diabetesjournals.org/content/20/7/1183.full.pdf

31. US Department of Health and Human Services (2004 Aug). *The Seventh Report of the Joint National Committee on Prevention, Detection, Evaluation, and Treatment of High Blood Pressure*. No. 04–5230. Available from:

    http://www.nhlbi.nih.gov/files/docs/guidelines/jnc7full.pdf

32. USAID *Health Systems Strengthening*. Available from:

    https://www.hfgproject.org/about-hfg/about-health-systems-strengthening/

33. Vati, J (2015). *Nursing Foundation: Concepts and Perspectives*. New Delhi: JAYPEE Publisher.

34. WHO (1999). *Definition, diagnosis and classification of diabetes mellitus and its complications: report of a WHO consultation. Part 1: Diagnosis and classification of diabetes mellitus*. Available from:

    http://apps.who.int/iris/bitstream/10665/66040/1/WHO_NCD_NCS_99.2.pdf?ua=1

35. World Health Organization (2000). The World Health Report 2000. Health systems: improving performance. Available at:

    http://www.who.int/whr/2000/en/whr00_en.pdf

36. WHO (2008). *The global burden of disease – 2004 Update*. Available from:

    http://www.who.int/healthinfo/global_burden_disease/GBD_report_2004update_full.pd

37. WHO (2013). *A global brief on Hypertension: Silent killer, global public health crisis*. Available from:

    http://apps.who.int/iris/bitstream/10665/79059/1/WHO_DCO_WHD_2013.2_eng.pdf?ua=1

38. WHO (2014). *Cancer Country Profiles-2014*. Available from:

    http://www.who.int/cancer/country-profiles/en/

39. WHO (2014). *Global status report on non-communicable diseases*. Available from:

    http://www.who.int/diabetes/en/

40. WHO (2014, May). *The top ten causes of death, fact sheet N°310*. Available from:

    http://who.int/mediacentre/factsheets/fs310/en/index2.html

41. WHO (2015). *About Diabetes*, 2015. Available from

   http://www.who.int/diabetes/action_online/basics/en/index1.html

42. WHO (2015). *Asthma*. Available from:

   http://www.who.int/mediacentre/factsheets/fs307/en/

43. World Health Organization (2015). *Burden of COPD*. Available from

   http://www.who.int/respiratory/copd/burden/en/

44. WHO (2015). *Chronic obstructive pulmonary disease (COPD Fact sheet Nº 315*. Retrieved from

   http://www.who.int/mediacentre/factsheets/fs315/en/index.html .

45. WHO (2015). *Global burden of stroke*. Available from:

   http://who.int/cardiovascular_diseases/en/cvd_atlas_15_burden_stroke.pdf?ua=1

46. WHO (2015). *Global Health Estimates (GHE): Estimates for 2000–2012*. Available from:

   http://www.who.int/healthinfo/global_burden_disease/estimates/en/index2.html

47. WHO (2015). *Global Health Observatory (GHO) data: Mortality and global health estimates*. Available from:

   http://who.int/gho/mortality_burden_disease/en/

48. WHO (2015). *India: first to adapt the Global Monitoring Framework on non-communicable diseases (NCDs)*. Available from:

   http://www.who.int/features/2015/ncd-india/en/

49. WHO (2015 Jan). *Global status of report on* non-*communicable diseases 2014.* Available from:

    http://apps.who.int/iris/bitstream/10665/148114/1/9789241564854_eng.pdf?ua=1

50. WHO (2015, Jun). *Chronic respiratory diseases. Global surveillance, prevention and control of chronic respiratory diseases: A comprehensive approach.* Available from:

    http://www.who.int/respiratory/publications/global_surveillance/en/f

51. Journal of Stroke. 2017 Sep; 19(3): 286–294, Stroke Epidemiology in South, East, and South-East Asia: A Review, Narayanaswamy Venketasubramanian, Byung Woo Yoon, Jeyaraj Pandian, and Jose C. Navarrod Published online 2017 Sep 29. doi: 10.5853/jos.2017.00234

Chapter V (A)

Preventive Strategies for Cardiovascular Diseases

Mrs. Shweta Pattnaik

Introduction

For many years, prevention strategies have been an important part of comprehensive efforts to reduce the burden of chronic diseases. Preventive healthcare consists of measures taken for disease prevention, as opposed to disease treatment. Just as health encompasses a variety of physical and mental states, so do disease and disability, which are affected by environmental factors, genetic predisposition, disease agents, and lifestyle choices. Health, disease, and disability are dynamic processes which begin before individuals realize they are affected. Disease prevention relies on anticipatory actions that can be categorized as primary, secondary, and tertiary prevention.

Even though public apprehension is more over the risks of developing cancer, in most countries the public has more to fear from cardiovascular disease (CVD). The first and second most common causes of death worldwide are Coronary heart disease (CHD) and stroke, the principal manifestation of CVD. The World Health Organization predicts that, by 2020, coronary heart disease will become the world's most vital cause of death and disability as well as premature death. Overall CVD thus leads to considerable patient morbidity through the management of stroke and heart failure, resulting in highest healthcare utilization costs for any disease in many of the countries. Strategies to prevent CVD have global significance hence, and should be given high priority for healthcare systems as discussed in previous chapters.

Incidence

On a global scale, the most common cause of death is cardiovascular diseases, 80% of which occur in low and middle-income countries. A recent report indicated that non-communicable diseases, particularly cardiovascular disease (CVD), have replaced contagious diseases as the leading cause of death in developing nations. The Registrar General of India's report confirmed this assertion that 42% of all deaths in the country are attributable to non-communicable disease, 19% of those being attributable to CVD.

Status in India

Rates of cardiovascular diseases are rapidly rising in India and other developing countries. 28% of all deaths in India are accounted for by cardiovascular diseases. Roughly 40 million deaths occur annually in India due to cardiovascular diseases. Mortality rates among working-age adults in India are higher than those in developed countries, contributing to a substantial loss of productive years of life. Coronary heart disease has the highest incidence of all diseases in India, affecting approximately 35.8 million people.

Accurate statistics for cardiovascular disease prevalence and incidence in rural areas of India are exceedingly challenging to establish. However, they are of great importance since over 70% of people in India reside in rural areas. The Framingham Heart Study (2010) reported that somewhere between 6.5% and 13% of people living in urban areas, and between 1.6% and 7.4% of rural dwellers in India are living with cardiovascular disease, and men and women are affected almost equally.

Joshi et al. (2009) conducted research in rural Andhra Pradesh and found that 32% of all deaths in that region were due to cardiovascular diseases, and that 6.6% of the population over 30 years of age had cardiovascular disease.

It is estimated that by 2020 cardiovascular disease will be the cause of over 40 per cent deaths in India as compared to 24 per cent in 1990. With over 3 million deaths owing to cardiovascular diseases every year, India is set to be the 'heart disease capital of the world' in a few years, said doctors on the eve of World Heart Day (September 29).

An estimate of about 17.5 million people died from CVDs in 2012, which represents 31% of all global deaths. Of these deaths, coronary heart disease was the reason for 7.4 million and 6.7 million were as a result of stroke. Over three quarters of CVD deaths take place in low and middle-income countries.

As earlier mentioned in the chapter III, out of 16 million deaths under the age of 70 due to non-communicable diseases, 82% are in low and middle-income countries and 37% are caused by CVDs.

Prevalence

Global

It has been assessed that chronic diseases accounted for about 60% of deaths worldwide in 2005, including cardiovascular diseases, cancer, respiratory diseases and diabetes. Cardiovascular diseases accounted for half of the total chronic disease deaths.

National

It was estimated that 29.8 million people in India out of a total estimated population of 1.03 billion were diagnosed with CHD in 2000. According to World Bank estimates, 31% share in the total burden of disease in 2015 was accounted for by CVD. On the basis of cross-sectional surveys in 2003, the prevalence was estimated to be 3–4% in rural areas and 8–10% in urban areas.

Regional

The overall prevalence of CAD in native South Indian population was found to be 11% whereas the age standardized prevalence was computed to be 9%. The figure of 11% represents around a 10-fold increase in the prevalence of CAD in urban India during the last 40 years. Unadjusted CHD rates range from 1.6% to 7.4% in rural populations and 1% to 13.2% in urban populations. Crude prevalence rate of CHD have a prevalence rate of 6–10% in urban areas of Northern states such as Jammu and Kashmir, Delhi and Uttar Pradesh and Western states such as Rajasthan. The rate is 6–7% in the rural areas in Jammu and Kashmir, 3–5% in Himachal Pradesh and Punjab among the Northern states, while in Rajasthan, it was 3–5%.

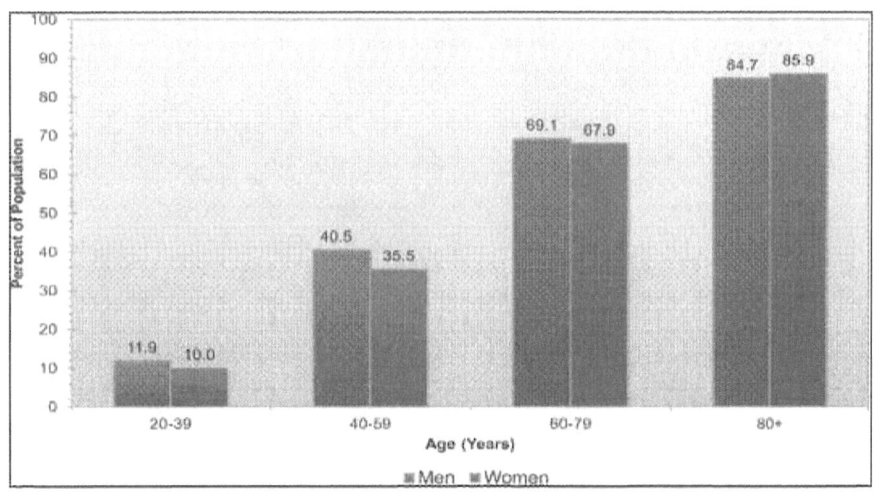

Fig. No. 5(a) 1: *Prevalence of cardiovascular disease in adults ≥20 years of age by age and sex*

Role of Prevention and Control Strategies

Health care requires 2 approaches, prevention and treatment where reduction in disease occurrence is required, and if disease occurs then comprehensive treatment is essential. Prevention or treatment programs and services should not only be effective, they should also be affordable to society and accessible, so that they reach the people who need them most.

In May 2000, the 53rd World Health Assembly adopted the WHO Global Strategy for the Prevention and Control of Non-communicable

Diseases. Since then the project was initiated in collaboration with Framework Convention on Tobacco Control and the Global Strategy for Diet, Physical Activity and Health.

More emphasis needs to be placed on the promotion of health and on preventing or delaying chronic diseases, disabilities, and injuries. Prevention is a priority to reduce the burden of the disease. Prevention is a hallmark of a quality health system. Prevention is the first step in management.

Greater risks in development of NCDs include poor nutrition during pregnancy and the first 2 years of life that cause individuals and populations to develop CVD and diabetes soon in life. Furthermore, HIV and tuberculosis are also linked with NCDs. Significant decline in the magnitude of NCDs would have a positive impact on the progress towards the achievement of Millennium Development Goals.

Risk Factors

Diseases of the heart, vascular diseases of the brain and diseases of blood vessels are included in CVDs. CVD represent a cluster of disorders, with complex interactions between the multiple risk factors. The different types of CVDs are listed below.

1. **CVDs due to atherosclerosis**
   - Ischemic Heart Disease or Coronary Artery Disease (Heart Attack)
   - Cerebrovascular Disease (Stroke)
   - Diseases of the aorta and arteries, including hypertension and peripheral vascular disease.

2. **Other CVDs**
   - Congenital Heart Disease
   - Rheumatic Heart Disease
   - Cardiomyopathies
   - Cardiac arrhythmias.

Atherosclerotic Disease

A disease process in the blood vessels that results in coronary heart disease and cerebrovascular disease is known as atherosclerosis. A large proportion of CVDs occur due to atherosclerosis. Out of the 17.3 million cardiovascular deaths, 7.3 million deaths occurred due to heart attacks and 6.2 million deaths occurred due to strokes in 2008.

Atherosclerosis is a complex pathological process in the blood vessels that develops over many years.

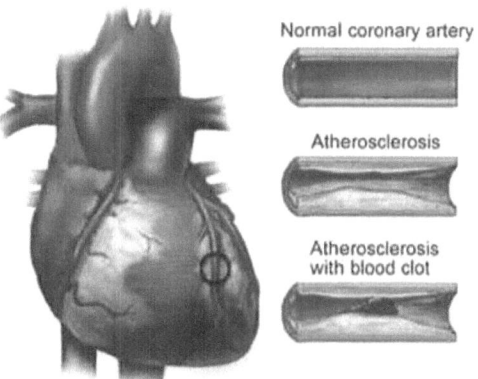

Fig. No. 5(a) 2: *Atherosclerosis*

In atherosclerosis, fatty material and cholesterol are deposited inside the lumen of medium and large blood vessels (arteries). These deposits are known as plaques which cause the inner surface of the blood vessels to become irregular and the lumen to become narrow, making it harder for blood to flow through it. Ultimately, the plaque ruptures, triggering the formation of a blood clot. If the blood clot develops in a coronary artery, it leads to heart attack; if it develops in the brain, it leads to stroke.

Factors that promote the process of atherosclerosis are previously mentioned in Chapter IV.

Rheumatic Heart Disease

When there is damage to the heart muscle and heart valves from rheumatic fever following a streptococcal infection causing pharyngitis/tonsillitis, we call it rheumatic heart disease.

Congenital Heart Disease

Malformations of heart structures present by birth are known as congenital heart defects.

They may be caused by:

i. A close blood relation between parents (consanguinity);

ii. Maternal infections (e.g. rubella);

iii. Maternal use of alcohol and drugs (e.g. warfarin); and

iv. Poor maternal nutrition (e.g. deficiency of folic acid).

Other CVDs

Disorders of the heart muscle (e.g. cardiomyopathy), disorders of the electrical conduction system (e.g. cardiac arrhythmias) and heart valve diseases are less common than heart attacks and strokes.

Assess

- CHD History
- Diet
- Body Mass Index
- Family history of CHD
- Blood Pressure
- Physical activity
- Smoking history
- Diabetes

1. **Measure fasting lipids (cholesterol, triglycerides, HDL).**

   Determine absolute risk of future coronary events

Table No. 5(a) 1: Risk assessment based management
(Adapted from www.heartjnl.com)

High risk	Medium Risk	Low Risk
▪ Establish lifestyle changes Dietary advice (low saturated fat, high fiber)	▪ Repeat fasting lipids ▪ Institute lifestyle changes ▪ Dietary advice	Review patient regularly
▪ Treat hypertension and diabetes ▪ Advise patient to stop smoking, exercise daily and maintain weight ▪ Treat with lipid lowering agent **Satisfactory results**	▪ Treat hypertension and diabetes ▪ Stop smoking, exercise daily and maintain weight If at 6 months **Unsatisfactory results** Treat with lipid lowering agent	

Prevention

In the developed countries the mortality rates have decreased significantly where primary prevention and individual healthcare intervention strategies have contributed enormously. Now it is time to work out in the developing countries for betterment of cardiac health. As per World Health Organization (WHO), Multinational Monitoring of Trends and Determinants of Cardiovascular Disease initiative (WHO MONICA Project), mortality from coronary heart disease and stroke declined dramatically in many of the 38 MONICA populations. The decline in mortality has been recognized to reduced incidence rates and improved survival after cardiovascular events due to prevention and treatment interventions. Across the populations there is a decline in coronary heart disease mortality and cardiovascular risk which contributed to 75% and 66% of the change in men and women, respectively, the remainder being attributed to providing healthcare resulting in improved survival in the first 4 weeks after the event.

Prevention strategies for CVD therefore have global significance and should be a priority for healthcare systems. Both primary as well as secondary prevention strategies are essential.

Primary Prevention

✓ **Who should assess their cardiovascular health risk?**

- All adults aged 40 or more
- Adults of any age who have:
    - A strong family history of an early cardiovascular disease.
    - A first degree relative (parent, brother, sister, child) with a serious hereditary lipid disorder. For example, familial hypercholesterolemia or familial combined Hyperlipidemia.
    - If you already have a cardiovascular disease or diabetes then your risk does not need to be assessed. This is because you are already known to be in the high-risk group.
    - Initial risk assessment should include lifestyle (smoking status, physical activity level, alcohol use/abuse, oral contraception use) and family history (relatives with premature CHD, hypertension, or diabetes). BMI, waist circumference, and blood pressure should be measured. For women, menopause is an additional risk factor causing CHD.

Secondary Prevention

This aims at the groups who are at greatest risk of CHD and for whom treatment will be cost-effective. The individuals who are at high risk are those who have a previous history of heart attack, angina or those with symptoms of arterial disease like stroke, transient ischemic attack, or peripheral vascular disease. Since all these people are affected with CVDs, therefore secondary prevention aims to prevent progression of the disease.

In order to maximize secondary prevention, rapid assessment and treatment of patients presenting with established CVD, formalizing their subsequent follow-up is necessary.

Fundamental strategies for hospitals include formal, protocol driven discharge or outpatient clinic policies that ensure patients have received the appropriate advice and secondary prevention interventions before discharge. It is also essential that the family doctor as well as the patient is aware of the follow-up arrangements for cardiac or stroke rehabilitation, smoking cessation, or treatment monitoring. The first step for secondary CVD prevention in primary care is accurate identification of those patients at maximum risk, by establishing disease registers for CHD and stroke. Having established registers, practices are needed to initiate, conduct, and repeat clinical audit routinely to ensure that the predetermined interventions are actually offered to those registered in CVD registers.

Multifactorial Global Risk Estimation

Individual global risk is determined through the method of Framingham equation. These tools include the Sheffield risk tables and the European coronary risk chart. In addition to these color charts (which classify risk by sex, age, systolic blood pressure, TC and HDL-C, and smoking status), and a number of computer based programs are available.

The total risk approach acknowledges that many cardiovascular risk factors tend to appear in clusters or in a combined form; accordingly combining risk factors to predict total cardiovascular risk is consequently a logical approach to decide who should receive treatment. There are many techniques for assessing cardiovascular risk status of individual patients. Most of these techniques use risk prediction equations derived from various sources, most commonly the Framingham Heart Study. The risk charts and tables created use different age categories, duration of risk assessment and risk factor profiles. Risk scores have different accuracy in different populations, tending to over predict in low-risk populations and under predict in high-risk populations. At least two-yearly risk factor updating and five-yearly global risk estimation is recommended by the American Heart Association.

Modification of Behavior

Reducing cigarette smoking, body weight, blood pressure, blood cholesterol, and blood glucose—all these have a valuable impact on major biological cardiovascular risk factors. Stopping smoking, engaging in regular physical activity and eating a healthy diet promote health and have no harmful effects. They also advance the sense of well-being and are usually less expensive to health care system than drug treatments which may also have adverse effects.

In order to lower blood pressure, a variety of lifestyle modifications have been suggested in clinical trials. Weight loss in the overweight, physical activity, self-control of alcohol intake, increased intake of fresh fruit and vegetables and reduced saturated fat in the diet, reduction of dietary sodium intake, and increased potassium intake are included in this.

More randomized trials, concerning a program of weight reduction, dietary manipulation and physical activity has also reduced the incidence of type 2 diabetes among people at high risk of developing it. Also, improvement in dyslipidemia and lowered risk of cardiovascular events are the result shown in trials of reduction of saturated fat and its partial replacement by unsaturated fats. Observational studies have found that cessation of smoking (other behavioral modifications) in particular, are associated with a reduction in cardiovascular disease mortality. The chances of developing cardiovascular disease in men have been reduced due to a healthy lifestyle and increased physical activity.

Tobacco

It is projected that there are presently one billion smokers in the world. The major form of smoked tobacco is manufactured cigarettes; 'bidis' (a type of filter-less hand-rolled cigarette), cigars, hookahs and chewed tobacco are the other forms of tobacco consumed. The utmost prevalence for smoking is estimated at nearly 31% in the WHO European Region, while the lowest is in the WHO African Region at 10%.

Exposure to secondhand smoke is also a risk to health from tobacco use followed by direct consumption of tobacco. Nearly 6 million people die from exposure to second hand smoke and tobacco use each year, accounting for 6% of all female and 12% of all male deaths in the world.

By 2030, there will be an increase in tobacco-related deaths to more than 8 million deaths. Smoking is strongly associated with mortality, largely because of an increased risk of CHD and stroke. Smoking cessation is associated with improved exercise tolerance and survival in patients with peripheral vascular disease or stroke. The most effective strategy to encourage smoking cessation is not clearly established even though the benefits of stopping smoking are evident. All patients should be given guidance and counseling on quitting, as well as support at follow-up.

There is evidence that advice and counseling on smoking cessation delivered by health professionals (such as physicians, nurses, psychologists, and health counselors) are advantageous and effective. Several systematic reviews have shown that onetime advice from physicians during routine consultation results in 2% of smokers quitting smoking for at least an year.

Likewise, nicotine replacement therapy can increase the rate of smoking cessation. Nicotine may be administered in a number of ways like nasal spray, skin patch or gum; no particular route of administration seems to be superior to the others.

Therefore, the important components to improve the health and well-being of a person is by policies and interventions focusing on prevention of tobacco use, promotion of smoke free environments and smoking cessation.

Exercise

There is strong observational evidence that moderate, regular physical activity reduces the risk of both CHD and stroke and that the risk is increased in people with a sedentary lifestyle, but there is limited evidence from randomized controlled trials (RCTs) of the value of exercise in primary prevention of cardiovascular disease. After Acute Myocardial Infarction, for secondary prevention, 2 meta-analyses of exercise-based rehabilitation in up to 14 RCTs have shown reductions in mortality of between 20% and 25% (absolute risk reduction [ARR], 3.1%) at 3-year follow-up.

Unhealthy Diet

Approximately 16 million (1.0%) DALYs and 1.7 million (2.8%) of deaths worldwide are due to low fruit and vegetable consumption. The amount of dietary salt consumed plays a vital role in determining the blood pressure levels and overall cardiovascular risk. Adequate consumption of fruit and vegetables can reduce the risk of CVD.

For the prevention of CVD, WHO recommends a salt intake of less than 5 grams/person/day. A correlation also exists between the magnitude of salt reduction and the magnitude of blood pressure reduction within the daily intake range of 3–12 grams/day; the lower the salt intake, the lower will be the blood pressure.

In addition, to decrease the relative risk of Acute Myocardial Infarction (AMI), a modest intake of fish (as little as 35 g daily) is needed. Following general advice to decrease the intake of saturated fats and cholesterol and increase the intake of polyunsaturated fats positively affects serum lipid levels and decreases the possibility of CHD. At last, weight maintenance education should be a part of routine advice for the general population, but is particularly important in patients at increased risk of cardiovascular events.

Stress

Stress also plays an important role in enhancing the cardiovascular risk. Stress may be related to physical, psychosocial, environmental, familial or economic factors. In recent times, an Expert Working Group of the National Heart Foundation of Australia undertook a review of the facts relating to major psychosocial risk factors where they concluded that there was no strong or consistent evidence for a causal association between chronic life events, work-related stressors (job control, demands and strain), type A behavior patterns, hostility, anxiety disorders or panic attacks and CHD. However, there are evidences which are strong and consistent of an independent and causal association between depression, social isolation and the prognosis of CHD. Hence it's crucial that these psychosocial factors are considered during individual CHD risk assessments.

Physical Inactivity

The fourth leading risk factor for mortality is insufficient physical activity. Approximately 3.2 million deaths and 32.1 million DALYs representing about 2.1% of global DALYs each year are attributable to inadequate physical activity.

The key determinant of energy expenditure and the fundamental thing to energy balance and weight control is physical activity. It improves endothelial function, which enhances vasodilatation and vasomotor function in the blood vessels.

Associations between physical activity and CVDs have reported reduced risk of death from coronary heart disease and reduced risk of overall CVDs, coronary heart disease and stroke in a number of studies. The prevalence of insufficient physical activity is more than double in high-income countries as compared to low-income countries for both men and women, with 41% of men and 48% of women being insufficiently physically active in high-income countries compared to 18% of men and 21% of women in low-income countries.

Berlin & Colditz assessed a relative risk of death from coronary heart disease of 1.9 (95% CI 1.6 to 2.2) for people with sedentary occupations compared with those with active occupations. A meta-analysis of studies in women showed that physical activity was related to a reduced risk of overall cardiovascular disease, coronary heart disease and stroke, in a dose–response fashion.

In summary, a sedentary lifestyle and increased risk of cardiovascular diseases are associated.

Obesity

At least 2.8 million people die each year as a result of being overweight or obese, and an estimated 35.8 million (2.3%) of global DALYs are caused by overweight or obesity worldwide. A growing health problem in both developed and developing countries is Obesity. Prospective epidemiological studies have revealed a relationship between overweight or obesity and cardiovascular morbidity, CVD mortality and total mortality. Obesity is strongly correlated to major cardiovascular risk factors, such as raised blood pressure, glucose intolerance, type 2 diabetes, and dyslipidemia. A weight reducing diet, combined with exercise, produces significant weight loss, reduces total cholesterol and LDL cholesterol, increases HDL cholesterol, and improves control of blood pressure and diabetes as shown by Meta-analyses of RCTs.

In a review of data from 24 prospective observational studies, **Blair & Brodney** found that many of the health risks associated with overweight and obesity are attenuated with regular physical activity. The level of obesity more than triples from 7% obesity for both males and females in lower-middle-income countries to

24% in upper-middle-income countries. Rising income is associated with rising rates of overweight among infants and young children in high-income countries. In contrast, in medium and low-income countries a positive relationship between socio-economic status and obesity in men, women and children has been seen.

Alcohol

There is a complex relationship between alcohol consumption and coronary heart disease and cerebrovascular diseases. A direct relationship also exists between higher levels of alcohol consumption and the pattern of binge drinking (defined as 60 or more grams of pure alcohol per day) with the risk of CVD. In general alcohol consumption is associated with multiple health risks that, at the population level, clearly prevail over potential benefits. High mortality from all causes and cardiovascular disease, including sudden death and hemorrhagic stroke can be seen in people who drink heavily. In addition, they may also suffer from psychological, social and other medical problems related to high alcohol consumption.

Hypertension

About 7 million premature deaths throughout the world and 4.5% of the disease burden (64 million DALYs) is estimated to be caused by raised blood pressure. It is a chief risk factor for cerebrovascular disease, coronary heart disease, and cardiac and renal failure. Treatment of raised blood pressure has been associated with a 35–40% reduction in the risk of stroke and a 16% reduction in the risk of myocardial infarction. Raised blood pressure often coexists with cardiovascular risk factors, such as tobacco use, overweight or obesity and dyslipidemia which increase the cardiovascular risk attributable to any level of blood pressure. Worldwide, these coexisting risk factors are often poorly addressed in patients with raised blood pressure, with the result that, even if their blood pressure is lowered, these people still have high cardiovascular morbidity and mortality rates.

In patients with diabetes, reduction of diastolic blood pressure to about 80 mmHg and of systolic blood pressure to about 130 mmHg is accompanied by a further reduction in cardiovascular events in comparison with patients with less stringent blood pressure control as seen in several trials. Blood pressure should be reduced to 130/80 mmHg or less in patients with high or very high cardiovascular risk, including diabetes or established vascular or renal disease. Policies to reduce salt consumption can change the population distribution of blood pressure so that there is a drop in cardiovascular risk. Through non-pharmacological (e.g. low salt diet, physical activity) and pharmacological measures, stroke and heart attack risk of people with high cardiovascular risk and/or raised blood pressure can be reduced. Primary care access to cardiovascular risk assessment and necessary medicines for reducing cardiovascular risk can improve health outcomes of people with hypertension.

Lipid Management

The benefits of cholesterol lowering therapy depend on the initial level of cardiovascular risk as shown in many studies. This happens because the relative reductions in risk as a consequence of lipid lowering are approximately the same at different levels of cardiovascular risk. Some systematic reviews and RCTs showed that cholesterol reduction improves cardiovascular outcomes in high-risk populations. The benefit is related to Baseline risk and extent of cholesterol reduction rather than initial cholesterol level.

In the Heart Protection Study (2002) a wide range of high-risk individuals aged 40–80 years, (n = 20536) were randomly allocated to receive 40 mg of Simvastatin daily or a placebo.

In this study it was found that about one-third of the participants were free of coronary heart disease where statin therapy reduced major vascular events.

Costa et al. (2006) evaluated the clinical benefits of lipid lowering drug treatment for primary and secondary prevention in patients with and without diabetes with systematic review and meta-analysis. Twelve randomized placebo-controlled double-blind trials, with a follow-up of at least 3 years were included in it. The analysis confirmed that patients, whether diabetic or not, benefit from lipid lowering in accordance with their complete cardiovascular risk.

Control of Diabetes

People with diabetes account for about 60% of all mortality in cardiovascular diseases. People with type 1 or type 2 diabetes are 2–3 times higher in the risk of cardiovascular events and the risk is disproportionately higher in women. Diabetic clients are often seen poorer than the nondiabetics in prognosis.

The first approach to control glycaemia should be through diet alone; if this is not sufficient, oral medication should be given, followed by insulin if necessary. Severe complications including heart attacks, strokes, renal failure, amputations and blindness occurs due to lack of early detection and care for diabetes. Health outcomes of people with diabetes can be improved with Primary care access to blood glucose measurement and cardiovascular risk assessment as well as essential medicines including insulin.

Hormonal Replacement Therapy

Hormone therapy has been used for prevention of cardiovascular disease, osteoporosis and dementia on the basis of data from observational studies.

Cochrane systematic review of 15 randomized double-blind trials (involving 35089 women aged 41 to 91 years) examined the effect of long-term hormone replacement therapy on mortality, cancer, gallbladder disease, fractures, heart disease, venous thromboembolism, stroke, transient ischemic attacks, and quality of life. They were placebo-controlled trials, in which perimenopausal or postmenopausal women were given estrogens, with or without progestogens for at least a year. Decreased incidences of fractures and colon cancer with long-term use were the only statistically significant benefit of hormone therapy. Long-term estrogen-only hormone therapy also considerably increased the danger of stroke and gallbladder disease.

Strategies to Control CVDs

In order to improve cardiovascular health, implementation of policies across different sectors is essential. It has an important role in the governance required for intersectoral action, even though it should not expect to lead all activities in other sectors. The health sector also works with other sectors and holds an important role to reduce differences in exposure and vulnerability to cardiovascular risk factors. Despite new insights into the impact on health of poor housing, built-up environment, lack of education and unemployment, systems in all countries remain insufficient to coherently execute whole-of-government strategies working between different sectors to address these issues. A significant obstacle to progress is the lack of development of the necessary governance and systems to implement coherent policies across government. The response needs to think about the impact of intersectoral policies on health as well as the profit of improvements in health for the goals of other sectors.

Need for a National Policy Framework

If health is a key consideration of sector-wide public policies in domains that have an influence on health, environments conducive to healthy behaviors can be created. The domains that influence health are transport, agriculture, education, finance, social services and trade. Only such a policy environment can provide people opportunities and reasonable choices to change and sustain healthy behaviors in relation to diet, physical activity and tobacco and alcohol use.

Effective Communication

Effective communication can initiate change. Bridging a gap between technical experts, policymakers and the general public is the core role of health communication.

How Is Effective Communication Beneficial?

- The aim of communication is to create awareness, improve knowledge and encourage long-term changes in individual and social behaviors.

- To act resourcefully on the opportunities at all stages of policy formulation and execution.

- Consumers will be better informed and capable of making healthier choices if sustained and well-targeted communication is present.

- The cost to the world of the present and expected epidemic of chronic disease associated to diet and physical inactivity dwarfs all other health costs. If society can be mobilized to recognize those costs, policymakers will ultimately start confronting the issue and they will become instruments of change.

Policies and Strategies for Tobacco Control

Chronic Care Foundation revealed that the Ministry of Health & Family Welfare has initiated the process of establishing a National Program for Tobacco Control to ensure availability of adequate resources for implementation of WHO FCTC (Framework Convention for Tobacco Control). The ministry is actively advocating with other stakeholder ministries for implementing effective tobacco control taxation and pricing policies.

The Tobacco Control Act, 2003 prohibits smoking in public places, direct or indirect advertisement of cigarettes and other tobacco products on billboards and in all media without point of sale. Rules prohibiting the sale of tobacco products to minors (less than 18 years), sale within a radius of 100 yards of any educational institution and rules for specified health warnings on the packages of all kinds of tobacco products have been issued. School teachers are the role model for students, conveyors of tobacco prevention and key opinion leaders for school tobacco control policy.

Many countries have effectively implemented the following articles of the WHO FCTC:

- Raising tobacco taxes and prices.
- Creating fully smoke free environments in indoor workplaces, public places and transportation.
- Counsel the population about the dangers of tobacco.
- Prohibition of tobacco advertising, promotion and sponsorship.
- Creating strong national tobacco control programs as a mechanism to exert governmental leadership in tobacco control.
- Protecting public health policies from commercial and other vested interests of the tobacco industry.

Policies and Strategies to Facilitate Healthy Eating

Increased consumption of snacks and drinks high in sugar, consumption of nutrient poor foods and increased caloric intake are associated with television advertising. To reduce CVDs and other NCDs, improvement of infant and young child feeding and the reduction in marketing of foods and non-alcoholic beverages high in salt, fats and sugar to children, are some of the cost-effective actions. For the implementation of food and nutrition policies a combination of national and local level actions in different sectors is beneficial. Maternity protection at work, improvement of family and community practices, improving skills in health workers, communication and information strategies, product labeling to help consumers make the right food choices and improving school food in combination with educational activities and interventions in workplace settings are included in this.

For maximum intake of salt for adults at 5 grams/day (i.e. 2000 mg/day of sodium) or lower, WHO has set a global target in terms of year by which the optimum will be reached. Steps to decrease salt intake by reducing salt in processed food are to be taken. Fried foods like samosa and kachori should be avoided. In rural areas, a public education campaign is required to support people to use less salt.

Policies and Strategies to Facilitate Physical Activity

For the prevention and control of CVD and in addressing overweight and obesity, physical activity can play a significant role. Areas for action on physical activity promotion include:

i. School-based programs.

ii. Transport policies that prioritize walking and cycling.

iii. Primary healthcare.

iv. Public awareness and mass media.

v. Community-wide programs.

vi. Sports system.

The participation of the sectors and leaders corresponding to each of these areas of action is critical as an effective approach requires the implementation of multiple concurrent strategies. Adequate levels of physical activity, like every day walking and cycling as a means of transportation, can best be achieved through an enabling environment. Thus, increasing physical activity is a public responsibility and not just an individual responsibility.

In urban settings, opportunities for physical activity are reducing due to the changing environment. City dwellers wish to have sedentary occupations, to use motorized means of transportation and are less interested to engage in physical activity during their leisure and recreation time.

The WHO Global NCD Action Plan (2008) urges Member States to promote physical activity through the implementation of school-based interventions and the provision of physical environments that support safe active commuting, safe transport and the creation of space for recreational activity. Therefore, facilitation of physical activities plays an important role in promoting a healthy lifestyle and reducing cardiovascular events.

Policies and Strategies for Alcohol Consumption

The Community Preventive Services Task Force recommends several strategies to prevent excessive alcohol consumption and associated harms from it. These strategies are based on systematic reviews of the scientific confirmation on intervention efficiency.

- Increasing alcohol taxes can decrease alcohol-related harms as well as revenue raising. Alcohol taxes are beverage specific and are implemented at the state and federal level. These taxes are generally based on the amount of beverage purchased.

- Maintaining restrictions on days of sale aims to prevent excessive alcohol consumption and related harms by regulating access to alcohol. Most policies are intended for weekend days (usually Sundays), and they may be relevant either to alcohol outlets in which alcohol may be legally sold, or to places where the buyer can drink at the place of purchase, like on-premises outlets, such as bars or restaurants.

- Maintaining limits on hours of sale is also planned, in part, to prevent excessive alcohol consumption and related harms by adaptable access to alcohol.

- Regulation of Alcohol Outlet Density is defined as applying state, country, city, or other type of governmental control to reduce or limit the number of places that can legally sell alcohol within a given area. Regulation is often implemented through licensing or zoning processes. An alcohol outlet is a place where alcohol may be legally sold for the buyer to drink there or elsewhere.

- Maintaining Minimum Legal Drinking Age (MLDA) Laws involves supporting legislation that specifies an age below which the purchase and consumption of alcoholic beverages are not allowed. MLDA laws have been shown to reduce alcohol-related crashes and associated injuries among 18 to 20-year-old drivers. All states currently have an MLDA of 21 years.

- Privatization of Retail Alcohol Sales is the repeal of state, country, city, or other type of governmental control over the retail sales of alcoholic beverages, thus allowing commercial retailing of those beverages. States with government control of alcohol sales are referred to as control states, and states with privatized sale are referred to as license states. The privatization of retail alcohol sales generally applies only to off-premises alcohol outlets and does not generally affect the retail sales of alcoholic beverages at on-premises alcohol outlets.

- Drink-driving countermeasures such as lowered blood alcohol concentration limits and "zero tolerance" for young drivers, random breath testing.

- Legal-based comprehensive restrictions on bans on advertising and promotion of alcoholic beverages.

- Treatment of alcohol use disorders and brief interventions for hazardous and harmful drinking.

To ensure mobilization of political will and the necessary resources for sustainable multi-sectoral action to guarantee the necessary resources and establish appropriate monitoring and evaluation mechanisms is the challenge to the implementation of these effective strategies.

Overcoming the Barriers

✓ **Participation of community members**

- Empowerment of the community is important, through effectively communicated health information.

- Integrating promotive and preventive care, early detection of risk factors and disease, as well as certain types of emergency care into the area of primary health care.

- A large mass of individuals can be energized to take on functions traditionally assigned to health care providers in a public health system with an objective to empower communities with information and skills.

- The outreach of services would be greatly enhanced through financial and technical resources and referral support provided by the public health system.

✓ **Care Providers in Primary Health Care**

- Services will extend outreach at a lower cost if the delivery of services is given by trained public health nurses, community health workers, and practitioners of complementary systems of medicine.

- To deliver the essential services, cadres of Community Health Workers (CHWs) are recruited from within the communities. The recruitment, training, and deployment of CHWs will help in providing chronic care by enhancing the number of trained paramedics with a clear mandate for chronic care.

- Similarly, the development of a cadre of public health nurses will help to increase the number of primary health care providers prepared with the skills for delivering essential chronic care.

- Practitioners of alternate (complementary) systems of medicine also need to be recruited into the delivery of chronic care on a particular country context.

✓ **Participation of Governmental and Non-Governmental Organizations**

- Professional associations must be comprehensively engaged in this effort, so that the private care providers are effectively addressed, in addition to government employees. Non-governmental organizations (NGOs) too can play a valuable role in creating educational resources as well as facilitating the training of various categories of care providers.

- In secondary and tertiary health care services the role of private sector has rapidly grown. In a number of states, the deliberate sector (represented by health NGOs) has also been contributing to primary and secondary care through direct services.

Literature Related to Current Trends in Controlling CVDs

➢ **Yoga**

A study was conducted by Roopa B Ankad et al. on the Effect of Short-term Pranayama and Meditation on Cardiovascular Functions in Healthy Individuals which concluded that there was a significant decrease in resting pulse rate and systolic and diastolic blood pressure after yoga practice, which is in harmony with the findings of other studies on physiological effects of yoga practice in healthy individuals. Similarly it was also reported about the reduction in resting PR and blood pressure after yoga practice in hypertensive patients, asthmatic patients and in diabetic patients.

Another study by **Pandurang Narhare** was done to know the effect of yoga on heart rate and blood pressure in healthy volunteers above the age of 40 years. The resting heart rate and blood pressure was assessed before the start of yoga practice and again after 6 months of yoga practice. The results were compared with respect to age, sex and BMI. The findings revealed that significant reduction in the heart rate occurs in the subjects practicing yoga (P<0.001). The systolic blood pressure was lowered to a highly significant level (P<0.001) and the diastolic blood pressure was reduced significantly (P<0.001). This revealed that the yoga provides significant improvement in aging to reduce the morbidity and mortality from cardiovascular diseases.

> **Meditation**

Department of Physiology, B.J. Medical College conducted a comparative study on respiratory functions, cardiovascular parameters and lipid profile of those practicing Raja Yoga meditation (short and long-term meditators) with those of non-meditators. The results revealed that vital capacity, tidal volume and breath holding were appreciably higher in short and long-term meditators as compared to non-meditators. Also meditators who did the meditation for a long time had significantly higher vital capacity and expiratory pressure than short-term meditators. Diastolic blood pressure was significantly lower in both short and long-term meditators as compared to non-meditators. A significant lowering of serum cholesterol in short and long-term meditators as compared to non-meditators can be seen in lipid profile.

> **Acupressure**

Kristina L et al. (2010) in her study investigated the effects of a type of acupressure, Jin Shin, on cardiovascular function in stroke survivors. A randomized, placebo-controlled, single-blind crossover design was utilized, in which 16 participants received 8 weeks of either active or placebo acupressure followed by washout and crossover into the opposite treatment condition. Heart rate and blood pressure measurements were taken throughout the treatments. Results revealed that active acupressure reduced heart rate significantly more than did placebo acupressure during treatments.

> **Foot reflexology**

A study conducted by **Vinaya Thomas (2015)** reveals the effective use of foot reflexology for hypertensive patients where a quasi-experimental study was adopted to assess the effect of foot reflexology on vital parameters among hypertensive patients. Findings of the study revealed that there was significant reduction between pretest scores of values of vital parameters and post test scores of values of vital parameters at the level of $p<0.001$. The mean difference in pulse rate between pretest score and post test score was 22.6. In the case of respiratory rate and blood pressure the calculated mean differences were 5.6 and 1.68 respectively which was found to be significant at $p<0.005$. This study results showed that the application of foot reflexology techniques reduces the increased vital parameters and help to keep the normal levels, especially the blood pressure. Foot reflexology is an adoptable intervention to holistic nursing.

Key Points

- Cardiovascular diseases are one of the major leading causes of death. Risk factors such as hypertension, diabetes and hyperlipidemia cluster together and are major risk factors for strokes and heart attacks.
- Investment in prevention is the most sustainable solution for the CVD epidemic.
- Smoking cessation and avoidance of second-hand smoke reduce the cardiovascular risk and thereby help to prevent CVDs.

- Physical activity is a key determinant of energy expenditure and thus fundamental to energy balance and weight control.

- Use of alcohol should be avoided as it damages the heart muscle, increases the risk of stroke and promotes cardiac arrhythmia.

- A modest reduction in salt intake reduces blood pressure in individuals with both normal and raised blood pressure.

- Early detection of hypertension and treatment to reduce cardiovascular risk is vital for prevention of strokes and heart attacks.

- Implementation of policies to promote healthy lifestyles in children and youth is therefore essential for prevention of CVD.

References

1. Katz, D, & Ather, A (2009). Preventive Medicine, Integrative Medicine & The Health of The Public. Commissioned for the IOM Summit on Integrative Medicine and the Health of the Public.

2. Hugh R Leavell and E Gurney Clark (1979). Preventive Medicine for the Doctor in his Community (3rd ed.). Huntington, NY: Robert E Krieger Publishing Company.

3. Ref.: Murray CJ, Lopez AD. The global burden of disease, 1990–2020. Nat Med 1998; 4: 1241–3.

4. World Health Organization (2005). National Cardiovascular Disease Database. Retrieved from http://www.whoindia.org/LinkFiles/NMH_Resources_National_CVD_database-Final_Report.pdf.

5. Gupta, R, Gupta, S, Joshi, R, Xavier, D (2011). Translating evidence into policy for cardiovascular disease control in India. Health Research Policy and Systems.

6. Government of India Ministry of Home Affairs: Office of the Registrar General and Census Commissioner, India (2011). Summary – Report on causes of death: 2001–03 in India. Retrieved from http://censusindia.gov.in

7. Reddy, K S. & Satija, A (2010). The Framingham heart study: impact on the prevention and control of cardiovascular diseases in India. Progress in Cardiovascular Diseases, 53, 21–27. Retrieved from http://www.sciencedirect.com

8. Government of India Ministry of Health and Family Welfare (2005). Burden of Disease in India. National Commission on Macroeconomics and Health, New Delhi.

9. Joshi, R, Chow, CK, Krishnam Raju, P, Raju, R, Reddy, K S, MacMahon, S, Lopez, A D, & Neal, B (2009). Fatal and nonfatal cardiovascular disease and the use of therapies for secondary prevention in a rural region of India. Circulation: Journal of the American Heart Association, 119, 1950–1955.

10. India set to be 'heart disease capital of world,' say doctors. Express: Sat Sep 29 2012, 04: 26 hrs.

11. Cardiovascular diseases (CVDs) Fact sheet N 317 Updated January 2015 http://www.who.int/mediacentre/factsheets/fs317/en/

12. International Journal of Scientific and Research Publications, Volume 3, Issue 10, October 2013 2 ISSN 2250-3153.

13. Dariush Mozaffarian, Emelia J Benjamin, Alan S. Heart Disease and Stroke Statistics 2015 Circulation Volume 131(4): 29–322 January 27, 2015.

14. Australia's health 2014 Preventing and treating ill health http://www.aihw.gov.au/australias-health/2014/preventing-ill-health/

15. WHO Library Cataloguing-in-Publication Data Prevention of cardiovascular disease: guidelines for assessment and management of total cardiovascular risk. World Health Organization. ISBN 978 92 4 154717 8 (NLM classification: WG 120).

16. Global atlas on cardiovascular disease prevention and control Policies, strategies and interventions Editors: WHO; World Heart Federation; World Stroke Organization Number of pages: 164Publication date: 2011.

17. F D R Hobbs 2004 Oct; 90(10): 1217–1223. doi: 10.1136/hrt.2003.027680PMCID: PMC1768505 Cardiovascular disease: different strategies for primary and secondary prevention?

18. Prevention of Cardiovascular Disease Guidelines for assessment and management of cardiovascular risk.

19. Tuomilehto J et al. Finnish Diabetes Prevention Study Group. Prevention of type 2 diabetes mellitus by changes in lifestyle among subjects with impaired glucose tolerance. N Engl J Med. 2001; 344(18): 1343–1350.

20. Hooper L et al. Reduced or modified dietary fat for prevention of cardiovascular disease. Cochrane Database Syst Rev. 2000; (2): CD002137.

21. World Health Organization. WHO Report on the Global Tobacco Epidemic, 2011: warning about the dangers of tobacco, WHO, Geneva, 2011.

22. Causes of death 2008, World Health Organization, Geneva, http://www.who.int/healthinfo/global_burden_disease/

cod_2008_sources_methods.pdf. World Health Organization. Global status report on non-communicable diseases 2010. Geneva, WHO, 2010.

23. Prevention of cardiovascular disease: an evidence-based clinical aid 2004 Greg R Fulcher, Greg W Conner and John V Amerena, Practical Implementation Taskforce for the Prevention of Cardiovascular Disease Med J Aust 2004; 181(6): 1–14.

24. Ashenden R, Silagy C, Weller D. A systematic review of the effectiveness of promoting lifestyle change in general practice. Fam Pract. 1997; 14(2): 160–176.

25. Bazzano LA, Serdula MK, Liu S. Dietary intake of fruits and vegetables and risk of cardiovascular disease. Current Atherosclerosis Reports, 2003, 5: 492–499.

26. World Health Organization. Global health risks: Mortality and burden of disease attributable to selected major risks. Geneva, WHO, 2009.

27. World Health Organization. Global status report on non-communicable diseases 2010. Geneva, WHO, 2010.

28. Oguma Y, Shinoda-Tagawa T. Physical activity decreases cardiovascular disease risk in women: review and meta-analysis. Am J Prev Med. 2004; 26(5): 407–418.

29. Avenell A et al. What are the long-term benefits of weight reducing diets in adults? A systematic review of randomized controlled trials. J Hum Nutr Diet. 2004 Aug; 17(4): 317–35.

30. Blair SN, Brodney S. Effects of physical inactivity and obesity on morbidity and mortality: current evidence and research issues. Med Sci Sports Exerc. 1999; 31(11 Suppl): S646-S662.

31. Wang Y. Cross-national comparison of childhood obesity: The epidemic and the relationship between obesity and socioeconomic status. International Journal of Epidemiology, 2001, 30: 1129–1136.

32. Roerecke M, Rehm J. Irregular heavy drinking occasions and risk of ischemic heart disease: A systematic review and meta-analysis. American Journal of Epidemiology, 2010, 171: 633–644.

33. Marmot MG. Alcohol and coronary heart disease. Int J Epidemiol. 2001; 30(4): 724–729.

34. Collins R et al. Blood pressure, stroke, and coronary heart disease. Part 2: Short-term reductions in blood pressure. Lancet. 1990; 335: 827–838.

35. Zanchetti A, Ruilope LM. Antihypertensive treatment in patients with type-2 diabetes mellitus: what guidance from recent controlled randomized trials? Journal of Hypertension. 2002; 20(11): 2099–2110.

36. Costa J et al. Efficacy of lipid lowering drug treatment for diabetic and nondiabetic patients: meta-analysis of randomized controlled trials. BMJ. 2006; 332(7550): 1115–1124 (Epub 2006 Apr 3).

37. Levitan EB et al. Is nondiabetic hyperglycemia a risk factor for cardiovascular disease? A meta-analysis of prospective studies. Arch Intern Med. 2004; 164(19): 2147–2155.

38. Farquhar CM et al., the Cochrane HT Study Group. Long term hormone therapy for perimenopausal and postmenopausal women. Cochrane Database Syst. Rev. 2005; (3): CD004143.

39. WHO Strategic directions and recommendations for policy and research.

40. Cecchini M et al. Tackling of unhealthy diets, physical inactivity, and obesity: Health effects and cost-effectiveness. Lancet, 2010, 376: 1775–1784.

41. Resolution WHA61.14. WHO 2008–2013 Action plan for the global strategy for prevention and control of non-communicable diseases. Geneva, World Health Organization, 2008.

42. Roopa Ankad Heart Views, Immediate effect of short duration of slow deep breathing on heart rate variability 04/2011; 12(2): 58–62. DOI: 10.4103/1995–705X.86016.

43. Effect of meditation on respiratory system, cardiovascular system and lipid profile. (PMID: 12683226) Department of Physiology, B.J. Medical College, Ahmedabad-380016. Indian Journal of Physiology and Pharmacology [2002, 46(4): 487–491].

44. Kristina L McFadden, M.A. and Theresa D Hernández, Ph.D Cardiovascular Benefits of Acupressure (Jin Shin) Following Stroke ObjectivesComplement Ther Med. 2010 Feb; 18(1): 42–48.

45. Vinaya Anjaly Thomas. Effect of foot reflexology on vital parameters among hypertensive patients, 2015, unpublished thesis, Choithram College of Nursing, Indore (M.P.).

Chapter V (B)

Preventive Strategies for Cancer

Dr. T. Sivabalan

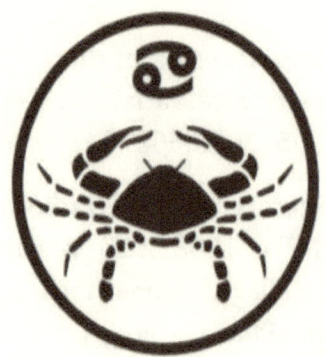 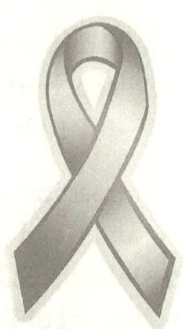

Introduction

'Never give up, life is worth living, there is life even after having cancer'

Cancer – a non-communicable disease – is emerging as one among the major public health problems in a developing country like India. Cancer affects everyone such as – the young and old, the rich and poor, men, women and children – and represents an enormous burden (physical, psychological, emotional, and financial) on patients, families and societies. The cancer impact is likely to increase substantially, causing lots of pain and suffering, and if not identified and treated properly on time with appropriate treatment, results in death.

Epidemiology

It is stated that approximately 80–90% of human cancers are attributable to the environmental and lifestyle factors such as use of tobacco and alcohol, and the dietary habits. World Health Organization estimated that worldwide 14 million new cases of cancer occurred, and 8.2 million cancer deaths occurred in 2012. It is expected that annual cancer cases may rise from 14 million in 2012 to 22 million within the next 2 decades. The most common causes of cancer deaths are cancers of lung (1.59 million deaths), liver (745000 deaths), stomach (723000 deaths), colorectal (694000 deaths), breast (521000 deaths) and esophageal cancer (400000 deaths).

Cancer is one among the top 10 leading causes of death in developing countries and the incidence of cancer in such countries is increasing alarmingly. In India cancer is an important public health problem with more than 9 lakhs cases occurring every year. Four lakhs deaths are estimated to occur every year due to cancer. The common cancer incidences in India were cervix uteri, breast, lip and oral cavity, lung and esophagus; however, the leading causes of cancer deaths were cervix uteri, lung, breast, lip and oral cavity, esophagus and pharynx.

Factors such as life style changes, modernization, urbanization, industrialization, population explosion and growing elderly population, all have contributed to epidemiological transition and development of cancers in the country. The risk of getting cancer before the age of 75 is 10% and the risk of dying from cancer is 7.5%. In India tobacco-related cancers constitute around 40% of all cancers in men, while among women high incidence rates were reported for breast, cervix and ovarian cancers which together accounted for 59% of all cancers in women.[10] Interestingly, more than 70% of patients report for diagnostic and treatment services in health care settings with advanced stages of disease, and this has led to a poor survival and high mortality rate.

> ### Box No: 1 Some Cancer Statistics
>
> **Tobacco use** – responsible for at least 30% of all cancer deaths, causing 87% lung cancer in men and 70% lung cancer in women
>
> **Overweight, obesity and physical inactivity** – responsible for 7 to 41% of all cancers **Harmful alcohol use** – responsible for 6% of death worldwide, 1 in 8 of which is due to cancer disease
>
> **Infections** (HPV/HIV) – responsible for 18% of global cancer burden
>
> **Air pollution** (outdoor and indoor) – responsible for 8% of lung cancer deaths
>
> **Occupational carcinogens** – responsible for 8% of lung cancer
>
> **(World Health Organization, 2012)**

Development of Cancer

Cancer is a group of more than 100 diseases, which originate from the cells that are abnormal in nature. All cancer cells have abnormal growth or out of control growth (i.e., abnormal proliferation and differentiation of cancer cells). There are 3 major types of cancers, such as, a) sarcoma – develops from the connective tissues (e.g., muscle and bone); b) carcinoma – develops from the epithelial tissues (e.g., lung, breast, prostate and colon); and c) lymphoma and leukemia – develops from the blood forming cells. Among these types, sarcoma is more prevalent in young persons and carcinoma is more common in older adults.

The human body is made up of various systems, these systems are comprised of a number of organs, organs are made up of a number of tissues and the tissues are composed of a number of cells. Cells are the basic unit of a human being and the body is made of trillions of live and viable cells. Normally the body cells grow, mature and break (divide) to form new cells, and after the life time a cell dies in an orderly way. In the early part of life (younger age) the cells divide faster and make the person grow. In middle part of life (adult), most of the cells divide slowly and divide only to replace the dying cells or to repair the tissue damage due to injuries/trauma. If the cells grow out of control, cancer occurs. In cancer, instead of dying, the cells continue to grow and form new abnormal cells, which are not regulated by the cell cycle. Alongside, the cancer cells have the ability of invading into other tissues and organs.

In every cell, deoxyribonucleic acid (DNA) is present in the nucleus which directs the functions of cells. In normal cell the damaged DNA dies off or repairs by itself. The damage may occur due to cellular damage from tobacco consumption, sunlight exposure and toxic agents, etc., or inheritance (it's passed on from their parents). If the damaged DNA does not die off, it produces new abnormal cells (which also have damaged DNA) that the body does not need.

Most of the times the causes of cancer are multifaceted and it's difficult to understand exactly what caused a cancer in the individual. Normally the cancer cells show cellular and nuclear changes, there is a loss of normal arrangement of cells, and changes in the cell membranes and organelles. The spreading of cancer form one place to another usually takes place through blood and lymph which is called as metastasis.

Risk Factors

Cancer is a complex group of diseases with many possible causes or risk factors. However many cancers develop without any apparent cause. Certain risk factors are known to increase the chance that one or more cells may become abnormal and this leads to cancerous changes. The risk factors for cancer include the following:

A. Age: Many cancers become more common as a person gets older. It is due to the accumulation of damage to cells over time, and the body's defense and resistance against abnormal cells become less effective than in younger age. Thus one damaged cell may manage to survive and multiply out of control, and develops into a cancer disease.

B. Genetic factors: Some types of cancer run in certain families, but most cancers are not clearly linked to the genes. The abnormal genes may trigger a cell to become abnormal and cancerous. The inherited mutations in a particular gene develop cancer (e.g., mutations in CDH1 gene – stomach cancer, mutations in BRCA1 and BRCA2 genes – breast cancer).

C. Immune system: People with poor immune system or problem in immune system have an increased risk of developing certain types of cancers. Individuals who had organ transplantation are suffering from HIV/AIDS and receiving immuno suppressive therapy, have higher risk of developing cancers. The chronic infection or transplanted organs can continually stimulate cells to divide, which may lead to genetic defect in the cells, and thus arises cancer.

D. Virus: Some viruses can cause cancer by causing the genetic changes in the cells which make the cells more likely to become cancerous. Viruses such as HPV – Cervical cancer and Oropharyngeal cancer, Hepatitis B and C virus – Liver cancer, Epstein Barr Virus (EBV) – Lymphomas, and T cell leukemia virus – T cell leukemia, cause various cancers as mentioned.

E. Bacteria: People who have Helicobacter pylori (H pylori) infection of stomach, develop inflammation, and have increased risk of stomach cancer.

F. Chemical carcinogens: Carcinogen is a substance (chemical – tobacco, radiation) which can damage a normal cell, and make it a cancerous cell. The more the exposure to carcinogenic agents, the greater is the risk of developing a cancer. The examples of carcinogens are:

a. tobacco – the smokers are more likely to develop cancer of lung, oral cavity, esophagus, bladder and pancreas. Smoking is thought to cause 1 in 4 of all cancers. The other forms of tobacco use like chewing tobacco, snuff, etc., also increase the risk of cancer, and

b. work place chemicals – like asbestos, benzene, formaldehyde, etc., increase the risk of developing certain cancers.

G. Lifestyle factors: Diet, physical activity and other lifestyle factors may increase the risk of developing cancers. Eating too much of fatty foods or red meat and processed meat, and having not enough fresh fruits and vegetables in the diet increases the probability of cancer occurrence in Gastro Intestinal Tract (colon, rectum). Drinking alcohol, lack of regular exercise and obesity can also increase the risk of developing some cancers. However eating lots of fruits and vegetables reduces the risk of cancers because these foods are rich in vitamins, minerals and antioxidants, etc., which protect against damaging chemicals that get into the body.

H. Radiation: Radiation is a carcinogen, and chronic exposure to the radioactive materials and nuclear fallout can increase the risk of leukemia and other cancers. Excessive exposure to sun light (Ultra Violet Rays – UV) increases the risk of developing skin cancers. Larger the exposure (dose), greater is the risk of cancer occurrence. Usually in the diagnostic procedures like X-ray and CT scan, the exposure is too meager to cause cancer.

I. Environmental factors: The environmental factors which are in and around the individuals may help to develop cancer. The factors such as tobacco smoke (passive smoking), sunlight, natural and manmade radiation, work place (occupational) hazards, etc., cause cancer. Usually these can be prevented and are avoidable; hence the risk of cancer is minimized.

Box No: 2 Risk Factors of Cancer

I. Non modifiable factors

- Age
- Family history (genetic factor)
- Female sex

II. Modifiable factors

- Infections (bacteria/virus)
- Radiation exposure
- Chemical carcinogen
- Risky sexual practices
- Environmental factors
- Exposure to sunlight
- Life style factors (diet, exercise, sedentary work, obesity, smoking, tobacco and alcohol)

Research Evidence: 01

The use of tobacco and its products causes around 31% of cancer deaths in men and 10% of cancer deaths in women worldwide, and it's a single most preventable modifiable cause of cancer. The research finding shows strong evidence of association between several nontobacco risk factors and the development of cancers. They are: a) consumption of alcohol and cancers of the oral cavity (mouth, pharynx, larynx, esophagus) and colorectum and breast, b) selected dietary factors and cancers of the liver (aflatoxins), lung (arsenic in drinking water and beta carotene supplements) and colorectum (red and processed meat), c) physical inactivity and colon cancer and d) adiposity and cancers of the esophagus, pancreas, colorectum, breast and kidney[1].

Research Evidence: 02

A systematic review of case control studies among Head and Neck Cancer patients showed that the family history (mainly first degree relatives) had increased risk of developing head and neck cancers. Alongside it revealed that the risk was higher when the affected relative was a sibling rather than a parent. It was noticed that the risk rose when the patients had history of alcohol and tobacco use. These results highlight that the family history plays a significant role in the etiology of Head and Neck Cancers[2].

Research Evidence: 03

A hospital based case control study on Human Papilloma Virus and other risk factors in development of cervical carcinoma in Southern India. A total of 205 cases and 213 age matched control women were included in the study. The polymerase chain reaction assay was used, and HPV infection was detected in all cases and in 27.7% of control women. Around 23 different HPV types were found, wherein HPV 16 was the most common type, followed by HPV 18 and 33, which showed a strong association. Other than HPV infection, the risk factors such as high parity, a woman's report of her husband's extramarital sexual relationships and early menopause were significantly associated with cervical carcinoma. It was recommended that the vaccine against HPV 16 and 18 may be effective in cervical cancers[3].

Research Evidence: 04

The scientific evidences proved that there is an association between infections (viral) and the development of cancer diseases. It was well supported by Harford JB, who found the significant associations between infections with Human Papilloma Virus, Epstein Barr Virus, Hepatitis C Virus and Kaposi Sarcoma Herpes Virus and cancers such as cervical cancer, Non Hodgkin and Hodgkin Lymphoma, hepatic carcinoma, and Kaposi Sarcoma respectively[4].

Research Evidence: 05

A study on association between alcohol intake and development of cancers of upper digestive tract highlighted that there was a strong dose dependent increase in risk of upper GIT cancer with increased alcohol intake. Compared with non-drinkers the risk of upper GIT cancer doubled among those drinking 7–21 drinks a week, whereas drinkers whose intake exceeded 69 drinks a week had a relative risk of 11.7. Compared with non-smokers, smokers of 1–19 g tobacco/day had a relative risk of 5.0 and smokers of >20 g tobacco/day had a risk of 7.5. It was evident that alcohol is a strong risk factor for oropharyngeal and esophageal cancer[5].

Research Evidence: 06

A study on risk factors of lung cancer in Chandigarh, highlights that the bidi smokers had a relative risk of 5.8 (95% CI: 3.4–9.7) and 11.6 (95% CI: 6.4–21.3), while cigarette smokers had values of 5.6 (95% CI: 3.15–10.1) and 7.7 (95% CI: 3.2–18.4). Smokers of more than 20 bidis per day had relative risk of 12.25 (95% CI: 4.15–36.1) and 33.2 (95% CI: 13.9–79.2) and smokers of more than 20 cigarettes daily, 5.8 (95% CI: 3.1–11.0) and 26.8 (95% CI: 6.0–120.2) respectively. It has been conclusively established that the prolonged exposure of tobacco smoke causes lung cancer[6].

Research Evidence: 07

The number of cancer cases caused by being obese is estimated to be 20% with the increased risk of malignancies being influenced by diet, body fat distribution and physical inactivity. Evidence have shown that the strongest association of obesity with the following cancers such as endometrial, esophageal adenocarcinoma, colorectal, breast, prostate, liver, pancreas and renal cancers. However obesity has weak association with malignancies like leukemia, lymphoma, multiple myeloma, malignant melanoma and thyroid tumors[7,8].

Warning Signs

Warning signs are an indication that something is wrong in the body, e.g., head ache is an early warning sign of increased blood pressure. Likewise the cancer disease also has certain warning signs which make the person more alert and help to seek professional medical help at appropriate time. The common warning signs of cancer are given below:

C. A. U. T. I. O. N

C – Change in bowel or bladder habits: In certain cancers there is a change in color, consistency, size or shape of stool (diarrhea/constipation), and presence of blood in urine or stool. These are commonly seen in colorectal cancer, bladder, kidney and prostate cancers.

A – A sore that does not heal: In some cancers there may be a sore that does not look better (healing) over a period of time, and will get bigger, more painful and start to bleed. These changes are commonly present in skin cancer, oral cancer, vaginal and penis cancers.

U – Unusual bleeding or discharge: There is a presence of blood in urine/stool, or discharge from nipple, penis, vagina, etc. which may suggest cancer diseases. These changes are commonly present in lung cancer, colon cancer, cervical cancer, breast cancer and bladder cancer, etc.

T – Thickening or lump in breast or other parts of body: There is a presence of thickening or lump in breast or scrotum (noticed when doing self-examination) and in any other part of the body, which suggests cancers. These changes are seen in breast and testicular cancers.

I – Indigestion or Difficulty in swallowing: Presence of feeling of pressure in the throat/chest which makes swallowing difficult and uncomfortable, and feeling of fullness with or without food. These manifestations are significantly present in esophageal cancer, stomach cancer and pharyngeal cancer.

O – Obvious change in mole or wart: Any alterations in Asymmetry, Border, Color and Diameter (ABCD) of the mole or wart indicate the signs of cancer (mainly the skin cancer/melanoma)

N – Nagging cough: Any obvious changes in voice or hoarseness of voice, and continuous cough which is not reduced/does not go away and presence of blood in the sputum. These manifestations are present in the lung cancer, laryngeal cancer or thyroid cancer.

> *'Warning signs – it's an indicator that gives a warning'*

Common Signs and Symptoms

The signs and symptoms are signals of injury, illness or disease. It's a signal that indicates something is not right in the body. A sign is a signal that can be seen by others – care giver, doctor or nurse. Example: fever and dyspnea, etc. A symptom is a signal that's felt or noticed by the person who has it, but may not be easily seen by others. Example: fatigue, pain and feeling of shortness of breath, etc. The common signs and symptoms are:

Table No. 5(b) 1: Signs and symptoms associated with cancers

SN	Site of cancer	Common signs and symptoms
1	Breast	Lump in the breast, asymmetry, skin retraction, recent nipple retraction, blood stained nipple discharge and eczematous changes in areola
2	Cervix	Post coital bleeding and excessive vaginal discharge
3	Colon and Rectum	Change in bowel habits, unexplained weight loss, anemia and blood in the stool
4	Oral cavity	White lesions (leukoplakia) or red lesions (erythroplakia) and growth or ulceration in mouth
5	Naso pharynx	Nose bleed, permanent blocked nose, deafness and nodes in upper part of neck
6	Larynx	Persistent hoarseness of voice
7	Stomach	Upper abdominal pain, recent onset of indigestion and weight loss

8	Skin melanoma	Brown lesion that is growing with irregular borders or areas of patchy coloration that may itch or bleed
9	Other skin cancers	Keratosis (lesion or sore on skin that does not heal)
10	Urinary bladder	Pain, frequent and uneasy urination and blood in urine
11	Prostate	Difficulty in urination and frequent nocturnal urination
12	Retinoblastoma	White spot in the pupil and convergent strabismus (in a child)
13	Testis	Swelling of one testicle (asymmetry)

Source: *Cancer Control 'Knowledge into action,' WHO guide for effective programs. Early Detection, World Health Organization, 2007*

Screening/Detection

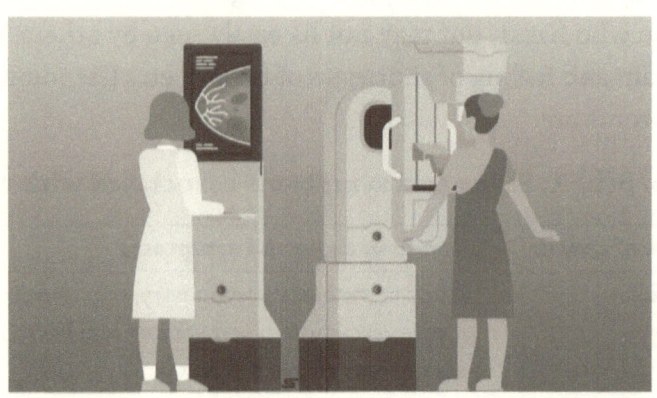

Screening refers to the use of simple tests among healthy population to identify individuals who have (risk of) cancer disease. The common examples of screening test for detection of cancers are: a) mammography (for breast cancer) and b) Pap smear test (for cervical cancer). The screening is usually carried out as mass screening (large population) and at times individual (selective) screening. The commonly used screening methods are: a) history and physical exam b) laboratory investigations c) imaging procedures and d) genetic tests.

The screening methods used to detect the common cancers are follows

I. Breast cancer

Perform the Breast Self-Examination (BSE) for women above 20 years of age (report any abnormality in breast like change in size, shape, presence of discharge, lump or tenderness, etc.) Figure No. 5(b) 1

Perform the clinical breast examination about every 3 years for women in their 30 years and every year exam for women 40 years and above

Perform the yearly mammograms (recommended) for the women above 40 years of age

Carry out MRI/CT scan, if the woman has family history or genetic predispositions

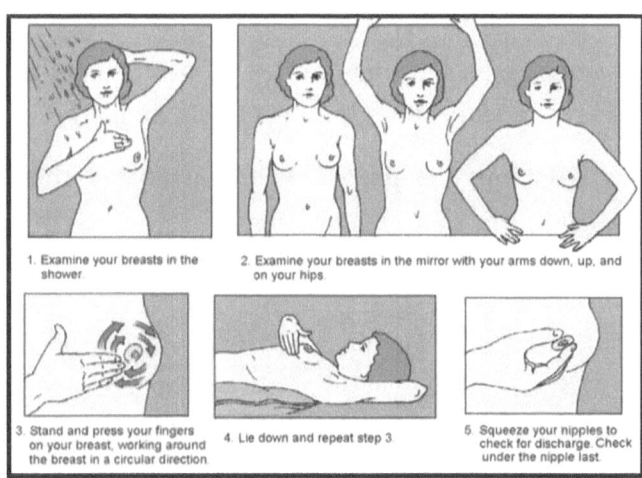

Fig. No. 5(b) 1: *Steps of Breast Self-Examination (BSE)*

II. Colorectal cancer

A person with 50 years of age and above needs to undergo the following tests such as:

Test to find the polyps: Perform the sigmoidoscopy, barium enema and CT colonoscopy once in every 5 years, and colonoscopy examination once in every 10 years.

Test to find the cancers: Perform the stool examination to assess the presence of occult blood once in a year, and fecal immunochemical test, fecal DNA test once in every 3 years; if the test is positive, a colonoscopy should be carried out.

III. Cervical cancer

Cervical cancer screening (testing) should begin at the age of 21 years, women between ages 21 to 29 should have a Pap smear test every 3 years. If abnormal results found, then test for HPV infection.

Women between the ages of 30 to 65 years must have a Pap smear test and HPV test every 5 years, or have a Pap test only in every 3 years.

IV. Uterine cancer

All the postmenopausal women should report the presence of symptoms such as unexpected bleeding or spotting, etc.

The endometrial biopsy is preferable for screening the uterine or endometrial cancers.

V. Lung cancer

The risk for lung cancer is mainly cigarette smoking (tobacco). Person who is above 55 years of age, with history of smoking for more than 15 years must be screened for malignancy.

VI. Prostate cancer

Men who are above 45 years must be tested for Prostate Specific Antigen (PSA) test with or without the Digital Rectal Examination (DSA), and it is very much essential for the men who have family history of prostate cancer.

'There can be a life after cancer, the prerequisite is early detection'

Diagnosis

The early screening and identification of cancer disease gives a better chance of its being managed and cured. The cancer treatment strategies, chemotherapy, radiation therapy and precise surgery provide solid base for the management of cancers. Some of the cancers such as cancer of skin, breast, mouth, testicles, prostate and rectum, etc., may be identified with routine assessment or self-examination before they become advanced disease or serious. The cancer disease is commonly diagnosed with the help of a thorough physical/clinical examination and a complete medical history. The laboratory investigations such as blood test, urine and stool examination may detect the presence of abnormalities that may suggest the development of cancer. After the initial assessment and screening, if tumor is suspected, then the diagnostic studies such as imaging tests like X-rays, CT scan, MRI, ultrasound (USG), endoscopy, Fine Needle Aspiration Cytology/Biopsy (FNAC) are carried out to determine the location, size and stage of cancer disease.

Management

The primary objective of cancer treatment was a) cure from disease b) prolonging the life and c) enhancement of quality of life (QOL) and longer survival. Treatment of cancer patients usually starts with recognition of disease by patient and health care professionals. The common cancer treatment strategies are chemotherapy, radiation therapy, surgery and hormonal therapy or a combination of these modalities.

A. Surgery: It's nothing but the removal of (cancer) tumor from the body, where surgery is used to diagnose, treat, cure or control the cancer disease. The impact of surgery is enormous if the cancer does not metastasize to other parts of the body. It's a most commonly used method of treatment for cancers.

B. Radiation therapy: It's a use of high doses of radiation (ionizing and non-ionizing) or energy particles to kill or destroy the cancer cells or shrink tumors. It is considered as local treatment where it focuses on the cancer site only. The radiation can be given internally, inside the organ (brachytherapy) or externally (teletherapy). This treatment is often used in combination with other treatment methods.

C. Chemotherapy: It's the use of drugs (anti-neoplastic agents) to kill or treat cancers. It is commonly administered intravenously (IV) where it has systemic effect (spread throughout body) on the body, and may be given as adjuvant (given after the main treatment like surgery) or neoadjuvant therapy (given before the main treatment like surgery, radiation).

D. Immuno therapy (biotherapy): It's a treatment that uses certain parts of a person's immune system to fight diseases such as cancer. This can be achieved by administering the immune system components, like manmade immune system proteins. The monoclonal antibodies and cancer vaccines are the examples of immunotherapy.

E. Gene therapy: It can be done outside the body (ex vivo) by extracting bone marrow or blood from the patient and growing the cells in a laboratory. The corrected/modified copy of the gene is introduced and allowed to penetrate into the cell's DNA before being injected back into the body. Gene transfers can also be done directly inside the patient's body (in vivo).

F. Targeted therapy: It's a newer type of cancer treatment where the drugs are used more precisely to attack the cancer cells, and the damage to normal cells is minimal.

G. Stem cell transplantation: It is used to replace stem cells in bone marrow when the bone marrow has been destroyed by disease or treatments like chemotherapy or radiation therapy. There are 3 types of stem cell transplants, which are classified, based on the sources from where the stem cells are collected. Autologous – the cells come from patient itself, Allogeneic – the cells come from a matched related or unrelated donor and Syngeneic – the cells come from the patient's identical twin.

Though these cancer treatment strategies are frequently very effective in controlling tumor progression, reducing cancer pain and discomfort, and extending life and quality of life, however, research evidences highlight that such therapies come with the risk of substantial side effects, some of which are short-term and time limited while others are long-term and serious side effects.

> **'Once an individual overcomes cancer, he doesn't need to be afraid of anything anymore'**

Prevention of Cancer

Prevention is an activity directed to prevent the illness, and promoting the health to reduce the need for secondary or tertiary health care. Majority (one-third) of all types of cancers are preventable. World Health Organization reported that more than 40% of all cancers (including breast, colorectal and cervical cancers) can be prevented and cured if they are identified and detected early. As prevention is better than cure, it is the key element in cancer control. Preventive strategies enhance the cost-effective long-term strategy for the control of cancer. People can follow and adhere to specific preventive strategies in their everyday lives to reduce the risk of developing cancers.

> **'Cancer is a Preventable Disease that Requires Major Lifestyle Changes'**

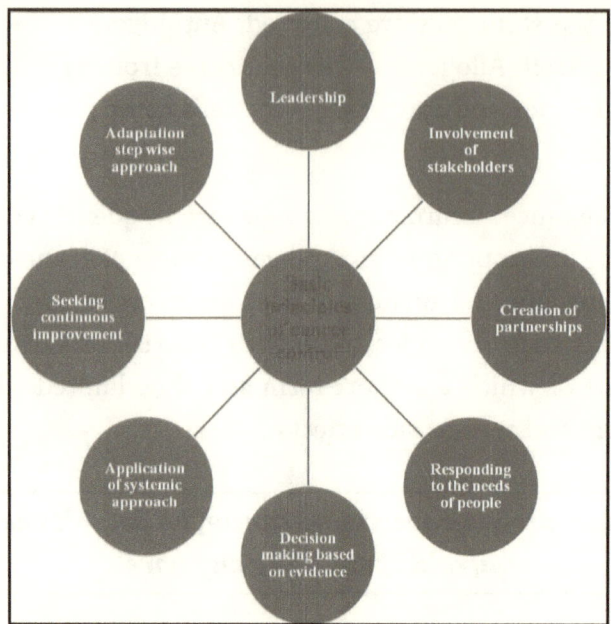

Fig. No. 5(b) 2: *Basic principles of cancer control*
Source: Cancer Control 'Knowledge into action,' WHO guide for effective programs. Palliative Care, World Health Organization, 2007

A. Individual Preventive Measures

The following below mentioned measures if followed diligently can result in the prevention of or reducing the chances of having cancer. The measures are:

1. Eat a healthy balanced diet: Regular consumption of a healthy balanced diet helps to reduce the risk of developing certain cancers. A healthy balanced diet consists of more of fruits and vegetables, plenty of bread, rice, potatoes, beans and wholegrain foods, etc. Alongside, eat some (small amount of) meat, fish and dairy products.

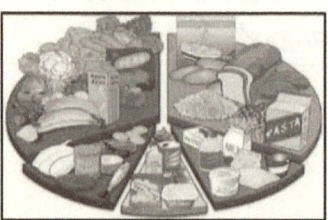
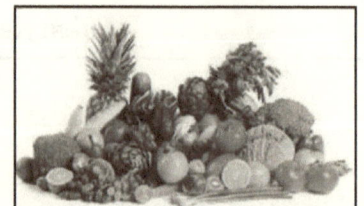

Consuming 4 to 5 cups of mixed fruits every day and eating healthy balanced diet helps to make sure that the body gets all the nutrients required. National Cancer Institute recommends a diet with large amounts of fruits and vegetables; these foods supply ample amounts of vitamin A, C and E as well as phytochemicals and antioxidants that help to prevent cancer.

2. Eat more fiber: Eating plenty of fiber rich food items reduces the risk of gastro intestinal cancers. Diet high in fiber helps to keep the bowel healthy and prevents constipation. The examples of fiber rich foods are whole grains, bread, cereals, rice, pulses, fruits and vegetables, etc.

3. Eat less red meat and processed meat: Though the non-vegetarian foods items such as meat and poultry are a good source of protein, vitamins, iron and zinc, the evidence suggests that the increased intake of meat (red and processed) enhances chances of the development of bowel cancer.

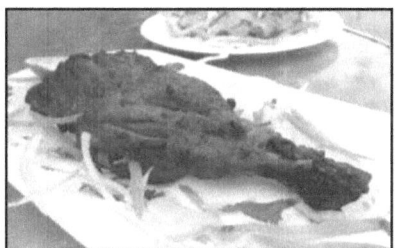 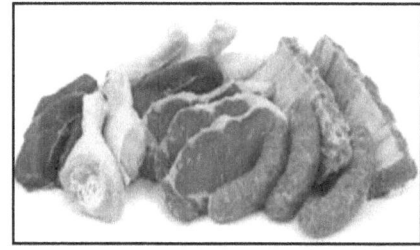

The reduced consumption or stoppage of use of red/processed meat like beef and pork drastically reduces the occurrence of gastro intestinal cancers.

4. Control or maintain a healthy weight: The excess overweight or obesity increases the risk of development of certain cancers such as bowel cancer, esophageal cancer, breast cancer and pancreatic cancer, etc. Maintenance of healthy body weight (normal Body Mass Index – BMI) and increased physical activities reduces the risk of cancer development. The significant and useful weight reduction measures are maintaining healthy diet, regular exercises (30–45 minutes) and avoidance of excessive weight gain. Include and practice regular exercise regimen in the day-to-day activities. Try to become more active on many days.

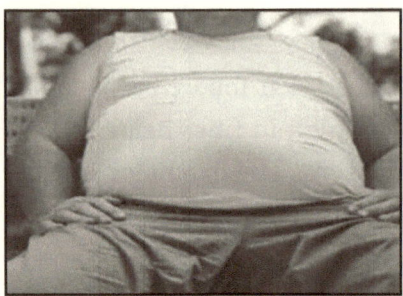 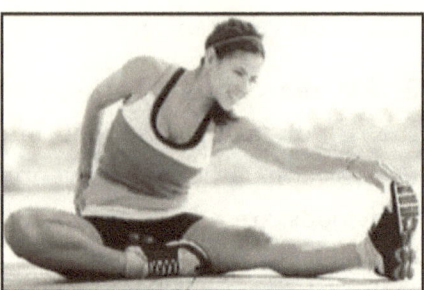

> **WHO defines Over Weight as a BMI equal to or more than 25, and obesity as a BMI equal to or more than 30**

5. Control or Drink less alcohol: There is strong evidence that suggests that alcohol consumption leads to certain cancers (head and neck cancers, liver cancer). It was found that the cancer risk declines after the person stops drinking alcohol or drinks less alcohol.

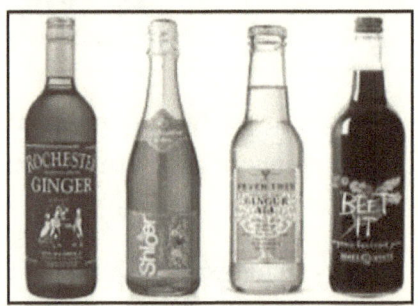 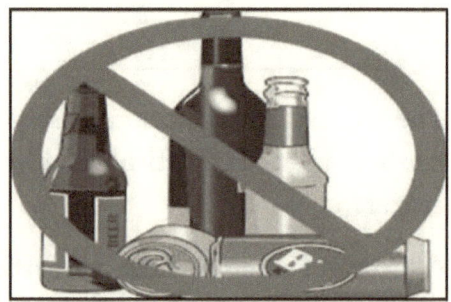

> **'An ounce of prevention is worth more than a million pounds of cure'**

The risk of developing cancer substantially increases when the person has drinking and smoking habits. If the person stops taking alcohol, the smoking also diminishes; thereby the combined effect on cancer development reduces drastically.

6. Stop smoking, avoid use of tobacco products: More than 70% of lung cancer is attributed to smoking alone. Alongside, smokeless tobacco (oral tobacco/chewing tobacco/snuff) causes oral, esophageal and pancreatic cancer. Stopping smoking greatly cuts the risk of developing lung cancers. The earlier a person stops, the greater the impact on health. But, it is never too late to quit smoking; the avoidance of tobacco carcinogen increases the survival and lessens the severity of cancer.

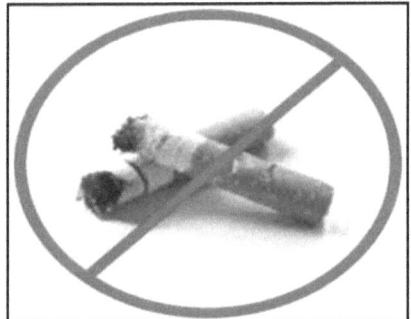
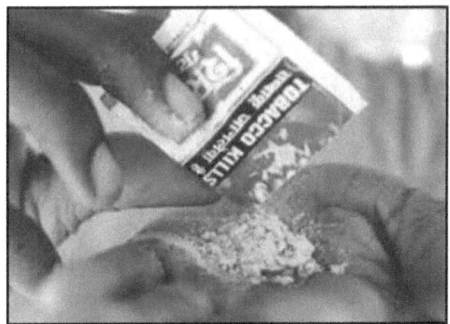

7. Protect the skin from sunlight: Avoid the sun during middle of the day, because the sunrays are strongest between 11: 00am to 03: 00pm. Plan and schedule your activities other times of the day. Cover the skin with dark, tightly woven clothing that covers the arms and legs. Use hat, sunglasses in day times, and apply sunscreen generously.

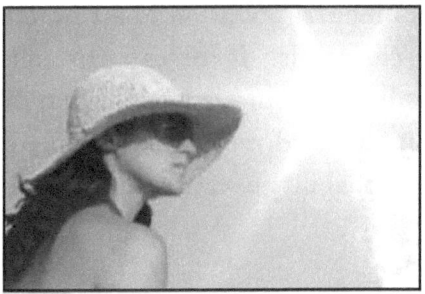
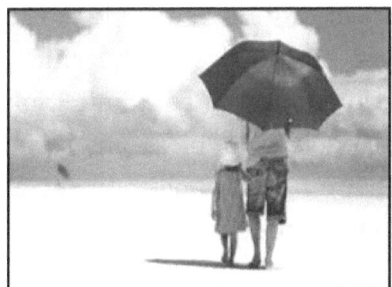

8. Avoid risky sexual practices: The practice of safe sexual practice is likely to reduce the sexually transmitted infections like HIV or HPV. The person having HPV or HIV has greater risk of getting cervical cancer, penis, and vagina cancers. Avoidance of sharing needles reduces the risk of hepatitis B and C which leads to liver cancer. In case of drug abuse or addiction get professional help to overcome the problem.

9. Get immunized against hepatitis B and HPV: Hepatitis B and C virus, HPV, H pylori and parasitic infection increase the risk of various cancers such as liver cancer, cervical cancer and bladder cancer, etc. Cancer prevention includes the protection from certain viral infections.

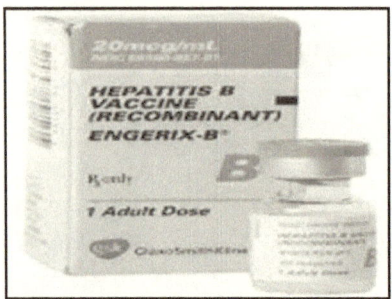
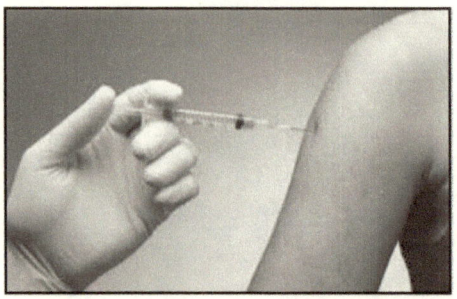

The hepatitis B vaccination is mandatory for those who have risky sexual behaviors and intra venous drug users; thereby it prevents the chance of getting cancerous diseases (liver cancer). Further, immunization against HPV infection protects against the cervical cancer and other genital cancers.

10. Control environmental pollution: Among the cancers around 5% of cancers occur due to the environmental pollution of air, water and soil with carcinogenic agents/chemicals. It occurs through drinking water, contamination of foods by chemicals or pollution of indoor and ambient air. Serious individualized measures to control environmental pollution decrease the probability of cancer occurrence in humans.

11. Avoidance of occupational carcinogens: In working areas around 40 agents and mixtures are carcinogenic to human beings, which are commonly termed as occupational carcinogens. The occupational carcinogens exposure commonly leads to cancer of lung, bladder, larynx, skin, and leukemia. Practicing the standard and specific safety measures during the working hours is the prime way to minimize the cancer risk among employees. The individual who are prone to development of occupational carcinogens, are requested to stop working in those areas or change the areas of work.

12. Avoid or minimize the radiation exposure: Ionizing radiation exposure may produce leukemia and other cancers. Ultraviolet (UV) radiation (sun light) is carcinogenic to humans, causing all major types of skin cancer (basal cell carcinoma, squamous cell carcinoma and melanoma). Reduce the chance of radiation exposure by proper planning and prescribing appropriately in relation to investigations using radiation or X-rays, etc. Avoid unnecessary radiation doses, particularly in children. Avoidance of radiation and utilization of protective clothing and sunscreen, etc. are the effective protective methods for skin cancers.

13. Check your body and get regular medical help: It is of paramount importance to identify any changes in the body like lumps, unexplained bleeding, discharge, changes in bowel and bladder functions, etc. (self-examination); and inform the health care professionals to detect the abnormality at the earliest for better treatment and survival.

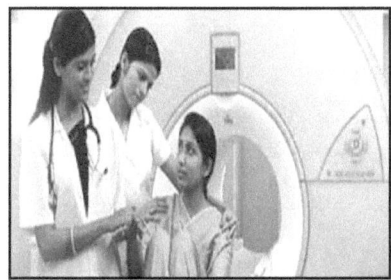
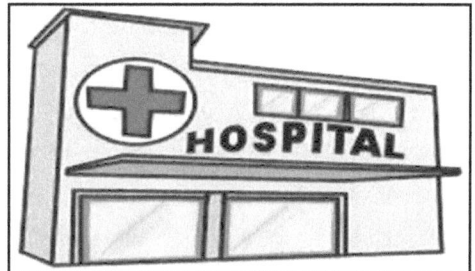

> *'The principal approach to cancer control is – Prevention, Early Detection, Diagnosis and Treatment'*

Research Evidence: 07

Cohort study by Hankinson SE, Colditx GA and Hunter DJ has shown that breast cancer risk was lowered by 50% in women who intentionally underwent weight loss higher than 10 kg after menopause. In addition, women who had bariatric surgery for obesity reported a significant reduction in cancer incidence in association with substantial weight loss.[9]

Research Evidence: 08

A use of single round of Visual Inspection with Acetic Acid (VIA) based screening led to a 25% reduction in cervical cancer incidence and a 35% reduction in mortality over seven years of follow up in Dindigul district of Tamil Nadu. Similarly the same results (31% reduction in mortality) were reported recently by a trial that offered multiple rounds of VIA based screening in Mumbai, Maharashtra.[10,11]

Research Evidence: 09

A systematic review on association between physical activity and breast cancer risk noticed that there was a 25% average risk reduction amongst physically active women as compared to the least active women; further the strongest associations were observed for recreational activity, for activity sustained over the lifetime, and for moderate to vigorous activity performed regularly. A greater decrease in breast cancer risk was observed with greater duration of activity (moderate to vigorous intensity). It was observed while participation in 2–3 hours per week was associated with an average risk reduction of 9%, women who reported 6–8 hours of activity per week or more had a decreased risk of 30%.[12]

B. Nutrition and Physical Activity for Cancer Prevention

Food plays an important role either in getting a cancer or for fighting against certain cancers in a human body. Good nutritional practices may help to prevent certain cancers.

Table No. 5(b) 2: List of cancer causing foods (to be avoided)

SN	Name of food	Cancer causing properties	Risk of cancers
1	Salted, Pickled and Smoked Foods	The salted and pickled products contain preservatives like nitrates which cause damage at cellular level and lead to cancer. The smoked foods are cooked at high temperature and have high level of acrylamide, and the nitrates are converted to much more dangerous nitrites	It increases the risk of developing colorectal cancer, stomach cancer and nasopharyngeal cancer
2	Processed meats	It contains the chemical preservatives like sodium nitrite and sodium nitrate (cancer causing ingredient), which influences the development of cancers	It increases the chance of developing colon and pancreatic cancer
3	Microwave popcorn	The microwave popcorn is lined with chemicals like perfluorooctanic acid and diacetyl linked to causing infertility and tumors	It enhances the development of lung cancer, liver, testicular and pancreatic cancers
4	Hydrogenated oils	It contains trans-fats, and it's commonly used to preserve processed foods, where it alters the structure and flexibility of cell membranes which leads to cancerous diseases.	It increases the risk of breast cancer, and prostate cancer

SN	Name of food	Cancer causing properties	Risk of cancers
5	Refined sugar	It contains fructose rich sweeteners (caramel color) and high fructose corn syrup which tend to increase insulin level and feed the growth of cancer cells and helps in proliferation. The food items containing this are candy, cakes, sodas, sauces and other cookies	It increases the incidence of bladder cancer, brain tumors, lymphoma and leukemia's
6	'Diet' foods	The foods which are 'low fat,' 'fat free,' 'sugar free' are replaced with chemicals. Diet foods are loaded with artificial sweeteners (saccharin), artificial colors and dyes (red 40, yellow 5 and 6) which are linked with cancers	It significantly increases the occurrence of renal cancer, bladder cancer and brain tumors
7	Refined white flour	The refined or bleached foods (with chlorine gas) contain traces of chemicals and high carbohydrate content which alter the blood sugar level and thus feed cancer cells and spread. The foods are white bread, white rice and soda, etc.	It enhances the occurrence of breast cancer in women

Preventive Strategies for Cancer

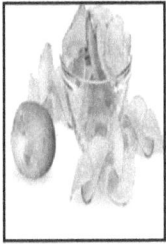 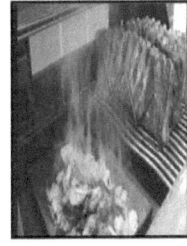 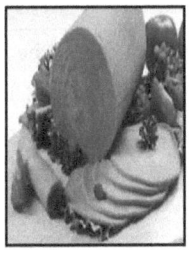 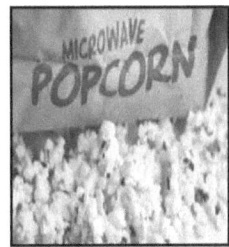

Salted foods   Smoked foods   Processed meats   Microwave popcorn

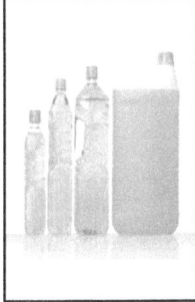 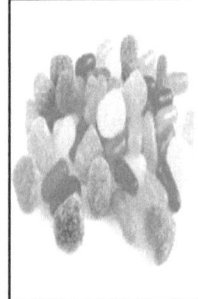 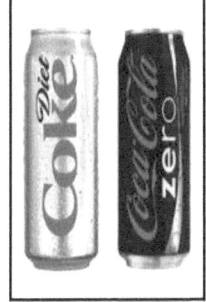 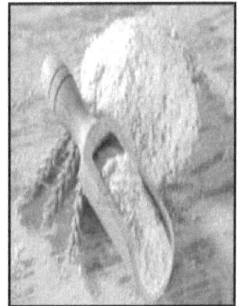

Hydrogenated oil   Refined sugar   'Diet' foods   Refined white flour

Fig. No. 5(b) 3: List of Foods to be avoided

Table No. 5(b) 3: Top cancer fighting foods

SN	Name of food	Cancer fighting properties	Name of cancers
1	Fish oil	It has long chain omega 3– a powerful anti-inflammatory in the body, which minimizes COX 2. It also has vitamin A, which fight against cancers	It helps to reduce the prostate, breast and colon cancer.
2	Carrots	It has carotenoids like beta – carotene which has an anti-cancer effect. The presence of falcarinol makes the cancer cells to grow slowly	It helps to reduce the lung, mouth, throat, stomach, intestine, bladder, prostate and breast cancers.

SN	Name of food	Cancer fighting properties	Name of cancers
3	Tomatoes	It has the prime active ingredient called lycopene which helps to reduce the bad fat level and is a strong antioxidant	It helps to fight against the prostate, lung, colon and breast cancers.
4	Green leafy vegetables	It has folic acid which helps in proper replication of DNA; the sulforaphanes have epigenetic (cancer correcting) benefits. Further, it helps the body to be more alkaline thereby it improves immune system and stops metastasis	It helps to fight against colorectal cancers, skin, lung and breast cancers.
5	Broccoli	It contains rich fiber which helps to eliminate toxins; further it has Indole 3 carbinol which modifies the estrogen action, thereby it fights against the estrogen driven cancers.	It aids in fighting the breast, prostate, brain and colorectal cancers.
6	Garlic	It has allicin which helps to stop the spread of cancer by stopping blood supply forming for tumors. It has selenium, tryptophan and sulphur based active agents that attack cancer cells.	It helps to reduce the incidence of stomach cancer, esophagus, colon and breast cancers.
7	Mushrooms	It contains Lentinan (polysaccharide) which help in building immunity, and lectin (protein) which attacks the cancerous cells and prevents the multiplication.	It is effective against breast cancer, prostate, bladder and colorectal cancers.

SN	Name of food	Cancer fighting properties	Name of cancers
8	Sweet potatoes	It contains beta carotene, which protects the DNA in the cell nucleus from cancer causing chemicals.	It reduces the risk of developing lung, skin, breast and prostate cancer.
9	Grapes	It contains the bioflavonoids and acts as antioxidants, further have resveratrol and ellagic acid which inhibit the enzymes that can stimulate cancer cell growth, thereby it slows the growth of cancer.	It is effective in acting against lung and prostate cancers.
10	Green tea and Black tea	It contains antioxidants (up to 40%) called as polyphenols which prevents cancer cells from dividing.	It reduces the risk of stomach, lung, colon, rectum, liver and pancreas cancer.
11	Red and Yellow peppers	It's a good source of capsaicin and vitamin C, which strengthens the immune cells and neutralizes toxins. It is also a good source of carotenoids.	It is effective against cancers of lung, pancreas and skin.
12	Orange and Lemon	It contains limonene which stimulates cancer killing immune cells (lymphocytes) to break down the cancer causing substances.	It is associated with low incidence of breast, lung, pancreas, colon and cervix cancers.

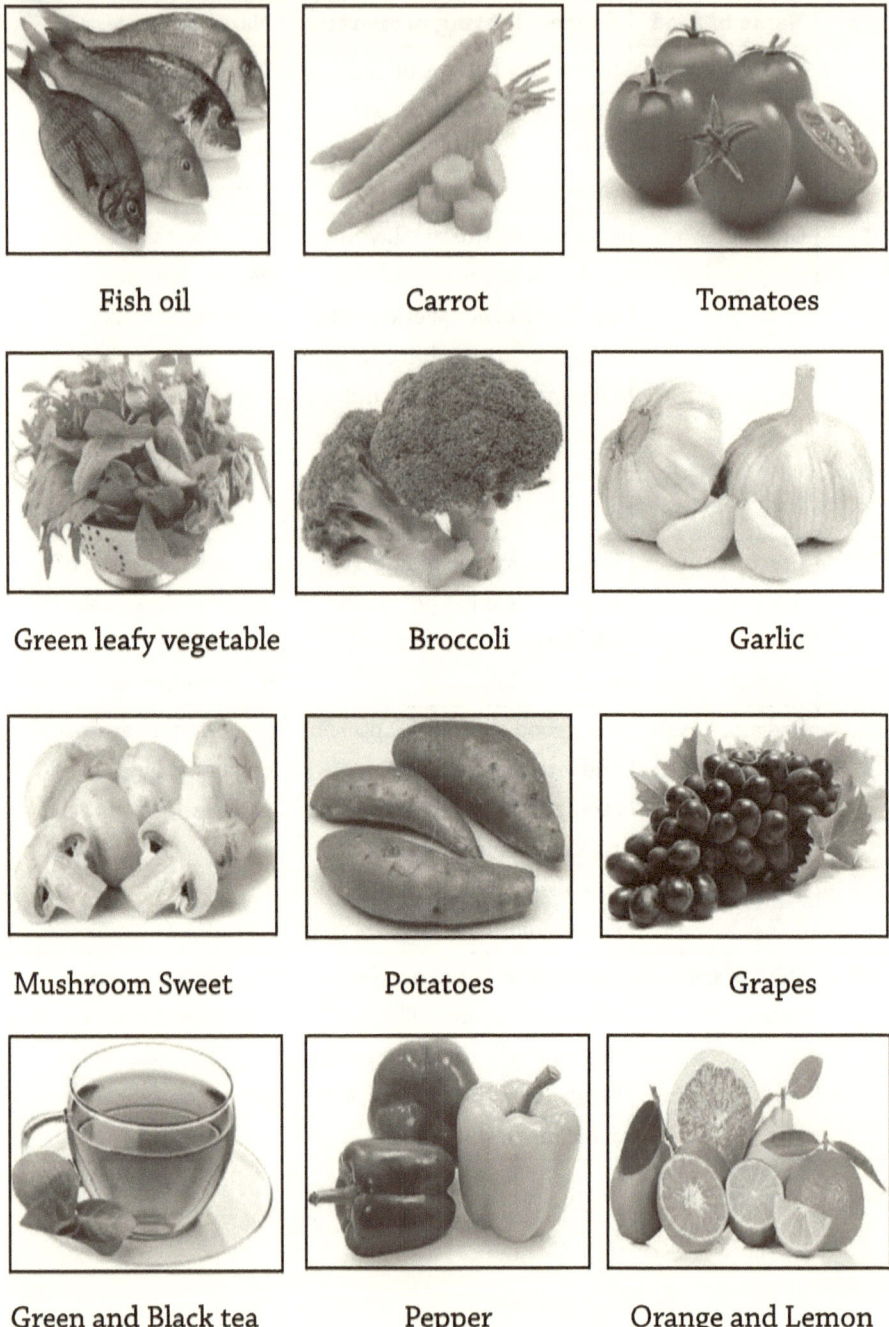

Research Evidence: 10

The cruciferous vegetables are rich in nutrients like beta carotene, vitamin C, E and K, and folate. The common examples are Broccoli, Cabbage, Cauliflower, Turnip and Radish, etc. The evidence from cohort studies has been reviewed. The intake of wide range of cruciferous vegetables found that the people who ate greater amounts of cruciferous vegetables had a lower risk of prostate cancer, colorectal cancer, lung cancer, and breast cancer.[13, 14]

Table No. 5(b) 4: Physical activities for prevention of cancers

Types	Moderate Intensity Activities	Vigorous Intensity Activities
Exercise and Leisure	Walking, dancing, bicycling, roller skating, horseback riding and yoga	Jogging or running, fast bicycling, circuit weight training, aerobic dance or exercise, jumping rope and swimming
Sports	Volleyball, golfing, softball, baseball, badminton and doubles tennis	Soccer, field hockey, singles tennis, racquetball and basketball
Home activities	Mowing the lawn, general yard and garden maintenance	Digging, carrying and hauling, masonry, carpentry
Occupational activity	Walking and lifting as part of the job (custodial work, farming, auto or machine repair)	Heavy manual labor (forestry, construction, firefighting)

'Small changes in your everyday life might help reduce your risk of cancer'

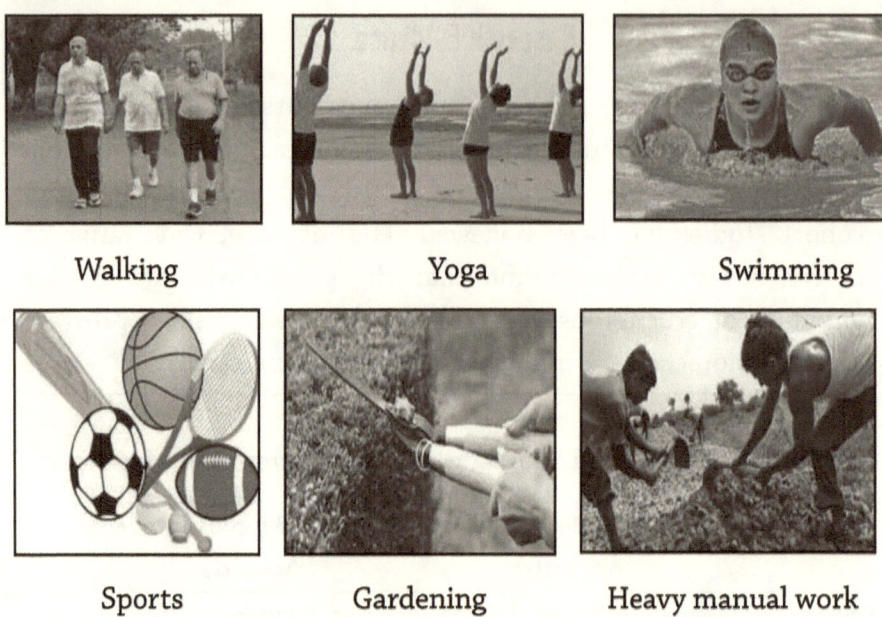

Fig. No. 5(b) 4: *Examples of Moderate and Vigorous Intensity Physical Activities*

C. Measures to Reduce the Sedentary Behavior

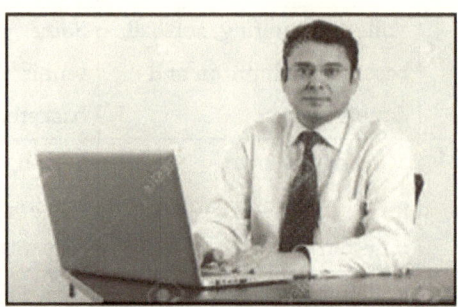

Sedentary behavior refers to activities that need very little physical movement and don't use much energy such as sitting for long periods of time. Sitting for a long period of time can increase the risk of cancer (the longer the person sits higher the risk). The sedentary behavior contributes to weight gain, diabetes, heart diseases, and along with it is linked to increased risk of colorectal cancer, ovarian, prostate and uterine cancers.

Evidence suggests that moving more to decrease the amount of time spent in sitting helps to reduce the risk of cancer and overall health. Following are the tips to help reducing sitting time which include:

> **'Sitting too much is a health hazard'**

Take frequent, short breaks from sitting (short standing or moving for 2 to 3 minutes is beneficial because the simple muscle movements have effect on cell process).

- Walk around while you are talking on the phone.
- Use stairs rather than a lift or elevator.
- Exercise at lunch with your coworkers, family or friends.
- Walk to visit coworkers instead of sending an e mail/phone.
- Plan active vacations rather than only driving trips.
- Join a sport team, and increase your daily steps every day.
- Spend more time playing with your kids, and walk briskly.
- Plan your exercise routine to gradually increase the days per week and minutes per session.
- Take regular desk breaks to reduce the sitting time while you are at work.
- Use a stationary bicycle or treadmill while watching television.
- Limit the amount of time spent watching television or videos and playing on computers.
- Follow the guidelines for physical activity for the age group and limit time spent in sedentary behaviors.

> **'Being active has many health benefits, including reducing the risk of cancers'**

D. Preventive Measures: National Cancer Control Program

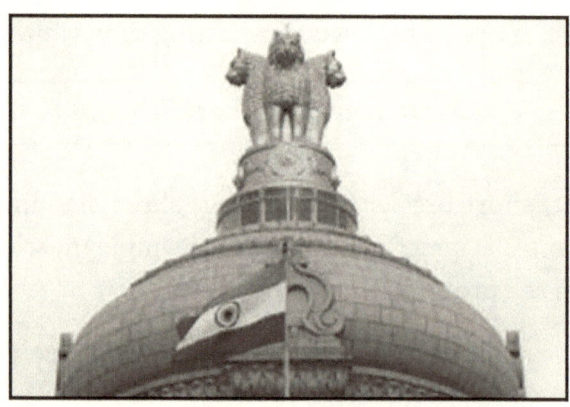

Cancer is one among the significant causes of morbidity, and the magnitude of the problem is enormous and gigantic. Its burden on the Indian economy for providing adequate health care is substantial. Thus, the Government of India launched the National Cancer Control Program (NCCP) in 1975–76 to tackle the increasing incidence of cancers in the country. This was later revised in 1984–85 stressing mainly on the primary prevention and early detection of cancers. The primary prevention focused on health education and awareness generation regarding hazards of tobacco consumption, genital hygiene, and sexual and reproductive health, etc.

> *'NCCP – An increased access in cancer care'*

The program created awareness among people regarding early symptoms of cancer, importance of observation of personal hygiene and healthy lifestyle, ill effects of tobacco consumption, etc. The project has 5 components a) health education, b) early detection, c) training of medical and paramedical personnel, d) palliative treatment and pain relief and e) coordination and monitoring. The National Cancer Control Program followed the following strategies for prevention of cancers:

Strategy 1: Control of tobacco-related cancers through primary prevention

- Extensive persuasive health education directed to control/reduce the tobacco habit (target group is teenaged students, as most of them pick up habits at this time).
- The school curricula made to involve messages for a healthy lifestyle and warn about the harmful effects of tobacco and alcohol.
- Appropriate legislative measures taken up for prohibiting sale of tobacco to youngsters, to help in protection of the nonusers of tobacco – 'passive smokers.'
- Initiated a ban on advertisement of cigarettes and cigarette smoking in various ways.
- Enacted laws and rigidly enforced them, that smoking in public places of entertainment and public transport is an offence/crime and imposed punishment/fine for the wrongdoing.
- Enacted laws to place the health warning labels on cigarette and bidi packets and on all tobacco products, advertisements, and on smokeless tobacco products.
- Increased the tax and prices for the cigarettes and other tobacco products.
- Provide training, assistance and counseling for women to quit smoking habits.
- Make sure that the home, work place and transport places are smoke free areas.

> *'Men are born to succeed, not to fail – Stop smoking'*

Strategy 2: Nutrition education for promoting good health and control of cancers

- Nutrition education is important for increasing public awareness, promoting good health and for control of cancers.

- Propogate the recommended dietary guidelines for human beings as per various age groups.

- Besides avoiding the risk factors, emphasize dietary intervention for cancer prevention in terms of lowering dietary fat content, increasing intake of fiber, fruits and vegetables.

- Public education and awareness about the beneficial effects of consuming plenty of fresh vegetables and fruits with spices such as turmeric in adequate amounts to prevent cancer.

> *'Good nutrition will prevent 95% of all diseases'*

Strategy 3: Life style and behavior modification for prevention of cervical cancer. The development of Invasive Cervical Cancer (ICC) has been strongly linked with early onset of sexual activity and multiple sexual partners.

- Hence the age for marriage for girls was raised beyond 18 years and for men beyond 21 years.

- Educated and adopted observing small family size, adopting safe sexual practices.

- Special attention was initiated towards personal hygiene of both males and females and use of obstructive methods of contraception which could help in primary prevention of cervical cancer.

- Introduced vaccination against hepatitis B virus into the vaccination program of infants, which would help in the control of liver cancer.

Followed the possible associated actions to prevent invasive breast cancer, such as:

a. Avoidance of breast irradiation particularly in young women
b. Avoidance of cigarette smoking, active or passive, particularly in adolescence
c. To have early first full term pregnancy
d. Delay in onset of menarche by avoiding over nutrition and by increased physical activity in adolescence
e. Prolonging the duration of lactation
f. Avoiding obesity especially in postmenopausal women

> **'Say no to risk factors, yes to life style modification'**

The above said cancer prevention strategies need to be followed/adhered for cancer prevention, as well as to minimize the impact of cancer disease on individual, family, and country.

E. World Health Organization Recommendations

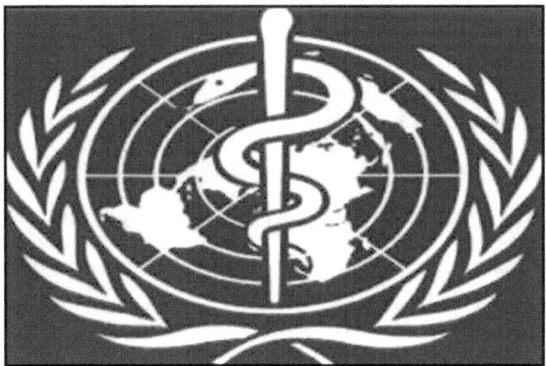

The following table highlights the core interventions to be followed for the prevention of cancer diseases which was recommended by the World Health Organization.

Table No. 5(b) 5: Core interventions for cancer prevention

I. Tobacco
Raise excise duties on tobacco to at least prevent tobacco products from becoming more affordable, and at best make them less affordable
Require by law and enforce 100% smoke free environments in all indoor workplaces and public places
Ban all advertising, promotion and sponsorship of tobacco products, brands and related trade, including promotion and sponsorship
Put health warnings on all tobacco packaging and ensure that product descriptions, packaging and labeling are in accordance with WHO Framework Convention on Tobacco Control
Work with appropriate media to build awareness among key groups, such as health professionals and policy makers, on the health impact of smoking and on the relevant tobacco control policies
II. Unhealthy diet, physical inactivity, overweight and obesity
Develop and implement national dietary guidelines and nutrition policies
Promote educational and information campaigns about reducing salt, sugar and fat consumption and eliminating cooking and preservation methods known to increase cancer risk
Develop and implement national guidelines on physical activity
Implement community-wide campaigns to promote the benefits of physical activity
Promote physical activity in workplaces
Introduce a national chronic disease prevention policy and action plans with specific reference to prevention and control of overweight and obesity
Promote public awareness campaigns about the links between overweight, obesity and cancer, recognizing that an unhealthy diet and physical inactivity are risk factors
III. Alcohol
Develop and implement an evidence-based national policy aimed at reducing or stabilizing the overall level of alcohol consumption

Raise public awareness, especially among young people about alcohol-related health risks, including cancer
Promote participation of non-governmental organizations and relevant stakeholders in reducing alcohol problems
IV. Hepatitis B virus
Implement universal infant immunization using recommended immunization schedules, based on epidemiological needs and programmatic considerations
V. Environmental exposure to carcinogens
Stop using all forms of asbestos
Provide safe drinking water
Reduce the use of biomass and coal for heating and cooking at home, and promote use of clean burning and efficient stoves
Implement food safety systems (i.e., legislation and monitoring) focusing on key contaminants
VI. Occupational exposure to carcinogens
Develop regulatory standards and enforce control of the use of known carcinogens in the Workplace
Avoid introducing known carcinogens into the workplace
Include occupational cancer in the national list of occupational diseases
Identify workers, workplaces and worksites with exposure to carcinogens
VII. Radiation
Provide information about sources and effects of all types of radiation
Establish national radiation protection standards
Ensure regular safety training of radiation workers
Establish technical guidelines for radiation sources, medical and industrial equipment
Promote UV risk awareness and UV protection actions

'Take action to prevent cancer'

F. Preventive Measures for the Specific Cancers

Prevention is the action of stopping something from happening or arising. It can be universal, selective and indicated preventive measures. Every case of cancer cannot be prevented; however the risk of developing these cancers may be greatly minimized by avoiding certain risk factors. The following are the specific prevention strategies for specific cancers.

I. Oral Cavity and Oropharyngeal Cancer

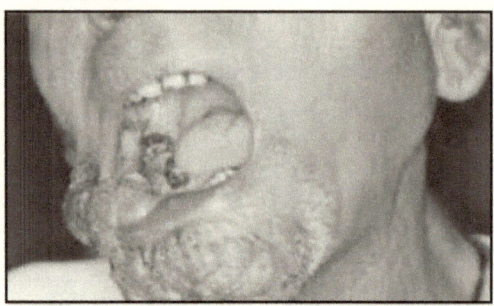

Oral cavity cancer is a cancer that starts in the mouth (oral cavity). The Oropharyngeal cancer starts in the oropharynx, which is the part of the throat just behind the mouth. Males are more commonly affected than females, and the common sites are: tongue, tonsils and oropharynx and gums, floor of the mouth, and other parts of the mouth.

Preventive measures

a. **Limit smoking and drinking:** Tobacco and alcohol consumption are the most important risk factors for oral cancers. To avoid this, not starting to smoke is the best way to limit/control the risk of getting these cancers. Quitting the use of tobacco significantly reduces the risk of developing oral cancers, even after long years of use. The same is applicable for alcohol consumption in individuals also; to prevent the occurrence of oral cancers do not drink, or at least limit the use of alcohol.

b. **Limit the exposure to ultraviolet light:** Ultraviolet radiation is a significant and avoidable/modifiable risk factor for cancer of lips and skin. Avoid or limit the time spent outdoors during the middle of the day, when the sun's UV rays are strongest. Use of sun protective measures such as hat, sunscreen and protective clothes, etc.is recommended.

c. **Use of properly fitted dentures:** Avoid the sources (i.e., ill fitted dentures) of mechanical irritation of oral mucosa which may lower the risk for development of oral cancer.

d. **Eat a healthy diet:** A diet with less fruits, vegetables and fiber has been very much linked to oral cancers; thus eating healthy foods (balanced diet including vitamin supplements) might be helpful in reducing the risk of development of these cancers.

e. **Avoid HPV infection:** Avoid the various risk factors (oral sex, multiple sexual partners and sexually transmitted diseases) for development of HPV infection. Vaccination against HPV infection lowers the risk of cervical and other cancers including oral cancer.

f. **Treatment of pre-cancerous growths:** Areas of leukoplakia or erythroplakia in the mouth may progress to cancer. After the biopsy exam, pre-cancerous area of leukoplakia or erythroplakia is removed surgically. After the surgical removal, continue to have a health checkup (follow-up visits) to look for cancer, and for new areas of leukoplakia or erythroplakia.

g. **Chemoprevention:** The use of medicines (e.g., retinoids) to help lower the risk of development of cancers is called chemoprevention; it is particularly needed for people who have a higher risk of developing these cancers, such as those with leukoplakia or erythroplakia.

II. Larynx and Hypo Pharynx Cancers

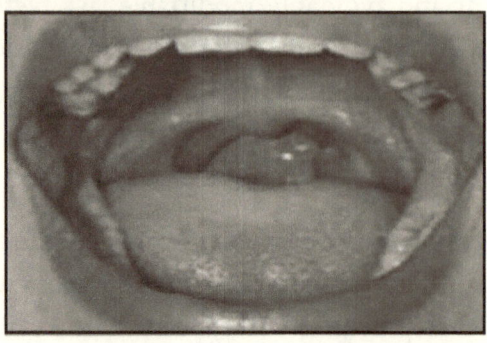

Cancers that start in the larynx are called laryngeal cancers. Cancers that start in the hypo pharynx are called hypo pharyngeal cancers. Laryngeal and hypo pharyngeal cancers are often grouped with other cancers of the mouth and throat (known as head and neck cancers). It is very common in men and those who have smoking habit.

Preventive measures

a. **Avoid smoking and drinking:** Avoiding the exposure to tobacco (by not smoking and avoiding secondhand, passive smoking) lowers the risk of these cancers. Alcohol consumption also greatly increases the cancer causing effect, so it is important to avoid the combination of drinking and smoking.

b. **Protection from occupational exposure:** Keep the work place well ventilated; use personal respiratory protectors (face mask), and other personal protective measures to minimize the chemical exposure at the work place.

c. **Eating a balanced diet:** Eating the well balanced (healthy) diet may help lower the risk of these cancers (and many others). It is recommended to eat plant foods, vegetables, fruits, cereals, whole grains and vitamin rich foods, etc. Further, try to avoid fat rich foods, processed foods and red meat, etc.

d. **Avoid HPV infection:** One of the risk factors for development of oral and throat cancer is HPV virus infection, and this infection commonly occurs due to the practice of oral sex and having multiple sex partners. The HPV vaccination is required to lower the risk of throat cancers.

III. Lung Cancer

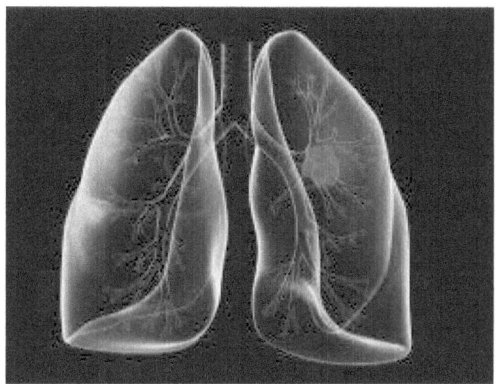

It's a cancer which starts from the respiratory tract, mainly the lungs. It usually starts in the cells (parenchyma) lining of bronchi and parts of the lung such as the bronchioles or alveoli. The types of lung cancers are: a) non-small cell lung cancer (85–90%) and b) small cell lung cancer (10– 15%). Smoking is a prime risk factor for the development of lung cancers.

Preventive measures

a. **Don't smoke:** The best way to minimize the risk of developing lung cancer is not to smoke (both active and passive smoking). Avoidance and cessation of smoking helps in repairing the damaged cells and tissues, thereby preventing lung cancer. Quitting the smoking habit helps to live longer without cancer and other chronic lung diseases.

b. **Avoid carcinogens at work:** Avoiding the areas which are known to cause cancer like the workplace and elsewhere, may also be helpful to minimize the cancer risk. Take precautions like using mask and other protective devices to minimize the chemical carcinogen exposure.

c. **Eat diet full of fruits and vegetables:** A healthy balanced diet with more fruits, vegetables and fiber rich foods also helps to reduce the chance of developing various cancers including lung cancer; this is well supported by scientific evidences.

d. **Exercise most days of the week:** Try to do exercises every day for a minimum of 30–45 minutes, and follow this by trying to increase the duration of the period of exercise. Perform the exercise for most days of the week.

IV. Stomach Cancer

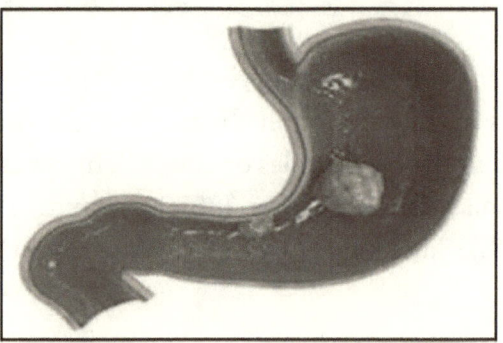

It is otherwise known as gastric cancer, and it arises in the inner layers (mucus membrane) of the stomach. After chronic exposure to risk factors (many years) the pre-cancerous growth develops followed by the occurrence of cancerous growth. However the pre-cancerous change does not manifest symptoms and often goes unnoticed. Stomach cancers can grow through the wall of the stomach and invade nearby organs, and also spread to the lymph nodes.

Preventive measures

a. **Reduce the amount of salty and smoked foods:** Food preservation methods such as salting, pickling, and smoking, etc. need to be minimized or stopped to avoid development of stomach cancers. However the use of refrigerators for food storage drastically minimizes the probability of cancer in stomach. Try to avoid a diet which contains smoked, pickled and salted meats/fish or food items.

b. **Eat more fruits and vegetables:** it was noticed that the consumption of diet rich in fruits and vegetables lowers the risk of stomach cancer (e.g., the citrus fruits – orange, lemon and grapes). Eating a healthy balanced diet is recommended to minimize the cancer risk (plant foods, vegetables and fruits, etc.) including stomach cancer.

c. **Eating a healthy diet:** Choose to eat whole grain breads and cereals instead of refined grains. Try to eat fish, poultry or red meat instead of processed meat which helps in lowering the risk of cancer. Consumption of food items rich in antioxidant property (vitamins A, C, and E and selenium) reduces the risk of stomach cancer.

d. **Physical activity and maintaining body weight:** Again being overweight/obese increases the percentage of risk of stomach cancer. On the other hand, being physically active (exercise) helps to lower the risk. Maintaining body weight and balanced calorie intake, and utilization of calories with physical activity minimizes the cancer risk.

e. **Avoid tobacco use:** Along with alcohol, consumption of tobacco may increase the risk of many cancers including stomach cancer (proximal stomach), and tobacco use is responsible for one-third of all cancer deaths. If you smoke, quit smoking immediately;

if you don't smoke, kindly don't start smoking because it increases the risk of stomach cancer.

f. **Treating H pylori infection:** As mentioned earlier, the H pylori infection causes cancer disease; treating the H pylori infection with appropriate antibiotics lowers the risk and development of pre-cancerous lesions, and minimizes the risk of developing stomach cancer.

g. **Aspirin use:** The use of Non-Steroidal Anti-Inflammatory Drugs (NSAIDs) such as Ibuprofen or Naproxen and aspirin lowers the risk of stomach cancer. Though these drugs lower the risk of cancer, they however cause the risk of bleeding disorders.

V. Colorectal Cancer

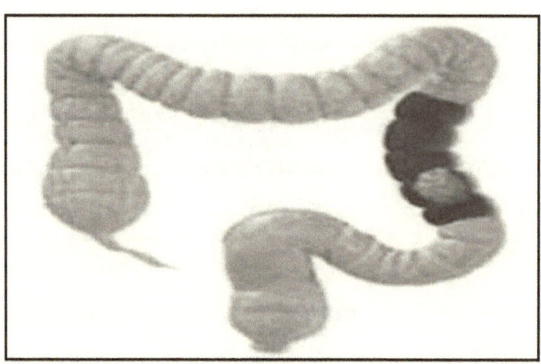

The cancer which arises/develops in the lower gastro intestinal tract especially in colon and rectum is called colorectal cancer. It is also called colon cancer or rectal cancer. Though they are named separately, their clinical manifestations are similar. As like other cancers, colorectal cancer also develops slowly and steadily (several years). Usually the formation of non-cancerous polyps occurs before the actual cancerous growth, and these polyps may turn into cancerous ones. The common types are: adenocarcinoma, carcinoid tumor, gastrointestinal stromal tumors, lymphomas and sarcomas.

Preventive measures

a. **Screening:** Screening is a primary step in detection of any kind of cancers, and the colorectal cancer is not exceptional. Individuals of middle age groups (mainly above 45 years) need or are recommended screening tests to detect the colorectal cancers. The transition of pre-cancerous polyps to the malignant growth needs longevity of duration (10–15 years), thus the regular screening helps to detect the development of cancer at the earliest.

b. **Eat variety of fruits, vegetables and whole grains:** Food items containing vitamins, minerals, fiber and antioxidants play a significant role in cancer prevention. Using a variety of fruits and vegetables in the diet helps to avoid the risk of developing colorectal cancers.

c. **Avoid/stop drinking:** It is recommended to limit the intake of alcohol to not more than 1 drink (1 ounce) a day for women and 2 drinks for men. Avoiding alcohol and tobacco minimizes the development of colorectal cancers.

d. **Maintain a healthy body weight:** Try to maintain the healthy body weight by performing regular exercises and following a healthy diet and life style practice. Alongside, gradually increase the amount/duration of exercise and reduce the number of calories intake to maintain a healthy body weight.

e. **Aspirin and Celecoxib use:** Use of aspirin (NSAID) and Celecoxib (COX 2 inhibitors) reduces the risk of pre-cancerous polyps and colon cancers.

f. **Genetic testing and screening:** Genetic counseling is required for the individual having family history of colorectal cancers. Alongside, the genetic testing/screening helps to identify the individual with abnormal gene (cancerous), and thus helps to take steps (like getting screened at early age or having surgery) to prevent the colon cancer.

VI. Liver cancer

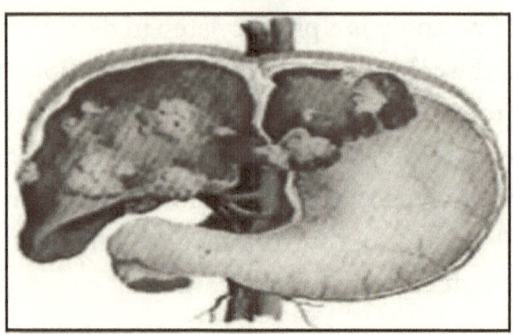

The cancers that start in the liver are called liver cancer. The different types of cells in the liver can form various malignant (cancerous) and benign (non-cancerous) tumors. A cancer that starts in the liver itself is called primary liver cancer. When the cancer of liver is started not from the liver, but the liver developed a cancer due to the metastasis (spread) of other cancers, it is called secondary liver cancer.

Preventive measures

a. **Avoiding and treating hepatitis infections:** Hepatitis B and C virus infection are the prime risk factors for development of liver cancer. These viruses can spread between individuals via sharing the contaminated needles and through unprotected sex. However these cancers may be prevented by not sharing needles and by using safer sex practices (use of condoms). Vaccination and treatment against HBV infection prevents the chance of HBV infection. The accidental exposure to HBV or HCV can be drastically controlled by following the standard safety practices of blood transfusion.

b. **Limiting alcohol and tobacco use:** Chronic alcoholism leads to liver diseases such as cirrhosis of the liver, which in turn, can lead to liver cancer. Quitting of drinking alcohol or limited drinking could help to prevent liver cancer. Along with drinking, smoking also increases the risk of liver cancer; hence the cessation of smoking is a mantra for the cancer prevention.

c. **Maintain healthy weight:** Avoidance of overweight/obesity might be another way to help or protect against liver cancer. People who are obese are more likely to have the disease called fatty liver and diabetes, both of which have been linked for development of liver cancer.

d. **Limit/avoid exposure to cancer causing chemicals:** Changing the way of storage of certain grains could reduce exposure to cancer causing substances such as aflatoxins. Limit the use of drinking water mixed with arsenic.

e. **Treating diseases that increase cancer risk:** The inherited disease like hemochromatosis may increase the chance of cirrhosis of liver and liver cancer. Early identification and timely appropriate management of these diseases could be able to lower this risk (cancer).

VII. Lymphoma

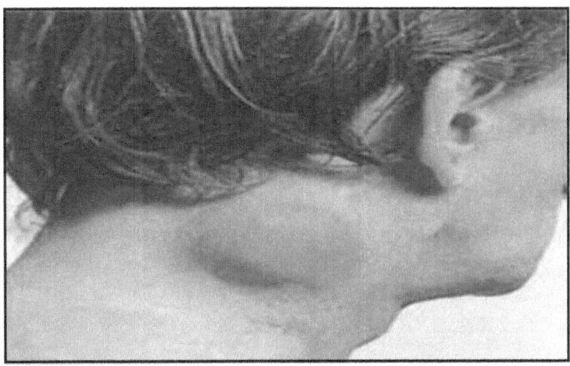

Lymphoma – It's a type of cancer that occurs in White Blood Cells called lymphocytes (immune cells). It has 2 categories such as: a) Hodgkin disease (named after Dr. Thomas Hodgkin, who first recognized it) and b) Non-Hodgkin lymphoma. Though it is common among children and adults, it is very common in early adulthood (15–40 years). Lymphoma commonly affects sites such as chest, neck, or under the arms, and often spreads to other parts of the body via lymph vessels.

Preventive measures

a. **Prevention of HIV infection:** Person suffering from HIV infection is known to have increased risk of lymphomas. The best way to limit the risk is to avoid the known risk factors for HIV/AIDS, such as intravenous (IV) drug use or unprotected sex with multiple partners. The management of HIV infection with anti-retroviral therapy lowers the chance of lymphomas. Further, along with HIV, the HBV, HCV and EBV infections need to be controlled.

b. **Treatment of H pylori infection:** H pylori infection has been linked to some lymphomas of the stomach. Treatment of H pylori infections with antibiotics and antacids may lower the risk of lymphomas in stomach.

c. **Immuno compromised state:** The individuals who are undergoing chemotherapy, radiation therapy or using immune suppressing agents for organ transplantation are prone to develop certain lymphomas. Utmost care needs to be taken while planning the cancer treatment with chemo/radiation to avoid (the risk of) occurrence of lymphomas.

d. **Maintain healthy body weight:** Overweight or obesity increase the risk of Non-Hodgkin's Lymphoma, and a diet rich in fat and meats also raises the probability of risk. Thus eating more of vitamin C, vitamin A rich foods, citrus fruits and green leafy vegetables, etc., helps to minimize the chance of lymphoma occurrence. Maintaining healthy weight and eating a healthy balanced diet helps to protect against the lymphoma.

VIII. Leukemia

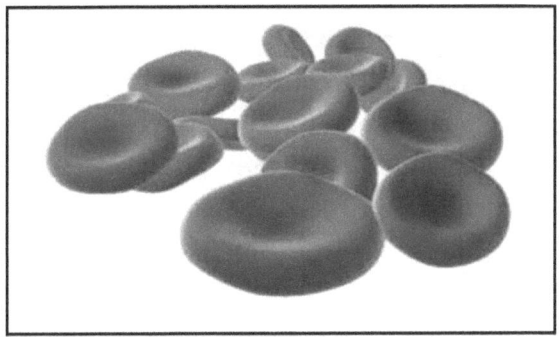

Leukemia – otherwise called as blood cancer, is a cancer of blood and blood forming cells of bone marrow and lymphatic system. It is broadly categorized as acute and chronic leukemia's. However based on the type of cells involved, it is classified as myelocytic and lymphocytic leukemia's. The person with leukemia often suffers from infection, anemia, bleeding disorders, weight loss, etc. It is often spread to the lymph nodes and other organs, and children are more commonly affected than adults.

Preventive measures

a. **Avoid or stop smoking:** Smoking makes a person at risk of developing many cancers including leukemia (AML—Acute Myelogenous Leukemia). One in every 4 cases of leukemia is associated with smoking. Quitting smoking is the best way to reduce the risk of leukemia.

b. **Control of chemical carcinogen exposure:** Benzene is a byproduct of coal and petroleum, which is present in a variety of forms like paints, plastics, pesticides, detergents, etc. People who are working in the manufacturing of these products have risk of leukemia. The avoidance of exposure to it and practicing the standard occupational safety measures controls the occurrence of leukemia.

c. **Cancer treatments:** Some forms of leukemia's may develop due to the treatment of cancers (such as chemotherapy, radiation therapy) or the use of immuno suppressing agents to avoid rejection in organ transplantation. Here the benefits over drawbacks of these treatments should be weighed and considered in treatment planning and the whole picture must be clarified with patients and their family members.

IX. Breast Cancer

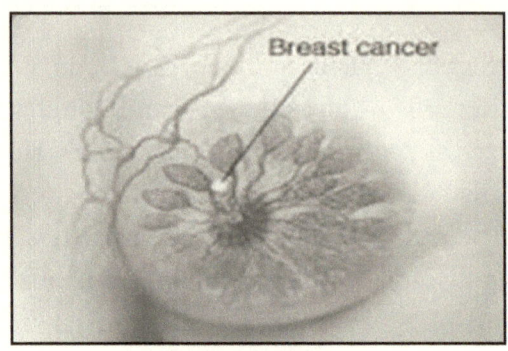

It's a malignant (cancer) tumor that arises in the cells of the breast, and among women breast cancer is the second commonest cancer leading to death. There are 3 categories of breast cancers, which are a) carcinoma – occurs in the lining layer of breast, b) adenocarcinoma – occurs in the gland tissues like ducts and lobules and c) sarcoma – occurs in the connective tissues like muscle, blood vessels of the breast. The death rates from breast cancer can be drastically reduced by the early screening and detection methods like breast self-examination and mammography.

Preventive measures

a. **Limit alcohol and don't smoke:** More the alcohol intake, greater is the risk of developing breast cancer among women. Limit the alcohol intake, i.e., not more than one drink (30 ml) a day. Scientific evidence highlights the association between smoking and risk of breast cancer, especially in premenopausal women.

b. **Control weight and be physically active:** Among women it is common that obesity occurs in the later part of life (after menopause). Obesity is one among the risk factors for breast cancer; hence the regular physical activity/exercise (minimum 30–45 minutes) helps to maintain an optimal weight, thereby helping to prevent breast cancer (i.e., above 30%).

c. **Breast feeding:** it was scientifically noticed that breast feeding has a role in prevention of breast cancer (the nullipara women have higher probability of breast cancer than the multipara mothers). The core aspect is duration of feeding. The longer she breastfeeds, the greater the protective effect.

d. **Limit dose/duration of hormonal therapy:** Women who are undergoing hormonal replacement therapy for the physiological or medical conditions (e.g. menopause) do have higher risk of breast cancer. The longer the duration, the higher is the risk of cancer. Here the benefits and drawbacks need to be considered before initiation of hormone replacement therapy.

e. **Avoid exposure to radiation:** Along with sunlight exposure, the routine imaging tests such as computerized tomography and X-ray have a link with breast cancer risk. It is expected to use the technology meticulously (if necessary only) to avoid the risk of cancer.

f. **Get regular breast cancer screenings:** Perform regular breast self-examination once in a month as instructed; and any abnormalities (lump, lesion, discharge, etc.) found needs to be informed to the health care professional immediately for the early diagnosis and management. Follow the health care provider's advice to decide type of screening needed and how often needed. If there is a family history of breast cancer, look for extra screening likes MRI, mammogram, ultrasound, etc.

X. Cervical Cancer

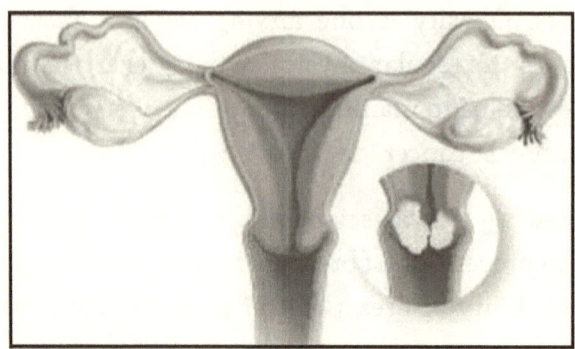

It occurs in the cells lining of the cervix (the lower part of uterus). It is otherwise called as cancer of uterine cervix. First the normal cells of cervix slowly change into pre-cancerous cells followed by turning into cancerous cells, which is called as dysplasia. Occurrence of this change may take many years, but sometimes can happen faster. The squamous cell carcinomas and adenocarcinomas are the 2 main types of cancers of the cervix. Among these the squamous cell carcinoma is more common, which starts from the squamous cells of the surface of the uterus.

Preventive measures

a. **Finding cervical pre-cancers:** A well proven way to prevent cervix cancer is to have screening to deduct pre-cancers before they can turn into invasive cancer. Pap smear test and HPV test are commonly used for this screening. If pre-cancerous growth is found it can be treated early and can stop the development of malignant cancer. The Pap smear test is a procedure used to collect cells from the cervix so that they can be looked at under a microscope to find cancer and pre-cancer. These cells can also be used for HPV testing. Pap test is usually done during a pelvic examination.

b. **Vaccinate against HPV infection:** Most of the cervical, vaginal and vulvar cancers are caused by HPV infection, and vaccination against HPV infection helps to protect against these types of cancers. A woman who has had vaccination still needs to undergo the Pap smear test for screening of cervical cancer.

c. **Safe sexual practices:** Things like use of condoms during sex and limiting the sexual partners (avoiding multiple sexual partners) help to control the spread of Sexually Transmitted Diseases (STD) and cervical cancer.

d. **Avoid smoking:** Avoidance of smoking (active or passive form) helps to control the risk of cancers including cervical cancers.

e. **Personal Hygiene:** Improvement in personal hygiene may lead to decline in certain types of cancer like cancer cervix.

XI. Ovarian Cancer

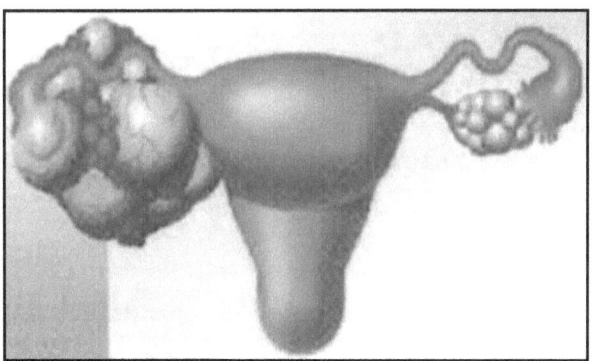

In females the ovaries are considered to be reproductive glands, and they produce eggs (ova) for reproduction, and female hormones like estrogen and progesterone. Cancer that occurs in the ovaries is known as ovarian cancer. The common types of ovarian cancer are: a) epithelial cell tumor – starts from cells of outer surface of ovary, b) germ cell tumor – starts from cells that produce eggs and c) stromal tumors – starts from structural tissues that hold the ovary together and produce female hormones.

Preventive measures

a. **Oral contraceptives:** The use of oral contraceptives (birth control pills) decreases the risk of developing ovarian cancer, mainly among women who use them for many years. Women who are on oral contraceptives for more than 5 years have 50% lower risk of developing ovarian cancer compared with women who have never used them. Apart from this, oral contraceptives use also reduces the risk for women with BRCA1 and BRCA2 mutations.

b. **Gynecologic surgery:** Surgical procedures such as tubal ligation and hysterectomy reduce the chance of developing ovarian cancer; however these surgeries must be performed for valid medical/surgical reasons and not for avoiding the risk of ovarian cancer.

c. **Genetic counseling:** Genetic testing and counseling must be considered, if the woman has family history of ovarian cancer. During genetic counseling, the woman's personal medical and family history needs to be reviewed, which helps to predict whether the woman is likely to have gene mutations associated with an increased ovarian cancer risk.

d. **Early/regular medical exams:** Women who had screening tests early will be able to identify the ovarian cancers at earlier age and have better prognosis and survival rate.

e. **Diet and lifestyle:** Ovarian cancer is linked to being overweight or obese. Losing weight through regular exercise and healthy balanced diet may reduce the risk of getting ovarian cancer.

XII. Uterine Cancer

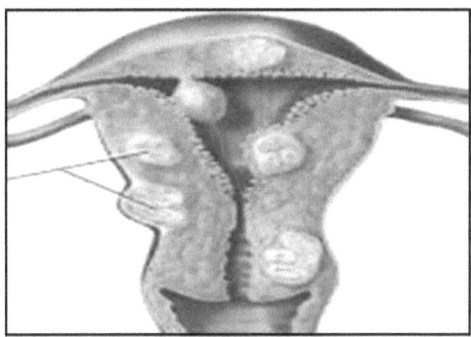

Endometrial cancer – It's a cancer that starts in the inner lining of the uterus. The inner lining is known as endometrium. Majority of uterine cancers occur in the endometrium, and these are called as endometrial carcinomas. Most of the endometrial carcinomas are adenocarcinoma – cancer starts in the cells lining glands of uterus. Cancers that start in the muscle layer of the uterus are called as sarcomas. Cancers that start in the cervix are different from cancers that start in the body of the uterus; they are described as cervical cancer.

Preventive measures

a. **Maintain healthy body weight:** Women who are overweight must ensure measures to control the weight to minimize the risk of endometrial cancer. Improvement in the physical activity increases the utilization of fats; thereby the fats will not have an effect of estrogen metabolism. Further it minimizes the chance of developing diabetes mellitus.

b. **Use of combined hormonal replacement therapy:** Evidence emphasizes that the use of combined (estrogen and progesterone) hormonal therapy helps to reduce the risk of uterine cancer more than the single drug therapy.

c. **Treatment of pre-cancerous disorders:** One of the risk factors for uterine cancer is pre-cancerous disorders of endometrium. Correcting or treating these disorders may lower the risk of uterine cancers, because the pre-cancerous condition may turn into malignant cancerous one.

XIII. Brain and Spinal Cord Tumors

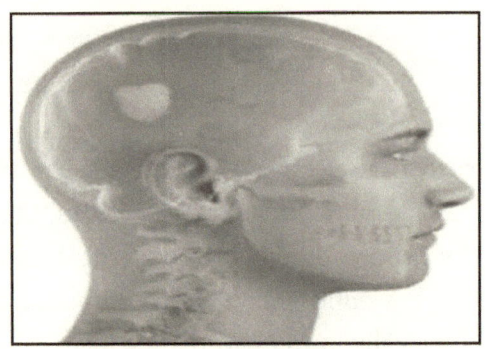

Brain and spinal cord tumors are masses of abnormal cells in the brain or spinal cord that have grown out of control. It may be a primary (that starts in the brain) or secondary tumor (that starts from other organs through metastasis/spread). In adults, metastatic tumors to the brain are more common than primary brain tumors and majority of brain or spinal cord tumors are malignant (cancerous) ones. The cancerous growth may cause damage or destroy tissues by growing and spreading into nearby areas. Unless they are completely removed or destroyed, most brain or spinal cord tumors will continue to grow and eventually be life-threatening. After leukemia, it is the second most common cancer in children.

Preventive measures

a. **Follow healthy life style practices:** The risk of many cancers including brain cancers can be reduced while following certain lifestyle changes (such as staying at a healthy weight, quitting smoking and alcoholism, eating balanced diet, etc.).

b. **Control/minimize the radiation exposure:** Radiation exposure is a prime contributing factor for the development of brain and spinal cord tumors. Hence it is recommended that the exposure to radiation sources must be limited or avoided as much as possible. The imaging tests (diagnostic use) such as X-rays or CT scans use also must be weighed for the benefits and drawbacks before advising for the tests; it is mandatory for the risk prevention.

c. **Use of protective devices:** Avoid the toxic chemicals associated with oil, rubber and other chemical industries. Constant use of lead apron or other protective devices and keeping a safe distance from radiation source helps to minimize the exposure to radiation.

d. **Treatment of cancers:** The early diagnosis and appropriate treatment strategies of other tumors helps to minimize the risk of metastasis (spread) of cancer to the brain and spinal cord.

XIV. Kidney (Renal) Cancer

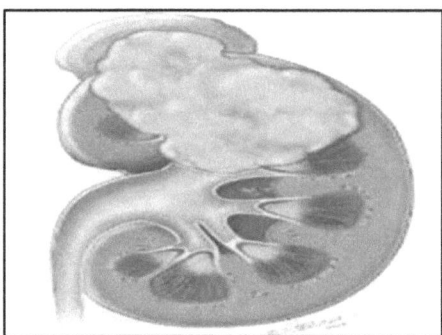

Kidney cancer – It's a cancer that starts in the cell/tissues of kidneys. The commonest renal cancer is renal cell carcinoma also termed as renal cell cancer or renal cell adenocarcinoma. About 9 out of 10 kidney cancers are renal cell carcinomas. The Wilms tumor (nephroblastoma), a type of renal cancer is more common in children than in adults, and men are more susceptible for renal cancer than their counterparts (women).

Preventive measures

a. **Quit smoking:** Cigarette smoking is responsible for a large percentage of cancers; hence stopping smoking (any form) may lower the risk of renal cancer.

b. **Maintain healthy body weight:** Maintaining a healthy weight by exercising (most days of the week) and using a diet rich in fruits and vegetables (reduce the intake of number of calories) helps to reduce the chance of getting this disease.

c. **Control of high blood pressure:** Regular monitoring of blood pressure, avoidance of alcohol consumption, and appropriate treatment for hypertension and follow-up helps to control renal cancers. In hypertension, the diet recommended is salt restricted diet and low fat diet to maintain the normal blood pressure level.

d. **Avoid the carcinogen exposure:** Avoiding workplace exposure to harmful substances such as cadmium and organic solvents may reduce the risk of renal cell cancer.

XV. Bladder Cancer

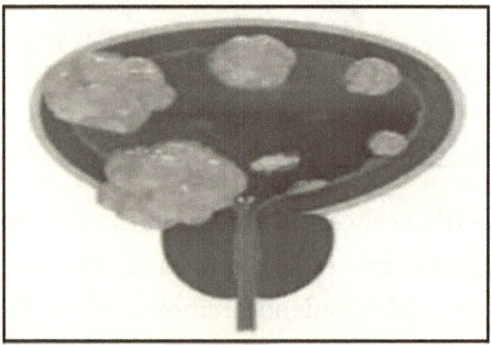

It is a cancer that occurs in the urinary bladder, and this is very much common in older people. Among the bladder cancers, the transitional cell carcinoma (occurs in the lining of bladder) is the most common type (9 out of 10 cases), while other types are less common.

Preventive measures

a. **Don't smoke:** Approximately 50% of bladder cancer develops among men and women due to the smoking habits. The bladder cancer can be largely prevented by quitting the smoking habits.

b. **Limit exposure to carcinogens in the workplace:** Follow the standard safety precautions while working at industries with aromatic amines.

c. **Drink plenty of fluids:** Evidence suggests that drinking more fluids (mainly water) lowers a person's risk of bladder cancer.

d. **Eat lots of fruits and vegetables:** Diet rich in fruits and vegetables might help to protect against bladder cancer. Eating such a diet has been shown to have great health benefits including lowering the risk of several types of cancer.

e. **Reduce the fat diet:** Evidence reveals that bladder and prostate cancer have association with increased intake of fat every day. To avoid these cancers, reduce or limit the use of foods that contain high fat like meat, nuts, oil, and dairy products such as milk, yogurt, cheese, etc.

XVI. Prostate Cancer

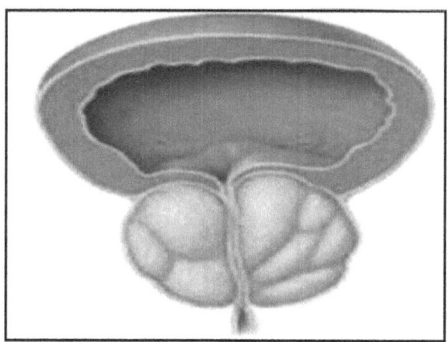

Prostate cancer is an occurrence of cancerous growth in the prostate gland. Majority of prostate cancers start in the gland cells, which is called as adenocarcinoma. Mostly these cancers grow slowly, and 1 in 7 men gets prostate cancer during his lifetime. Prostate cancer is the second leading cause of cancer death in men, and 1 man in 38 will die because of this disease.

Preventive measures

a. **Body weight, physical activity, and diet:** The effects of body weight, physical activity, and diet on prostate cancer risk are not clear; however the following measures can be carried out to reduce the risk of prostate cancer. They are: eating of variety of vegetables and fruits, being physically active, staying at a healthy weight, etc.

b. **Vitamins, minerals, and other supplements:** Studies had suggested that taking supplements of vitamin E or the mineral Selenium might lower prostate cancer risk.

c. **Medicines:** Two drugs used to treat benign prostatic hyperplasia (BPH) such as Finasteride and Dutasteride have been studied, and it has been found that these drugs help lower prostate cancer risk.

Conclusion

Cancer disease in all forms causes 12% of deaths throughout the world. It is a second leading cause of death (21%) in developed countries and in developing countries cancer ranks as the third cause of death (10%) among all deaths. Though cancer has larger impact on various dimensions of health, prevention and risk reduction strategies can greatly lower the physical, emotional and financial burden of cancer and improve the overall health of cancer survivors, including lowering the risk of recurrence of cancer. The risk reduction strategies like lifestyle modifications such as smoking, alcohol, diet and sedentary behavior, play a significant role in drastic reduction of incidence of cancer diseases. Not all cancers are preventable; however avoiding risk factors can prevent certain types of cancers. Prevention is crucial for stopping the alarming spread of cancer diseases. Delaying the onset of the disease could reduce half (50%) of the cancer diseases. Thus the famous quote that 'prevention is better than cure' is vindicated.

Key Points

- World Health Organization estimated that around 84 million people will die in the next 10 years if action is not taken to prevent/control cancer.

- Interestingly, majority (70%) of all cancer deaths occur in low and middle-income countries, where resources available for the prevention, diagnosis and treatment of cancer are scarce and limited.

- However, the fact that a large extent of the cancer disease is avoidable/preventable (>40%), highlights that the cancer prevention should be an essential component of all comprehensive cancer control plans.

- Most common cancers are curable if they are screened and detected early, and treated with appropriate treatments. Even at the late stage of cancer, the suffering of patients can be relieved with the help of good palliative and hospice care.

- The vital components of cancer control strategies include prevention, early detection, treatment and palliative care.

- Cancer prevention should coincide with other chronic disease prevention programs because important cancer risk factors – such as tobacco use, unhealthy diet, physical inactivity and obesity – are risk factors for other chronic non-communicable diseases.

- Systematic planning and following the principles of cancer control helps to control the giant disease in cost-effective and inexpensive manner.

- Implement the World Health Organization Global Strategy on diet, physical activity and health, add the hepatitis B vaccine to the national immunization programs, and control and eliminate the most widespread occupational and environmental carcinogens.

- Great impact to reduce the burden of cancer comes from the way of primary prevention, where the extensive comprehensive health awareness education is needed.

- Regular screening for uterine, cervix, oral and breast cancers could have a significant effect on reducing the mortality from cancer.

- Reduce sedentary behaviors by sitting less and moving more; because sitting too much is a health hazard.

- Regardless of resource availability, every country should take appropriate measures to curb the cancer epidemic, save lives and prevent sufferings.

Box No: 3 Simple Tips to Reduce Your Cancer Risk

- Don't consume tobacco in any form (smoking, powder, pan)
- Avoid or stay away from tobacco contents
- Avoid or limit the alcohol consumption
- Maintain steady and healthy body weight
- Perform regular physical activities/exercises
- Eat well balanced diet, plenty of fruits and vegetables
- Protect the skin or avoid excessive exposure to sun
- Regular health check-up/screening for cancers

> *'Healthier lifestyle leaves cancerous file'*
> – *Jenny Hope*

References

1. Parkin DM, Boyd L and Walker LC. The fraction of cancer attributable to lifestyle and environmental factors in the UK in 2010. Br J Cancer 2011; 105(2): 77–81.

2. Negri E, Boffetta P, Berthiller J, Castellsague X, Curado MP, Maso LD et al. Family History of Cancer: Pooled Analysis in the International Head and Neck Cancer Epidemiology (INHANCE) Consortium. Int J Cancer. 2009, 15; 124(2): 394–401.

3. Franceschi S, Rajkumar T, Vaccarella S, Gajalakshmi V, Sharmila A, Snijders P et al. Evaluate the role of HPV and other risk factors in the etiology of invasive cervical carcinoma (ICC) – A hospital based case control study. Int J Cancer. 2003; 107: 127–133.

4. Harford JB. Viral infections and human cancers: the legacy of Denis Burkitt. Br J Haematol 2012; 156: 709–18.

5. Gronback M, Becker U, Johansen D, Tonnesen H, Jensen G and Sorensen IA. Population-based cohort study of the association between alcohol intake and cancer of the upper digestive tract. BMJ, 1998; 317: 844–47.

6. Gupta D, Boffeta P, Gaborieau V and Jindal SK. Risk factors of lung cancer in Chandigarh, India. Indian J Med Res 2001; 113: 142–50.

7. International Agency for Research on Cancer. Weight control and physical activity. IARC Handbook of Cancer Prevention. IARC Press, Lyon, France, 2002.

8. World Cancer Research Fund. Food, Nutrition, Physical Activity and the Prevention of Cancer: A Global Perspective, American Institute for Cancer Research, Washington, DC, USA, 2nd edition, 2007.

9. Hankinson SE, Colditz GA and Hunter DJ. Reproductive factors and family history of breast cancer in relation to plasma estrogen and prolactin levels in postmenopausal women in the nurse's health study. Cancer Causes and Control, 2009; 6(3): 217–224.

10. Sankaranarayanan R, Rajkumar R and Theresa R. Initial results from a randomized trial of cervical visual screening in rural South India. Int J Cancer 2004; 109: 461–467.

11. Sankaranarayanan R, Shastri SS and Basu P. The role of low level magnification in visual inspection with acetic acid for the early detection of cervical neoplasia. Cancer Detect Prev 2004; 28: 345–351.

12. Lynch BM, Neilson HK, and Christine FM. Physical Activity and breast Cancer prevention, Recent Results in Cancer Research. 2011; 186: 13–44.

13. Kolonel LN, Hankin JH and Whittemore AS. Vegetables, fruits, legumes and prostate cancer: a multiethnic case control study. Cancer Epidemiology, Biomarkers and Prevention, 2000; 9(8): 795–804.

14. Flood A, Velie EM and Chaterjee N. Fruit and vegetable intakes and the risk of colorectal cancer in the Breast Cancer Detection Demonstration Project follow up cohort. The American Journal of Clinical Nutrition, 2002; 75(5): 936–943.

15. Bairwa KS. Effectiveness of an information booklet on cancer risk factors, Nursing Journal of India. 2002, LXXXXIII(10): 227–228.

16. World Health Organization. World Cancer Statistics, 2005, available at http://who.worldcancerreport/cancerretrieved on 21.07.2014.

17. GLOBOCAN 2008. Cancer Statistics Database (version 1.2), available at http://globocan.iarc.fr retrieved on 24.09.14.

18. Global and Regional Burden of Disease and Risk factors. 2001. available at http://cancerjournal.org retrieved on 13.06.14.

19. World Health Organization. Cancer control – Knowledge into action, WHO guide for effective action, Module 2. 2007: 1–45.

20. Indian council of medical Research. Annual report of population-based cancer registries of the National Cancer Registry programme, ICMR, 2003. New Delhi, available at http://www.medind.nic.in/ibd/t06/il/ibdt06ilpl5.pdf retrieved on 12.7.2014.

21. Lipscomb J Patient – reported outcomes in cancer; a review of recent research and policy initiatives, Cancer Journal of clinicians. 2007; 57: 278–300.

22. Kanavos P. The rising burden of cancer in the developing world. Ann Oncol. 2006; 17(8): 15–23.

23. Cancer risk factors and risk reduction, Module 5. 2005: 1–10. Available at www.cancer.gov retrieved on 28.05.2015.

24. Patel AV. Leisure time spent sitting in relation to total mortality in a prospective cohort of US adults. American Journal of Epidemiology, 2010; 172(4): 419–29.

25. Chaudhry K. Tobacco control in India. In 50 Years of Cancer Control in India, Director General of Health Services, Govt. of India, 2001, pp. 196–211.

26. Pandey M, Mathew A and Nair, M K. Cancer vaccines: a step towards prevention and treatment of cancer. Eur. J. Surg. Oncol., 1999, 25, 209–214.

27. Murthy NS and Mathew A. Cancer epidemiology, prevention and control. Current Science, 2004, 86(4): 518–527.

28. Varghese C. Cancer prevention and control in India. 50 years of cancer control in India. Current Science, 2004, 86(4): 48–59.

29. Sankaranarayanan R, Ramadas K and Thara S. Clinical breast examination: preliminary results from a randomized controlled trial in India. Journal of the National Cancer Institute, 2011, 103: 1476–1480.

30. Gandini S, Merzenich H and Robertson C. Meta-analysis of studies on breast cancer risk and diet: the role of fruit and vegetable consumption and the intake of associated micronutrients. Eur J Cancer, 2000; 36: 636–646.

31. National Institute of Health and Family Welfare. National Cancer Control Programme, 2009, available from http://www.nihfw.org retrieved on 30.11.14.

32. American Cancer Society. Cancer information, 2015 available at www.cancer.org retrieved at 30.05.2015.

33. Government of India. Annual Report 2005–2006. New Delhi: Ministry of Health and Family Welfare, 2006.

34. Mayo Foundation for Medical Education and Research. Patient care and Health information, 2015 available at www.mayoclinic.org retrieved on 29.05.2015.

Chapter V (C)

Respiratory Diseases: Management and Preventive Strategies

Mrs. Shweta Pattnaik

Introduction

Respiratory diseases are an emerging problem in developing countries. At present chronic respiratory diseases are a challenge to human health because of their increasing frequency and severity rates and economic impact.

In recent decades, the overall incidence of respiratory diseases has grown manifold due to overcrowding and urbanization, high levels of pollution, tobacco smoking and the HIV epidemic. Up to one-third of patients attending primary health care (PHC) settings seek health care for respiratory problems.

Incidence

According to the WHO World Health Report 2000, 17.4% of all deaths are accounted for by respiratory diseases. Among them are lower respiratory tract infections, chronic obstructive pulmonary disease (COPD), tuberculosis and lung cancer. Changes in the health care systems, schooling, income, and tobacco use are leading to lessen the burden of Non-communicable diseases, while the load of chronic respiratory diseases (CRDs) with asthma, COPD, and lung cancer will worsen because of tobacco use and population aging.

Chronic respiratory diseases are defined as chronic diseases of the respiratory tract and other structures of the lung. The most common diseases are asthma and chronic obstructive pulmonary disease. More than 3 million people died of COPD in 2012, which is equal to 6% of all deaths globally that year. More than 90% of COPD deaths occur in low and middle-income countries.

Why Chronic Respiratory Diseases are becoming a burden?

- ✓ The burden of CRDs is numerous. The principal risk factor for the development of CRDs is tobacco smoke which can be direct or indirect exposure towards it. Heavy exposure to air pollution, occupational health disorders, malnutrition, low birth weight, and multiple early lung infections follow as the other reasons for CRDs.

- ✓ Because of rapid urbanization, prevalence of asthma is increasing day by day. The contributing factors for asthma prevalence are contact with tobacco smoke, housing with poor aeration, indoor allergens, viral infections, outdoor air pollution, and chemical irritants. On the other hand, evidences exist that show that modern cities having cleaner environments under stimulate postnatal immune systems which leads to over-sensitization.

- ✓ In developing countries proper consideration and services are not being given to CRDs to supervise and handle them. Increasing magnitude of the disease is due to the absence of taking steps against it.

- ✓ A large population of the world is facing poverty which is determined by the type of housing, nutritional level, educational level and the types of occupations available to people, which have a negative impact on the health status. The disease prevalence and severity increases due to socio-economic factors which may lead to adverse health outcomes caused by the lack of access to proper health care.

Respiratory System

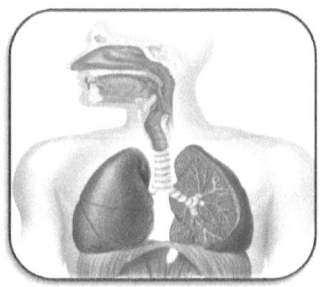

Fig. No. 5(c) 1: *Respiratory System*
(Adapted from http://www.wisegeek.com/)

The cells of the human body require a constant stream of oxygen to stay alive. The main function of the pulmonary system is gas exchange where oxygen is delivered and carbon dioxide is removed out. This adequacy is measured by partial pressure of arterial oxygen (PaO_2) and partial pressure of arterial carbon dioxide ($PaCO_2$). The whole system is divided into 2 parts mainly, Upper respiratory Tract that includes the nose, pharynx, adenoids, tonsils, epiglottis, larynx and trachea, and the Lower respiratory Tract that is made up of bronchi, bronchioles, alveolar ducts and alveoli.

Respiratory disorders: These are mainly classified as follows:

Table No. 5(b) 1: List of disorders affecting respiratory system

Acute Infections	Chronic Infections
<ul><li>Respiratory failure</li><li>Acute respiratory distress syndrome(ARDS)</li><li>Acute bronchitis</li><li>Empyema</li><li>Pneumonia</li><li>Tuberculosis</li><li>Pulmonary embolism</li></ul>	<ul><li>Asthma</li><li>Chronic obstructive pulmonary disease</li><li>Bronchiectasis</li><li>Cancer of lung</li></ul>

Acute Disorders

Acute respiratory infection is a serious infection that prevents normal breathing function. It usually begins as a viral infection in the nose, trachea (windpipe), or lungs. If the infection is not treated, it can spread to the entire respiratory system. The disease is quite widespread. It is particularly dangerous for children, older adults, and people with immune system disorders. According to the World Health Organization (WHO), acute respiratory infections kill an estimated 2.6 million children annually every year worldwide.

Respiratory Failure

A disorder of pulmonary function where an alteration in the gas exchange system occurs, i.e., inadequacy in maintaining arterial blood levels of oxygen and carbon dioxide. A PaO_2 below 60mm Hg is considered as Hypoxemic respiratory failure (Type I) whereas a $PaCO_2$ of more than 50 mm Hg is Hypercapnic Respiratory failure (Type II).

Causes

- ARDS including shock, sepsis and pneumonia
- Obstructive sleep apnea
- Cardiogenic pulmonary edema
- COPD, asthma
- Central nervous system disorder like drug overdose, brain tumor, cerebral injury or hemorrhage
- Neuromuscular disorders involving Myasthenia Gravis and Guillain Barre Syndrome

Health Promotion Strategies

- Education is the primary strategy to prevent respiratory failure.

- Teach all clients and the public health about the risks of smoking, water safety and measures to prevent smoke inhalation in a fire.
- Discuss the importance of pneumococcal vaccine and annual influenza immunization for those at risk, over age 65 and people with chronic diseases.
- Work with clients addicted to narcotic drugs to attain and maintain drug free status.
- Encourage patients at risk, especially older adults and those suffering with lung disease to get immunized with pneumococcal pneumonia vaccine which gives protection against streptococcus pneumonia bacteria.
- Ensure annual immunization for influenza in persons 6 months and older.
- The Center for Disease Control and Prevention recommends immunization for-
    a. Chronic pulmonary, renal, hepatic, neurologic, hematologic or metabolic disorders
    b. Are or will be pregnant during the influenza season
    c. Age 6 months to 18 years and receiving long-term Aspirin therapy
    d. Morbidity obese (BMI 40 or greater)
    e. Immunocompromised
    f. Residents of nursing homes or chronic care facilities
        - Health care workers
        - Cardiovascular diseases
        - Household contacts of those at risk of influenza

Acute Respiratory Distress Syndrome (ARDS)

This is a clinical syndrome resulting from acute lung injury at the level of alveoli causing severe hypoxemia and decreased compliance of the lungs. Characteristic features include severe hypoxemia, decreased lung compliance, bilateral pulmonary infiltrates and absence of cardiogenic pulmonary edema. Acute respiratory distress syndrome and pneumonia are always connected with each other. 7.1% and 16.1% of all patients admitted to an intensive care unit and patients on mechanical ventilation accordingly develop acute lung injury or acute respiratory distress syndrome. The mortality rate related to these conditions is between 34 and 55%, and most deaths occur due to multiorgan failure. Mortality is 55% and is improved with early intervention.

Causes

- Hemorrhaghic shock or septic shock.
- Some inhalation injuries.
- Infections.
- Trauma and drug overdose.
- Disseminated intravascular coagulation, air emboli, CABG.

Health Promotion Strategies

Maximal respiratory functions following ARDS are usually achieved within 6 months. Respiratory function may remain impaired which may necessitate changes in occupation, lifestyle and family roles.

- Avoiding smoking and second hand smoke and environmental pollutants is vital to prevent lung damage.
- Obtain immunization for pneumococcal pneumonia and influenza.

- Provide referrals to home health and respiratory care services as indicated as well as for occupational therapy and counseling as needed.

- Such patients should essentially be provided with continuing services which must be initiated, coordinated and monitored by primary care physicians. Physicians should assess functional status at hospital follow-up and evaluate subsequent visits, making sure that the resources of the multidimensional health care team (e.g., physical and occupational therapy, rehabilitation nursing, home health care, subspecialty colleagues) are used effectively for the promotion of optimal health.

Acute Bronchitis

It is the inflammation of the bronchi in the lower respiratory tract due to infection seen usually as a sequel to upper respiratory tract infection. It causes a cough that often brings up mucus. It can also cause shortness of breath, wheezing, a low fever, and chest tightness.

Causes

- Mostly viral (rhinovirus, influenza) but also bacterial like Streptococcus pneumonia, Hemophilus influenza.

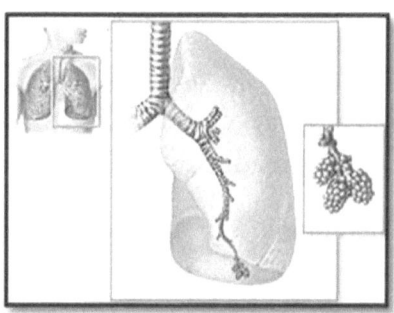

Fig. No. 5(c) 2: *Inflamed bronchial tubes*
Adapted from - www.nlm.nih.gov/medlineplus/acutebronchitis.html

- Exposure to irritants may also trigger bronchitis.

Health Promotion Strategies

- Encourage patients to take prompt treatment regarding shortness of breath and worsening condition.

- Avoid being exposed to dry environment as a dry cough may still be present after bronchitis.
- Initiate mobilization of secretions with an increase in the hydration status.
- Promote chest physiotherapy and coughing.
- Be cautious against over the counter usage of cough suppressants, anti-histamines and decongestants that may cause drying and retention of secretions.
- Complementary and alternative therapies can be used after discussing with health care providers. Echinacea, eucalyptus and thyme are some herbs beneficial for Asthma and bronchitis. However, there are no definitive studies proving their usefulness.

Pneumonia

Pneumonia is the inflammation of the lung parenchyma, i.e., the respiratory bronchioles and alveoli, making breathing painful and limiting oxygen intake. It is mostly caused by infectious agents and can be spread in different ways such as coughing and sneezing.

Pneumonia can be mentioned as the primary infectious reason of death in children worldwide, accounting for 15% of all deaths of children under 5 years old. Pneumonia led to the death of an estimated 935000 children under the age of 5 worldwide in 2013.

Worldwide pneumonia causes 15% of all deaths in children under the age of 5 years, out of which 2% are newborns. Children in poor and rural communities are most affected. Despite available interventions, pneumonia claimed the lives of 1.3 million children in 2011 and was responsible for 18% of child deaths globally.

Causes

Table No. 5(c) 2: List of various micro organisms leading to respiratory infection

Community Acquired	Hospital Acquired	Opportunistic
Streptococcus pneumonia	Staphylococcus aureus	Pneumocystis carinii
Mycoplasma pneumonia	Pseudomonas aeruginosa	Mycobacterium tuberculosis
Haemophilus influenza	Klebsiella pneumonia	Cytomegalovirus
Influenza virus	Escherichia coli	Fungi
Chlamydia pneumoniae		

Health Promotion Strategies

- Make the client's aware about benefits of immunization against influenza and pneumococcal pneumonia. But vaccine coverage must be improved, and lower cost vaccines are needed where the burden of pneumonia is highest.

- Regular assessment of the pulmonary function is required especially for older adults.

- Restoring and maintaining mobility plays a vital role in improving ventilation and helps to mobilize the secretions.

- Promoting adequate hydration helps to expectorate out the secretions.

- Avoid smoking and exposure to second hand smoke so as to prevent irritation of the lungs.

- Development of immunization for mothers to protect them and their newborns from pathogens that bear a disproportionate mortality burden in the neonatal period.

Pulmonary Tuberculosis

Tuberculosis is a chronic recurrent infectious disease affecting the lungs and also other parts of the body. It remains one of the major primary causes for mortality and morbidity worldwide. In 2014, 9.6 million people were diagnosed to have TB and 1.5 million died due to this disease. More than 95% of deaths related to TB occur in low and middle-income countries, and it is said to be one of the top 5 causes of death for women aged between 15 and 44. In 2014, an estimated 1 million children were diagnosed with TB and 140000 children died of TB. In 2014, an estimated 480000 people developed multidrug resistant TB (MDR-TB) globally.

India is the highest TB burden country in the world with 20% of cases occurring globally. Every year 1.8 million people develop TB, of which 0.8 million are new smear positive highly infectious cases. Two out of 5 Indians are infected with TB bacillus. The average annual risk of infection is estimated to be 1.5%. Everyday 5000 people develop this disease. It is estimated that in India nearly 0.37 million people die of TB every year.

Poor urban areas are affected the most wherein injection drug use, homelessness, malnutrition and poor living conditions are present. People residing in slum areas with unhygienic conditions and overcrowding are found to have maximum suspected cases. Transmission can be seen in hospitals, homeless shelters, prisons, residential facilities and drug treatment centers.

Immunocompromised patients having altered immunity, such as those with silicosis, diabetes mellitus, chronic renal failure, leukemia, lymphoma and those suffering from AIDS are at particular risk to be affected with tuberculosis.

One of the greatest challenges to public health is Multi-drug-resistant TB (MDR-TB) and extensively drug-resistant TB (XDR TB). Resistance to isoniazid and rifampin, 2 most effective first line antibiotics leads to MDR-TB. Resistant to the 2 most effective first line drugs along with resistance to the best second-line medications, any fluoroquinolone and at least one of the 3 injectable drugs leads to XDR TB which is rare, but often fatal. Once a strain of M. tuberculosis develops resistance to 2 of the most potent first line antituberculous drugs (e.g., Isoniazid, Rifampin) we call it multidrug resistant tuberculosis (MDR-TB).

Health Promotion Strategies

Tuberculosis today presents an emerging threat not only to an individual but to the entire public health. Therefore, the ultimate goal aims at eradicating TB worldwide. Education and Screening programs play an essential role in detecting the number of TB cases. Individuals with a diagnosis of TB must be reported to the public health authorities for identification and assessment of contacts and risk to the community.

Public health teaching includes creating awareness to prevent the spread of TB by covering their mouths when coughing or sneezing and disposing off sputum properly. Programs to address the social determinants of TB are necessary to decrease transmission of TB.

Teaching should comprise strict adherence with the prescribed regimen. This may be worked out with the help of teaching sessions, counseling, contracts, reminder system, incentives or rewards and Direct Observed Treatment (DOT). Here the public health nurse plays an important role in maintaining the follow-up on household contacts and assessment of the adherence towards drug regimen.

Prevention depends on the early diagnosis of infection and treatment to achieve cure. In countries where tuberculosis is predominant, BCG vaccination for infants is recommended. The government should avail the facility of smoking cessation clinics, alcohol treatment facilities and support groups to ensure the minimization of TB cases.

Importance of good nutrition and dietary guidelines should be recommended for patients with TB for early recovery.

Public Health Intervention

Mainly focuses on testing, surveillance, prevention, and control of TB. The government is responsible for rural, state and local public health in collaboration with the private sectors should focus on the implementation of strategies to control TB.

- Quick recognition and reporting of persons who have tapered TB.
- Prevent close contacts of patients with contagious TB.
- Take steps to prevent TB among Latent Tuberculosis Infection (LTBI) by identifying those who are more at risk for development of TB disease through targeted testing and administration of a curative course of treatment.
- Identifying settings at high risk for transmission by applying effective infection-control measures to reduce the risk.

Implementation will still remain a challenge. The variable latency period between infection and the progression to active TB disease can slow down control efforts. Moreover, testing and screening programs must differentiate LTBI from active TB disease, where LTBI is asymptomatic and non-contagious and active TB disease is contagious.

The most widely utilized test for LTBI is the Montoux tuberculin skin test, which involves injecting purified protein derivative under the skin and measuring any subsequent reaction. However, the test may not detect TB infection for up to 10 weeks after exposure, and the results are subject to broad interpretations and false readings due to immunosuppression among TB patients with other chronic diseases or who are malnourished.

An alternative test, the Quanti FERON test, approved for use in 2005, involves testing a patient's white blood cells for evidence of TB infection.

Chronic Infections

In industrialized and developing countries, a major public health challenge represented is chronic respiratory diseases because of their frequency and economic impact. In emergent countries most patients have poor access to health care, where poverty and non-communicable respiratory disease are very common. An additional problem in the developing countries is limited resources with health planners. The burden and trend of chronic respiratory diseases and their impact on economy are highlighted in this paper, and a suggestion for improving practical strategies for patient management in developing countries.

Obstructive lung disease, the most common chronic pulmonary disease is characterized by increased resistance to airflow due to airway obstruction or narrowing of the airways. It is constituted by asthma, COPD, cystic fibrosis and bronchiectasis.

The epidemiology of asthma differs in many ways from that of chronic bronchitis and emphysema, for example, in its age and sex incidence, relationships to social class, allergy, and time trends. But many of the clinical features are common to all 3 diseases with the result that diagnosis may be difficult.

Asthma

Another important chronic inflammatory disease of the airways is asthma which leads to recurrent episodes of wheezing, breathlessness, chest tightness and coughing. Inflammation causes increased responsiveness of the airway to multiple stimuli. According to WHO approximately 235 million people are currently suffering from asthma. Asthma is a public health problem which can be seen in high-income countries as well as in low and lower-middle-income countries were most deaths occur.

Asthma creates significant burden to individuals as well as families and restricts individuals' activities for a lifetime. Many clients develop the disease in the absence of risk factors. However, the strongest risk factor for the development of asthma is a combination of genetic predisposition with environmental exposure to inhaled substances and particles that may aggravate allergic reactions or irritate the airways, such as:

- Indoor allergens (for example, house dust mites in bedding, carpets and stuffed furniture, pollution and pet dander).
- Outdoor allergens (such as pollens and molds).
- Tobacco smoke.
- Chemical irritants in the workplace.
- Air pollution.

Additional triggering factors include cold air, extreme emotional stress such as anger or fear, and physical exercise. Even certain medications like aspirin and other non-steroid anti-inflammatory drugs, and beta-blockers have been associated with trigger to asthma.

Health Promotion Strategies

> **WHO strategy for prevention and control of asthma**

WHO recognizes that asthma is of major public health importance. The aim of its strategy is to support Member States in their efforts to reduce the disability and premature death related to asthma. Who's program objectives are:

- Survey to figure out the extent of asthma, analyze its determinants and monitor trends, with an emphasis on poor and destitute populations.

- Reduce the level of exposure to common risk factors, mainly tobacco smoke, frequent lower respiratory infections during childhood, and air pollution (indoor, outdoor, and occupational exposure) by primary prevention.

- Improving access to interventions like medicines, upgrading standards and accessibility of care at different levels of the health care system cost effectively.

Although complementary therapies have not been proven to completely cure asthma but to some extent they are beneficial. Dietary therapies include elimination of certain foods or food additives (sulphite) from the diet. Some studies suggest that an increased intake of ascorbic acid, an antioxidant, zinc and magnesium may help alleviate manifestations of asthma. Those suffering with mild asthma may be benefitted from addition of omega-3 polyunsaturated fatty acids to the diet, which will help them to experience less severe and fewer attacks **(Spencer & Jacobs, 2003).** Refer clients interested in using natural preparations to a CAM therapist and emphasize the importance of talking to the physician before using these preparations along with conventional treatment. In addition to this other therapies like biofeedback, yoga, breathing techniques, acupuncture, homeopathy and massage have been found to control asthma symptoms. Promoting asthma support groups in communities would be helpful for such patients.

Measures applicable to reduce asthma attacks can be:

- Warm up slowly before exercising in cold weather; wear a mask or scarf to retain the air warmth and humidity while exercising.

- Promote adequate rest, hydration, and good nutrition to maintain immune function.

- Use techniques to reduce or manage physical or psychological stress.

- Avoid furred animals as allergen of pets may also be one of the factors causing asthma. Some people are allergic to cockroach remains and the dried droppings so measures to control these insects are important.

- Prompt diagnosis and treatment of upper respiratory tract infections and sinusitis may prevent an exacerbation of asthma.

Chronic Obstructive Pulmonary Disease

COPD is a preventable and treatable disease characterized by airflow restriction that is not completely reversible. The airflow limitation is usually progressive and is associated with an unusual inflammatory response of the lung to noxious particles or gases (typically from exposure to cigarette smoke). Proper treatment for COPD can minimize the symptoms and improve the quality of life.

Experts from the Global Initiative for Obstructive Lung Diseases (GOLD) have defined the disease on the basis of spirometric criteria by using the post-bronchodilator forced expiratory volume in one second (FEV1) and its ratio to the forced vital capacity (FVC).

Chronic Obstructive Pulmonary Disease (COPD) is not one single disease but also includes chronic lung diseases that cause limitations in lung airflow. The terms 'chronic bronchitis' and 'emphysema' are no longer used, but they comes within the COPD diagnosis.

COPD is the fourth leading cause of death in the United States. In almost 8 out of 10 cases, COPD is caused by exposure to cigarette smoke. In addition, other environmental exposures (such as those in the workplace) can also lead to COPD.

Obstructive lung disease typically affects middle-aged and older adults. Cigarette smoking is clearly implicated as the primary cause of COPD. Another factor that influences the development of COPD is Genetic factors. An example of this is that all smokers do not develop COPD. Progression of the disease can be slowed down by quitting smoking. Women and men are affected equally, but more women have died of COPD than men since 2000.

Burden of COPD

65 million people have moderate to severe chronic obstructive pulmonary disease (COPD) according to WHO. Globally more than 3 million people died of COPD in 2005, which corresponds to 5% of all deaths. Most of the information existing about COPD prevalence, morbidity and mortality comes from high-income countries. Even in those countries, it's difficult and expensive to collect the accurate epidemiologic data on COPD. Almost 90% of COPD deaths occur in low and middle-income countries as well.

Once COPD was more common in men, but as tobacco use among women increased in high-income countries, and due to the higher risk of exposure to indoor air pollution (such as biomass fuel used for cooking and heating) in low-income countries, the disease now affects both men and women equally.

Who's Role and Activities: COPD

According to WHO, chronic obstructive pulmonary disease (COPD) is a major public health issue. The Organization plays a key role in coordinating international efforts against the disease. The aim of this is to support the Member States in their efforts to reduce the number of disease cases, disability and premature death related to COPD.

Immediate actions supposed to be taken are:

- Public awareness of the disease should be enhanced to make sure that the patients and health professionals identify the disease and are aware of the severity of problems associated with it.
- Global epidemiological surveillance should be organized and coordinated to monitor global and regional trends in COPD.

- An optimal strategy should be developed and implemented for management and prevention of COPD.

For reducing the cases of COPD patients and channelizing the strategies, a few important organizations have been formed and among them are:

Global Alliance against Chronic Respiratory Diseases (GARD): Global Alliance against Chronic Respiratory Diseases (GARD) is a voluntary alliance working towards a common goal of improving global lung health. GARD promotes an integrated approach that capitalizes upon synergies of chronic respiratory diseases with other chronic diseases. The main focus is on the needs of low and middle-income countries and vulnerable populations. The Global Initiative for Chronic Obstructive Pulmonary Disease (GOLD) is a part of GARD.

WHO Framework Convention on Tobacco Control (WHO FCTC): WHO Framework Convention on Tobacco Control (WHO FCTC) was developed in response to the globalization of the tobacco epidemic, with the aim to protect billions of people from the devastating impact of tobacco consumption and exposure to tobacco smoke.

WHO's Program on Indoor Air Pollution

High levels of indoor air pollution are caused by cooking and heating with solid fuels on open fires or traditional stoves. Indoor smoke contains a variety of health-damaging pollutants, such as small particles and carbon monoxide, and particulate pollution levels may be 20 times higher than accepted guideline values.

WHO aims to conduct a comparative evaluation of intervention experiences in different settings. The effectiveness of interventions as well as the enabling factors that facilitate long-term, sustained adoption and use of suitable improved technologies will be investigated in this evaluation.

Health Promotion Strategies

Not smoking – never starting or quitting is the best preventive measure for COPD. The client and family have the primary responsibility for disease management. Teaching is vital to promote optimal health and slow disease progression. Teaching for home care focuses on effective coughing and breathing techniques, preventing exacerbations, and managing prescribed therapies. The incidence of COPD would decrease noticeably if people would not begin smoking or would stop smoking.

- Avoiding exposure to occupational and environmental pollutants and irritants is an important preventive measure to maintain healthy lungs.

- Counseling the patient in smoking cessation is vital because it is the only way to slow down the progression of COPD.

- Early diagnosis and treatment of respiratory tract infections and exacerbations of COPD help prevent progression of the disease.

- COPD patients should avoid contacts with the sick, practice good hand washing techniques, take medications as prescribed, exercise regularly, and maintain a healthy weight.

- Postural drainage and endurance of muscle training exercises should be promoted.

- Influenza vaccine and pneumococcal vaccine are recommended for patients with COPD. Families with a history of COPD as well as alpha-1 anti-trypsin deficiency should be aware of the genetic nature of the disease. Regular screening by a pulmonologist should be done.

- An evidence-based intervention to reduce symptoms and improve quality of life is pulmonary rehabilitation and it acts as an effective intervention to improve exercise capacity and decrease hospitalizations, anxiety and depression.

- A study by **Yang and Chen (2005)** looked at change processes involved in moving from inactivity to activity in clients with COPD. This study found that those who adopted more behavioral change processes like counter conditioning, helping relationships, reinforcement management and self-liberation were more likely to engage in and maintain regular exercise, (defined as at least 20 minutes of exercise of any intensity performed more than 3 times a week) usually walking. Thus we can observe that this study and others support programs of regular physical activity to maintain functional status and reduce symptom progression.

- CAM therapies may be useful to manage symptoms of COPD. Dietary measures such as minimizing intake of dairy products and salt may help to reduce mucus production and keep mucus more liquefied. Herbal tea made with peppermint and yarrow or comfrey may act as expectorants to help relieve congestion. Licorice root also has expectorant and anti-inflammatory effects that may be beneficial. Refer to a herbalist before taking any such treatment. **(Spencer and Jacobs, 2003).**

- Research findings of **Joseph M (2014)** suggest that pursed lip breathing and expiratory muscle training are effective in relieving exertional dyspnea among COPD patients.

- Acupuncture, hypnotherapy and guided imagery may help the client with smoking cessation. This will also help in reducing anxiety and breathing patterns. **(Fontaine, 2005).**

Occupational Lung Disease

These are a group of disorders where the persons are exposed to inhalation of noxious substances in the work environment. This may be mainly classified as,

Pneumoconiosis: Chronic fibrotic lung disease caused by inhalation of inorganic dusts and particulate matter, and

Hypersensitivity pneumonitis: Allergic pulmonary disease caused by exposure to inhaled organic dusts.

Health Promotion Strategy

- Prevention is the key strategy for all Occupational Lung Diseases.
- Using protective barriers (PPE) that limit the amount of inhaled particles is essential for people who work in industries with known risks.
- Eliminating exposure to offending agents is an important part of disease management.
- Teaching about the dangers of Occupational Lung Diseases and ways to reduce the risk needs to begin early before the disease develops.
- Avoiding cigarette smoking and heavy air pollution.
- Immunization against pneumococcal and annual influenza vaccine to be promoted.
- Facilities of yearly tuberculin testing for clients with silicosis should be provided.
- Other aspects include increased amount of fluid intake for liquefying the secretions and deep breathing and coughing exercises.

Health strategy for Respiratory Diseases Can Be Formed As

Standard protocols are not available for assessing and managing chronic non-communicable respiratory disease in most developing countries. The services that exist do not get in touch with most of the population afflicted by "human poverty." These people are usually illiterate without any access to health services, and die before the age of 40 years.

Health promotion facts:

- Avoid cigarette smoking as well as passive smoking.
- Thoroughly perform hand washing to prevent cross infection.
- Avoid exposure to air pollutants, allergens.
- Immunize yourself with Pneumococcal and Flu vaccine after physician's reference.
- Protect yourself properly when working in an environment exposed to dust, smoke and fumes.

As per WHO the following are the objectives of the strategy through which implementation of the program can be done.

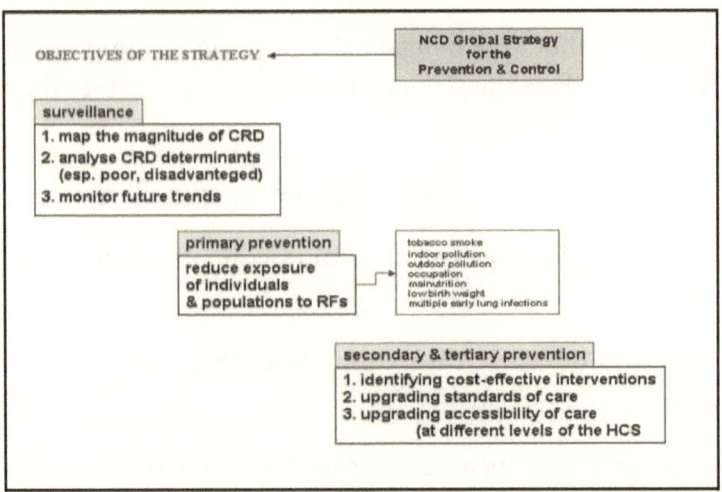

(RF–Risk Factor; HCS–Health Care System)

Fig. No. 5(c) 3: *WHO strategy for respiratory diseases (Adapted from www.who.in)*

Surveillance

It's important that the healthcare leaders should primarily focus on monitoring the factors in terms of magnitude for knowing the reasons of disease occurrence, cases admitted, deaths occurred and measures taken to resolve it. Standard indicators should be adopted. They should be aware of the functioning of health workers at rural areas.

To evaluate the quality of care, the elements of health care structure that can be monitored include drug availability, cost and quality, existence of local guidelines and policies, and level of training of health professionals.

Primary Prevention

Prevention is the best cure for CRDS. Laying stress in the immunization aspect plays a key role in preventing respiratory disorders in the developing countries. Prevention of active and passive smoking is one of the major features in reducing the burden of CRDs as well as for other chronic diseases. Avoiding exposure to risk factors should be initiated at the time of pregnancy and childhood. Other risk factors that should be given importance include low birth weight, poor nutrition, and acute respiratory infections of early childhood, indoor and outdoor air pollutants, and occupational risk factors.

Other sectors within a community must be actively engaged for effectiveness of primary prevention. Proper education to promote healthy lifestyle should be given such as healthy nutritional habits, regular exercise and avoidance of tobacco, airway irritants and allergens.

More researches have to be carried out to promote evidence-based strategic implementation. The rural areas have to be specifically taken note of where the delivery of care is not very prompt. The health workers need to be given education and training regarding preventive aspects of respiratory infections so that further channelizing to the distant areas may be conducted. ***Many cases go unnoticed;***

therefore health workers need to perform screening at individual level as many people may take the symptoms very casually.

Working in collaboration with NGOs may be helpful in carrying out the functioning and implementing the strategies. Proper referrals should be made so as to provide the best care available and in turn reducing the mortality rates. Taxes and rates for products that are associated with risk should be highly increased so that they are consumed less. Advertisements promoting such products should be totally avoided.

Secondary and Tertiary Prevention

To prevent further progression and to ensure cost-effective management, early detection of occupational asthma is vital. Programs for early detection of COPD have been recommended but their cost-effectiveness has yet to be fully evaluated. Effective management including smoking cessation, pulmonary rehabilitation and reduction of personal exposure to noxious particles and gases can reduce symptoms, improve quality of life, and increase physical fitness, although long-term decline in lung function may not be reversible. Evidence indicates influenza vaccination is a cost-effective intervention for patients with COPD.

Asthma is a treatable disease with preventable morbidity but not curable. Avoidance of allergens and non-specific triggers is included in secondary and tertiary prevention. Optimal pharmacological treatment, including the use of anti-inflammatory medication, has been shown to be cost-effective in controlling asthma, and preventing the development of chronic symptoms, which also reduces mortality.

What can we as nurses do in controlling respiratory infections?

- ✓ Promoting education in rural as well as urban areas at the primary level to decrease the incidence of respiratory diseases.

- ✓ Creating awareness regarding preventive aspects of respiratory infections.

- ✓ Carrying out activities like organizing health camps, distribution of pamphlets, screening out the ones with risk are important.

- ✓ Screening out the cases of respiratory infections with the help of nursing students posted in communities and then reporting it to higher authorities.

- ✓ Nurses in industrial and public health settings can begin by recognizing potential dangers and teaching workers about measures to reduce dust in their work area and the use of Personal Protective Devices such as masks.

- ✓ Nurses working with affected families have an excellent opportunity to begin educating children about the risks associated with occupation.

- ✓ Teaching the Primary Health Care workers, school teachers and others must be promoted as they are the main persons who remain in touch with the community people.

- ✓ Promotion of isolation for known cases of Tuberculosis, and furthermore, guidance should be given for preventing its spread to others.

- ✓ Carrying out researches to promote healthy living and thus implementing those evidence-based findings.

- ✓ Co-coordinating the implementation policies in collaboration with NGOs and also governmental organizations.

- ✓ Communicating the findings of the researches conducted to the higher authorities and taking action accordingly.

With such interventions an initiation from nurses can be done to promote healthy and happy living, thereby preventing respiratory diseases from becoming a burden.

Key Points

Prevention and management of chronic respiratory disease may be attained by:

- o Reducing tobacco smoking in the whole population
- o Encouraging smoking cessation
- o Improving the quality of services through standardized case management
- o Improving access to affordable essential medications
- o Improving efficiency by avoiding ineffective and costly care
- o Promoting pulmonary rehabilitation
- o Enhancing the quality of life of persons suffering from CRDs
- o Comprehensive care is of utmost importance in controlling the spread of the disease

References

1. Nadia At-Khaled, Donald Enarson & Jean Bousquet. Chronic respiratory diseases in developing countries: the burden and strategies for prevention and management, Bulletin of the World Health Organization, 2001, 79: 971–979.

2. Ottmani, S E et al. (eds). Respiratory Care in Primary Care Services: A Survey in 9 Countries, World Health Organization, Geneva, 2004; WHO/HTM/TB/2004.333; http://whqlibdoc.who.int/hq/2004/WHO_HTM_TB_2004.333.pdf

3. Christine Di Maria and Matthew Solan. Healthline acute respiratory infection, July 25, 2012.

4. CDC, 2012, Morbidity And Mortality Annual Report, 61 (32, 61–618).

5. Aaron Saguil, Matthew Fargo, 2012. Acute Respiratory Distress Syndrome: Diagnosis and Management, American Family Physician, Feb 15; 85(4): 352–358.

6. Lewis, 2015. Assessment and Management of clinical Problems, 2nd Edition, Published by Elsevier Pg. no.497–587

7. CDC 2007. Atlanta, GA: Department of Health and Human Services, CDC, September 2006. http://www.cdc.gov/tb/statistics/reports/2007/pdf/fullreport.pdf.

8. CDC, Trends in Tuberculosis—United States, 2007. MMWR 2008; 57(11): 281–285. http://www.cdc.gov/mmwR/preview/mmwrhtml/mm5711a2.htm.

9. Swigart and Kolb (2004) Le Mone burke, medical surgical nursing critical thinking in client care, 4th edition Dorling Kindersley (India) Pvt. ltd.2008.1209–1367

10. American Thoracic Society, Centers for Disease Control and Prevention, and Infectious Diseases Society of America. Controlling Tuberculosis in the United States. Am. J. Respir. Crit. Care Med. 2005; 172: 1169–1227

11. CDC, Division of Tuberculosis Elimination. Fact Sheet: QuantiFERON-TB Gold Test. http://www.cdc.gov/tb/pubs/tbfactsheets/QFT.htm. Accessed August 24, 2008.

12. Nadia Aït-Khaled, Donald Enarson & Jean Bousquet. Chronic respiratory diseases in developing countries: the burden and strategies for prevention and management, Bulletin of the World Health Organization, 2001, 79 (10)

13. Spencer & Jacobs, 2003. LeMone & Burke, medical surgical nursing, critical thinking in client care, 4th edition Dorling Kindersley (India) Pvt. ltd.2008.1209–1367

14. Global Initiative for Chronic Obstructive Lung Disease (GOLD). Strategy for the diagnosis, management, and prevention

of chronic obstructive pulmonary lung disease: Executive summary [Internet]. [Cited 2010 Mar 12.] Available from: http://www.goldcopd.com

15. Centers for Disease Control and Prevention (CDC), National Center for Health Statistics. Compressed mortality file 1999-2006. CDC WONDER online database, compiled from Compressed Mortality File 1999-2006 Series 20 No. 2L. Atlanta: CDC; 2009 [cited 2010 Mar 5]. Available from: http://wonder.cdc.gov/cmf-icd10.html

16. WHO, strategy for prevention and control of chronic respiratory diseases, 2014 WHO reference number: WHO/MNC/CRA/02.1 http://www.who.int/respiratory/publications/crd_strategy/en

17. Pomidori L, Contonoli M, Mandolesi G et al. A simple method for home exercise training in patients with chronic obstructive pulmonary disease; I year study; Journal of cardiopulmonary rehabilitation\prev 32: 53, 2012

18. Harrison S, Greeining N, Wlliams J, et al. Have we underestimated the efficacy of Pulmonary Rehabilitation in improving mood? Resp. medicine, 106: 838. 2012

19. Yang and Chen (2005). LeMone & Burke, medical surgical nursing critical thinking in client care, 4th edition Dorling Kindersley (India) Pvt. ltd.2008.1209-1367

20. Joseph M (2014) Effectiveness of Pursed lip breathing and Expiratory muscle exercise among COPD patients, Indian Journal of Nursing Studies, Vol.5 no.1, Jan-June 2014

21. Fontaine, 2005 LeMone & Burke, medical surgical nursing critical thinking in client care, 4th edition Dorling Kindersley (India) Pvt. ltd.2008.1209-1367

Chapter V (D)
Preventive Strategies in Diabetes

Dr. Nancy Fernandes

India, a country experiencing rapid socio-economic progress and urbanization, carries a considerable share of the global diabetes burden. Studies in different parts of India have demonstrated an escalating prevalence of diabetes not only in urban populations, but also in rural populations as a result of the urbanization of lifestyle parameters. The prevalence of prediabetes is also high. Recent studies have shown a rapid conversion of impaired glucose tolerance to diabetes in the southern states of India, where the prevalence of diabetes among adults has reached approximately 20% in urban populations and approximately 10% in rural populations. Because of the considerable disparity in the availability and affordability of diabetes care, as well as low awareness of the disease, the glycemic outcome in treated patients is far from ideal. Lower age at onset and a lack of good glycemic control are likely to increase the occurrence of vascular complications. The economic burden of treating diabetes and its complications is considerable. It is appropriate that the Indian Government has initiated a national program for the management and prevention of diabetes and related metabolic disorders. Lifestyle modification is an effective tool for the primary prevention of diabetes in Asian Indians. The primary prevention of diabetes is urgently needed in India to curb the rising burden of diabetes.

What is Diabetes?

Diabetes mellitus is a group of metabolic diseases characterized by high blood sugar (glucose) levels that result from defects in insulin secretion, or its action, or both. Diabetes mellitus, commonly referred to as diabetes (as it will be in this chapter) was first identified as a disease associated with 'sweet urine,' and excessive muscle loss in the ancient world. Elevated levels of blood glucose (hyperglycemia) lead to spillage of glucose into the urine, hence the term sweet urine.

Normally, blood glucose levels are tightly controlled by insulin, a hormone produced by the pancreas. Insulin lowers the blood glucose level. When the blood glucose elevates (for example, after eating food), insulin is released from the pancreas to normalize the glucose level. In patients with diabetes, the absence or insufficient production of, or lack of response to insulin causes hyperglycemia. Diabetes is a chronic medical condition, meaning that although it can be controlled, it lasts a lifetime.

It is the commonest form of condition, caused by a deficiency of the pancreatic hormone insulin, which results in a failure to metabolize sugars and starch. Sugars accumulate in the blood and urine, and the by-products of alternative fat metabolism disturb the acid-base balance of the blood, causing a risk of convulsions and coma.

Impact of Diabetes on Other Systems

Over time, diabetes can lead to blindness, kidney failure, and nerve damage. These types of damage are the result of damage to small vessels, referred to as micro vascular disease. Diabetes is also an important factor in accelerating the hardening and narrowing of the arteries (atherosclerosis), leading to strokes, coronary heart disease, and other large blood vessel diseases. This is referred to as macro vascular disease. Diabetes affects approximately 26 million people in the United States, while another 79 million have prediabetes condition. An estimated 7 million people in the United States have diabetes and do not even know it.

From an economic perspective, the total annual cost of diabetes in 2012 was estimated to be 245 billion dollars in the United States.

This included 116 billion in direct medical costs (health care costs) for people with diabetes and another 69 billion in other costs due to disability, premature death, or work loss. Medical expenses for people with diabetes are over 2 times higher than those for people who do not have diabetes. Remember, these numbers reflect only the population in the United States. Globally, the statistics are staggering. Diabetes was the 7th leading cause of death in the United States listed on death certificates in 2007.

Magnitude of Diabetes

According to Whiting in 2000, India (31.7 million) topped the world with the highest number of people with diabetes mellitus followed by China (20.8 million) and the United States (17.7 million) in second and third place respectively. According to Wild et al. the prevalence of diabetes is predicted to double globally from 171 million in 2000 to 366 million in 2030 with a maximum increase in India. It is predicted that by 2030 diabetes mellitus may afflict up to 79.4 million individuals in India while in China it is likely to affect 42.3 million and 30.3 million in the United States.

India leads the world with the largest number of diabetic subjects, earning the dubious distinction of being termed the 'diabetes capital of the world.'

As per the International Diabetes Federation (2013), approximately 50% of all people with diabetes live in just 3 countries: China (98.4 million), India (65.1 million) and the USA (24.4 million). The so-called 'Asian Indian Phenotype' refers to certain unique clinical and biochemical abnormalities in Indians which include increased insulin resistance, greater abdominal adiposity, i.e., higher waist circumference despite lower BMI, lower adiponectin and higher sensitive C-reactive protein levels. This phenotype makes Asian Indians more prone to diabetes and premature coronary artery disease. At least a part of this is due to genetic factors. However, the primary driver of the epidemic of diabetes is the rapid epidemiological transition associated with changes in dietary patterns and decreased physical activity as evident from the higher prevalence of diabetes in the urban population. Even though the prevalence of micro vascular complications of diabetes like retinopathy and nephropathy are comparatively lower in Indians, the prevalence of premature coronary artery disease is much higher in Indians compared to other ethnic groups. The most disturbing trend is the shift in age of onset of diabetes to a younger age in the recent years. This could have long-lasting adverse effects on the nation's health and economy. Early identification of at-risk individuals using simple screening tools like the Indian Diabetes Risk Score (IDRS) and appropriate lifestyle intervention would greatly help in preventing or postponing the onset of diabetes and thus reducing the burden on the community and the nation as a whole.

Risk Factors

Apart from the conventional risk factors propelled by urbanization, industrialization, globalization, aging, increasing obesity, and falling levels of physical activity are all contributing to increases in diabetes worldwide. Other factors may also contribute. It has been proposed that obesity, regional adiposity, higher percentage body fat, early life influences including fetal programming and genetic factors contribute to increased risk. The variables independently associated with diabetes in adults include age, BMI, WHR, income and family history of diabetes. Indians tend to have more body fat and a higher risk of diabetes for the same BMI as compared to Western populations. In view of this, the WHO recommends that for public health action, BMI of 23–27.5 kg/m^2 be considered at increased risk for type 2 diabetes and cardiovascular disease; and 27.5 kg/m^2 or higher be considered as high risk.

Insufficient production of insulin (either absolutely or relative to the body's needs), production of defective insulin (which is uncommon), or the inability of cells to use insulin properly and efficiently leads to hyperglycemia and diabetes. This latter condition affects mostly the cells of muscle and fat tissues, and results in a condition known as insulin resistance. This is the primary problem in type 2 diabetes. The absolute lack of insulin, usually secondary to a destructive process affecting the insulin producing beta cells in the pancreas, is the main disorder in type 1 diabetes. In type 2 diabetes, there also is a steady decline of beta cells that adds to the process of elevated blood sugars. Essentially, if someone is resistant to insulin, the body can, to some degree, increase production of insulin and overcome the level of resistance. After time, if production decreases and insulin cannot be released as vigorously, hyperglycemia develops. When blood glucose levels fall, for example during exercise, insulin levels fall too.

While Indians share several high risk alleles for diabetes with Caucasians, a recent Genome Wide Association Study (GWAS), has reported a new susceptibility locus at 2q21. It is however clear that in a complex disorder such as diabetes, the known genetic loci contribute approximately 10% to the risk of disease development.

Reasons for the Rise in Prevalence of Diabetes Among Indians

Urbanization vs. Rural

The International Diabetes Federation (IDF) Diabetes Atlas states that in low and middle – income countries, the number of people with diabetes in urban areas is 181 million, while 122 million live in rural areas. The data from the ICMR-INDIAB study also shows that prevalence of diabetes in urban areas ranged from 10.9–14.2% while in rural areas the range was 3.0–8.3%. A rural-urban gradient has also been observed in a study from Tamil Nadu, where the prevalence of diabetes in periurban villages and cities in the state of Tamil Nadu reported as 9.2% and 16.4% respectively.

In the urban areas, the increase in prevalence of diabetes is evident from findings of periodic population-based studies performed in the city of Chennai in South India in the last 2 decades. In these studies, the prevalence of diabetes increased from 8.3% in 1989 to 18.6% in 2006. Similar observations have been reported from Delhi, North India, wherein the urban prevalence of diabetes in studies conducted 2 decades apart (1991–1994 to 2010–2012) increased from 14.2 to 23.0%. Also, the age at detection of diabetes had decreased over this period, with urban metropolitan data suggesting nearly 5% diabetes prevalence in the age group 25–34 years.

In studies from Rajasthan, Vellore and Mysore, prevalence in rural areas has been reported to be as low as 1.8%, 2.1% and 3.8% respectively. This contrasts with the extremely high prevalence of 19.8% reported from a rural hilly area in North-Eastern India. A trend of increasing prevalence in rural areas is noticeable with several studies done in the past decade showing prevalence ranging from 9.2–13.3%. The rural areas of economically backward states have a lower prevalence as reported in the ICMR-INDIAB study (2011). The prevalence in rural areas of the economically better regions of Chandigarh, Tamil Nadu and Maharashtra was 8.3%, 7.8% and 6.5% respectively. On the other hand, in the economically less advantaged state of Jharkhand, the prevalence was only 3.0%. Table no.1 depicts the Indian scenario of diabetes in the country based on documented research finding. (Refer Table 1)

Table No. 5(d) 1: Studies show prevalence of diabetes in India (urban and rural)

Year	Author	Place	Prevalence (%) Urban	Prevalence (%) Rural
2008	Mohan et al.	Nationwide; self-reported	7.3	3.1
2008	Ramachandran et al.	Tamil Nadu	18.6	9.2
2011	ICMR INDIAB (Anjana et al.)	Chandigarh	14.2	8.3
2011	ICMR INDIAB (Anjana et al.)	Tamil Nadu	13.7	7.8

Year	Author	Place	Prevalence (%) Urban	Prevalence (%) Rural
2011	ICMR INDIAB (Anjana et al.)	Maharashtra	10.9	6.5
2011	ICMR INDIAB (Anjana et al.)	Jharkhand	13.5	3.0
2012	Prasad et al.	Orissa	15.7	
2012	Rajput et al.	Haryana		13.3
2012	Singh et al.	Delhi (age >60 urban slum)	18.0	
2013	Shah et al.	Manipur (Muslims only)		16.6
2013	Kumar et al.	West Bengal (Policemen)	15.0	
2014	Walia et al.	Chandigarh	16.4	
2014	Zaman et al.	Arunachal Pradesh		19.8

Genetic Predisposition

Several studies on migrant Indians across the globe have shown that Asian Indians have an increased risk for developing type 2 diabetes and related metabolic abnormalities compared to other ethnic groups. Although the exact reasons are still not clear, certain unique clinical and biochemical characteristics of this ethnic group collectively called as the 'Asian Indian phenotype' is considered to be one of the major factors contributing to the increased predilection towards diabetes. Despite having lower prevalence of obesity as defined by BMI, Asian Indians tend to have greater waist circumference and waist to hip ratios thus having a greater degree of central obesity. Again, Asian Indians have more total abdominal and visceral fat for any given BMI and for any given body fat they have increased insulin resistance which is second cause of type 2 diabetes.

Yajnik et al. in their study stated that low birth weight is a contributor to insulin resistance among Indians. Their hypothesis was that small Indian babies have smaller abdominal viscera and low muscle mass, but preserve body fat during intrauterine development, which may predispose to insulin resistance state. Misra and Vikram in their study concluded that high prevalence of excess body fat, adverse body fat patterning, hypertriglyceridemia, and insulin resistance beginning at a young age have been consistently recorded in Asian Indians irrespective of their geographic locations. These data suggest that primary prevention strategies should be initiated early in this ethnic group. In a study conducted by Kostecka M it is stated that nutrient excess and nutrient deficiency in the diets of preschool children can lead to permanent modification of metabolic pathways and increased risk of diet-dependent diseases in adults. Children are most susceptible to the adverse consequences of bad eating habits. The study was conducted to evaluate the eating habits and the diets of preschool children as risk factors for excessive weight, obesity, insulin resistance and the metabolic syndrome.

The study was conducted on randomly selected 350 preschool children attending kindergartens in south-eastern Poland. Three-day dietary recalls were processed and evaluated. The analyzed dietary content indicated alarmingly low consumption of vegetables, raw fruits, dairy products and whole grain products. The study concluded that diets characterized by excessive energy value and nutritional deficiency can lead to health problems. In most cases, excessive weight gain in children can be blamed on parents and caretakers who are not aware of the health consequences of high-calorie foods rich in fats and sugar.

In India third major cause is environmental factor, with increase in urbanization resulting in dramatic change in lifestyle from traditional to modern, leading to physical inactivity due to technological advancement, affluence leading to consumption of diet rich in fat, sugar and calories and high level of mental stress. All this could adversely influence insulin sensitivity and lead to obesity.

Preventive Strategies in Diabetes

Diabetes mellitus is of 3 types:

i. Type 1 is insulin-dependent diabetes mellitus (IDDM),
ii. Type 2 is Noninsulin-dependent diabetes mellitus (NIDDM), and
iii. Type 3 is gestational diabetes found in some women during pregnancy.

Fig. 5(d) 1 and Fig. 5(d)2 provide a quick understanding of the pathogenesis of diabetes and of the metabolic syndrome seen in type II diabetes.

Type 1 IDDM: It is characterized by loss of the insulin producing beta cells of islet of Langerhans of the pancreas. Sensitivity and responsiveness to insulin are usually normal. This type of diabetes mellitus comprises up to 10%. Type 1 IDDM can affect children (juvenile onset diabetes mellitus) or adults. Common causes: Loss of beta cells leading to type 1 IDDM is autoimmune destruction or by antibodies directed against insulin and islet proteins. Three main factors involved in type 1 diabetes are: i. genetic, ii. environmental, and iii. autoimmunity.

Type 2 NIDDM: It is due to combination of defective insulin secretion and defective responsiveness to insulin or reduced insulin sensitivity. It is quite common, comprising 90% or more of cases in many populations.

Type 3 gestational diabetes: It involves combination of inadequate insulin secretion and responsiveness.

Pathophysiology

Diabetes occurs when there is a disbalance between the demand and production of the hormone insulin.

When food is taken, it is broken down into smaller components. Glucose is a simple sugar found in food. Glucose is an essential nutrient that provides energy for the proper functioning of the body cells. Carbohydrates are broken down in the small intestine and the glucose in digested food is then absorbed by the intestinal cells into the bloodstream, and is carried by the bloodstream to all the cells in the body where it is utilized. The liver is also able to manufacture glucose. However; glucose cannot enter the cells alone and needs insulin to aid in its transport into the cells. Without insulin, the cells become starved of glucose energy despite the presence of abundant glucose in the bloodstream. In certain types of diabetes, the cells' inability to utilize glucose gives rise to the ironic situation of 'starvation in the midst of plenty.' The abundant, unutilized glucose is wastefully excreted in the urine. There are 4 different types of islets and their secretory products as seen in Table no. 5(d) 2.

If due to any reason a specific islet cell is damaged, it ceases or there will be reduction in the secretory product thereby impairing metabolism.

Table No. 5(d) 2: Endocrine cell types in pancreatic islets of Langerhans

Islet Cell Type	Secretory Products
A cell (alpha)	Glucagon
B cell (beta)	Insulin
D cell (delta)	Somatostatin
F cell	Pancreatic Polypeptide

Insulin is a hormone that is produced by specialized cells (beta cells) of the pancreas (the pancreas is a deep-seated organ in the abdomen located behind the stomach). In addition to helping glucose enter the cells, insulin is also important in tightly regulating the level of glucose in the blood. After a meal, the blood glucose level rises. In response to the increased glucose level, the pancreas normally releases more insulin into the bloodstream to help glucose enter the cells and lower blood glucose levels after a meal. When the blood glucose levels are lowered, the insulin release from the pancreas is turned down. It is important to note that even in the fasting state there is a low steady release of insulin that fluctuates a bit and helps to maintain a steady blood sugar level during fasting. The main action of insulin is to promote storage of ingested nutrients as shown below in Table no. 5(d) 3. The Table also helps to understand the anti-catabolic effect during fasting and anabolic effect during post prandial period. In normal individuals, such a regulatory system helps to keep blood glucose levels in a tightly controlled range. As outlined above, in patients with diabetes, the insulin is either absent, relatively insufficient for the body's needs, or not used properly by the body. All of these factors cause elevated levels of blood glucose (hyperglycemia).

Table No. 5(d) 3: Anti-catabolic and Anabolic effects

	Anti-catabolic Effects – require low insulin (e.g. fasting)	**Anabolic Effects – require high insulin (e.g. post prandial)**
Muscle	inhibits gluconeogenesis and glycogen breakdown	stimulates glucose uptake (via GLUT-4 receptors) and glycogen synthesis stimulates amino acid uptake and protein synthesis
Liver	inhibits gluconeogenesis and glycogen breakdown promotes triglycerides synthesis	stimulates glycolysis and glycogen storage stimulates chylomicrons and VLDL uptake
Adipose	Inhibits intracellular breakdown of triglycerides	Increases glucose transport (via GLUT-4 receptors) Induces activity of Lipoprotein Lipase which hydrolyzes circulating triglycerides leading to uptake of FFA and glycerol

In normal persons the hormone insulin, which is made by the beta cells of the pancreas, regulates how much glucose is in the blood. When there is excess of glucose in blood, insulin stimulates cells to absorb enough glucose from the blood for the energy that they need.

Insulin also stimulates the liver to absorb and store any excess glucose that is in the blood. Insulin release is triggered after a meal when there is a rise in blood glucose.

High insulin will promote glucose uptake, glycolysis (breakdown of glucose), and glycogenesis (formation of storage form of glucose called glycogen), as well as uptake and synthesis of amino acids, proteins, and fat (Table 4D.1).

Low insulin will promote gluconeogenesis (breakdown of various substrates to release glucose), glycogenolysis (breakdown of glycogen to release glucose), lipolysis (breakdown of lipids to release glucose), and proteolysis (breakdown of proteins to release glucose). Insulin acts via insulin receptors (Table 4D.1)

Table No. 5(d) 4: Insulin level and synthesis in liver, adipose tissue and muscle

Type of insulin	Liver	Adipose or fat tissue	Muscle
High insulin	Glycolysis Glycogenesis	Triglyceride synthesis	Amino acid uptake Protein synthesis
Low insulin	Gluconeogenesis Glycogenolysis	Lipolysis	Proteolysis

Normal Responses to Eating and Fasting

After eating: There is increased insulin secretion, causing glycolysis, glycogen storage, fatty acid synthesis/storage, and protein synthesis.

After an overnight fast: There is low insulin and high glucagon that can cause glycogen breakdown, hepatic gluconeogenesis, and lipolysis.

After a prolonged fast: There is extremely low insulin and low glucagon, this causes lipolysis to take over. Lipids are the main fuel source. Gluconeogenesis is minimized, as it causes nitrogen wasting, ammonia build-up, and loss of muscle mass.

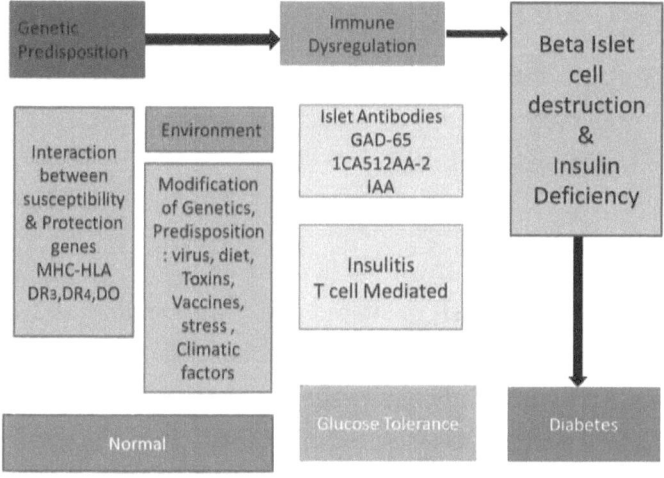

Fig. No. 5(d) 1: *Pathogenesis in Type 1Diabetes*

Pathophysiology of Type 1 Diabetes

In autoimmune diseases, such as type 1 diabetes, the immune system mistakenly manufactures antibodies and inflammatory cells that are directed against and cause damage to patients' own body tissues. In persons with type 1 diabetes, the beta cells of the pancreas, which are responsible for insulin production, are attacked by the misdirected immune system resulting in beta cell deficiency which in turn leads to complete insulin deficiency. Therefore it is termed also as autoimmune disease. It is believed that the tendency to develop abnormal antibodies in type 1 diabetes is, in part, genetically inherited, though the details are not fully understood. (Refer Fig. 5(d) 1). Causes as follows:

Genetic Factors

It accounts for about $1/3^{rd}$ of the susceptibility. In a genetic susceptibility person, there is a development of autoantigen receptors lead to destruction of beta cells.

Environmental Factors

Exposure to viral infection like mumps, etc. is mainly involved. The environmental factors changes structure features with beta cell and leads to destruction of beta cell.

Autoimmunity Factors

Type 1 IDDM is a slow T cell mediated autoimmune disease. Destruction of the insulin secretion cell in the pancreatic islets takes place over many years. The pathological changes in the prediabetic pancreas in Type 1 IDDM are characterized by insulinitis. It is the infiltration of islet with mononuclear cells containing activated macrophages, helper cytotoxic T-lymphocytes, natural killer cells, B-lymphocytes.

Exposure to virus or other environmental toxins may serve to trigger abnormal antibody responses that cause damage to the pancreas cells where insulin is made. Some of the antibodies seen in type 1 diabetes include anti-islet cell antibodies, anti-insulin antibodies and anti-glutamic decarboxylase antibodies seen in the blood. These cause lymphocytic infiltration and destruction of islets. The destruction may take time but the onset of the disease is rapid and may occur over a few days to a few weeks. These antibodies can be detected in the majority of individuals having diabetes, and may help determine which individuals are at risk for developing type 1 diabetes.

At present, the American Diabetes Association does not recommend general screening of the population for type 1 diabetes, though screening of high risk individuals, such as those with a first degree relative (sibling or parent) with type 1 diabetes should be encouraged. Type 1 diabetes tends to occur in young, lean individuals, usually before 30 years of age; however, older individuals do present with this form of diabetes on occasion. This subgroup is referred to as latent autoimmune diabetes in adults (LADA). LADA is a slow, progressive form of type 1 diabetes. Of all the people with diabetes, only approximately 10% have type 1 diabetes and the remaining 90% have type 2 diabetes.

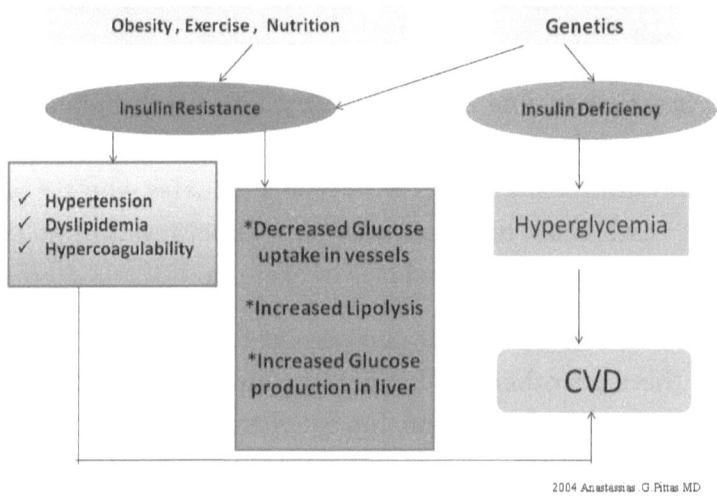

Fig. No. 5(d) 2: *Pathogenesis in type 2 Diabetes and the Metabolic Syndrome*

Pathophysiology of Type 2 Diabetes

Type 2 diabetes was also previously referred to as noninsulin-dependent diabetes mellitus (NIDDM), or adult onset diabetes mellitus (AODM). In type 2 diabetes, individuals can still produce insulin, but it is inadequate for their body's needs, particularly in the face of insulin resistance. In many cases this actually means the pancreas produces larger than normal quantities of insulin.(See Fig. No.5(d) 2) A major feature of type 2 diabetes is a lack of sensitivity to insulin by the cells (fat and muscle cells) of the body.

In addition to the problems with an increase in insulin resistance, the release of insulin by the pancreas may also be defective and suboptimal.

In fact, there is a known steady decline in beta cell production of insulin in type 2 diabetes that contributes to worsening glucose control, which is a major factor for these individuals who ultimately require insulin therapy. Finally, the liver in these individuals continues to produce glucose through a process called gluconeogenesis despite elevated glucose levels. The control of gluconeogenesis becomes compromised.

While it is said that type 2 diabetes occurs mostly in individuals over 30 years old and the incidence increases with age, there is an alarming increase in number of patients with type 2 diabetes who are barely in their teen years. Most of these cases are a direct result of poor eating habits, higher body weight, and lack of exercise.

While there is a strong genetic component to developing this form of diabetes, there are other risk factors, the most significant of which is obesity. There is a direct relationship between the degree of obesity and the risk of developing type 2 diabetes, and this holds true in children as well as adults. It is estimated that the chance to develop diabetes doubles for every 20% increase over desirable body weight.

Module on Preventive Strategies for Non-Communicable Diseases

Regarding age, data shows that for each decade after 40 years of age regardless of weight there is an increase in incidence of diabetes. The prevalence of diabetes among individuals 65 years of age and older is around 27%. Type 2 diabetes is also more common in certain ethnic groups. Compared with a 7% prevalence in non-Hispanic Caucasians, the prevalence in Asian Americans is estimated to be 8%, in Hispanics 12%, in Blacks around 13%, and in certain Native American communities 20–50%. Finally, diabetes occurs much more frequently in women with a prior history of diabetes that develops during pregnancy and is referred to as gestational diabetes.

Other Non-Communicable Conditions Associated with Diabetes

Gestational diabetes: Diabetes can occur in other conditions temporarily as in pregnancy due to hormonal changes resulting in elevated sugar levels. This resolves after child birth, though there remains a risk as 35–60% of the women with gestational diabetes may develop type 2 diabetes over 10–20 years if they required insulin or remain overweight. Therefore it is important that these women undergo glucose tolerance test end of 6 months to identify if the condition persisted beyond pregnancy.

Pancreatitis: It is inflammation of the pancreas due to toxins, trauma, alcohol or result of surgical removal of pancreas.

Hormonal disturbance: Excessive growth hormone production resulting due to pituitary tumor at base of brain, causing acromegaly leading to hypoglycemia or Cushing's syndrome where excess production of cortisol by adrenal gland can result in promoting blood glucose elevation. Hormones that raise blood sugar include glucagon, epinephrine and norepinephrine, cortisol, growth hormone, etc. These hormones are released due to stress. Thus during phases of stress, diabetes control worsens and blood sugar rises.

Infection and drugs: Drugs like prednisone and HIV infection are known to unmask latent diabetes.

Dietary habits: Nutrient excess and nutrient deficiency in the diets of children can lead to permanent modification of metabolic pathways and increased risk of diet-dependent diseases in adults. Children are at risk factors for excessive weight, obesity, insulin resistance and the metabolic syndromes as there is alarmingly low consumption of vegetables, raw fruits, dairy products and whole grain products due to consumption of fast foods. Diets characterized by excessive energy value (high-calorie foods rich in fats and sugar) and nutritional deficiency can lead to health problems. Table 5 D.2 provides a comparison at a glance between Type 1 and Type 2 diabetes.

Table No. 5(d) 5: Comparison between Type I and Type II diabetes

	Type 1 diabetes	Type 2 diabetes
Etiology	Autoimmune	Peripheral insulin resistance
Formerly known as	IDDM	NIDDM or 'adult onset' diabetes
Age of onset	Younger	Older
Obesity	Rare	Common
Family history	Rare	Common
HLA association/genetic association	Yes	No
Ketosis	Yes	No
Insulin resistance	No	Yes
Presence of body's own insulin	No	Yes
Respond to oral agents	No	Yes

Clinical Manifestations in Diabetes

The early symptoms of untreated diabetes are related to elevated blood sugar levels, and loss of glucose in the urine. High amounts of glucose in the urine can cause increased urine output and lead to dehydration. Dehydration is manifested by increased thirst and water consumption.

- The inability of insulin to perform normally has effects on protein, fat and carbohydrate metabolism. Insulin is an anabolic hormone, that is, one that encourages storage of fat and protein.

- A relative or absolute insulin deficiency eventually leads to weight loss despite an increase in appetite.

- Some untreated diabetes patients also complain of fatigue, nausea and vomiting.

- Individuals with diabetes are prone to developing infections of the bladder, skin, and vaginal areas.

- Fluctuations in blood glucose levels can lead to blurred vision. Extremely elevated glucose levels can lead to lethargy and coma. Refer table no 5. D.2 to understand the clinical difference between type I and type II diabetes

Pathophysiology behind Symptoms and Complications of Diabetes

- Polydipsia or increased thirst is due to high blood glucose that raises the osmolarity of blood and makes it more concentrated.

- Polyuria or increased frequency of urination is due to excess fluid intake and glucose induced urination.

- Weight loss occurs due to loss of calories in urine.

- Polyphagia or increased hunger due to loss or excess glucose in urine that leads the body to crave for more glucose.

- Poor wound healing, gum and other infections due to increased blood glucose providing a good source of nutrition to microbes and due to a diminished immunity.

- Heart disease occurs due to changes in the large blood vessels leading to coronary, cerebral, and peripheral artery diseases, atherosclerosis, dyslipidemia, etc.

- Eye damage is termed diabetic retinopathy and occurs due to damage of the fine blood vessels of the retina in the eye due to long-term exposure to high blood sugar.

- Kidney damage is similar damage to small and large blood vessels of the kidneys. Initially there is proteinuria or increased outflow of protein and may lead to end stage renal disease (ESRD).

- Nerve damage can affect the arms and legs and is called stocking-glove numbness/tingling. It can also affect autonomic functions leading to impotence, erectile dysfunction, difficulty in digestion or gastroparesis, etc.

- Diabetic foot occurs due to peripheral nerve damage as well as blood vessel affliction due to long-term diabetes. Little trauma, sores and blisters go unnoticed due to lack of sensation and peripheral vascular disease impairs healing and allows infection.

- Diabetic ketoacidosis is caused in type 1 diabetes where there is complete lack of insulin and reliance on fatty acids for energy. This uncontrolled lipid breakdown leads to formation of ketones and causes acidosis and ketonemia. This is a medical emergency.

- Non-ketotic hyperosmolarity is caused due to extreme rise of blood sugar. This is seen in type 2 diabetics. There is just enough insulin to suppress ketone synthesis. The high blood sugar leads to excessive concentration or osmolarity of blood which in turn leads to dieresis and collapse of the blood vessels and cardiovascular shock. This is a medical emergency.

- Individuals at risk should test their blood glucose levels for random, fasting, postprandial, hemoglobin A1C test and especially to rule out pregnancy-induced or infection-induced diabetes, and undertake an oral glucose tolerance test. (Refer table 5).

Table No. 5(d) 6: Diagnosing Diabetic Mellitus.

Glucose Intolerance	Diabetes
	Classic symptoms of diabetes PLUS casual plasma glucose/ Random blood glucose ≥ 200mg/dL or
100 < Morning < FPG 126 mg/dL (IFG)	Morning FPG ≥ 126 mg/dl or
140 < 2-hour PG < ß ß200 mg/dL (IGT)	2-hour Post prandial/PG ≥ 200 mg/dl
A diagnosis of diabetes must be confirmed by repeating any of the tests on another day. Unless unequivocal hyperglycemia with metabolic decompensation is present.	
IFG = impaired fasting glucose, IGT = impaired glucose tolerance. Casual is defined as any time of the day without regard to time since last meal. FPG = fasting plasma glucose, defined as no consumption of food or beverage (other than water) for at least 8 hours. 2-hour PG = 2 hour post load glucose during a 75-gram oral glucose tolerance test.	

Oral Glucose Tolerance Test

This test is most commonly performed during pregnancy. Blood is drawn once, and then a syrupy glucose solution is given to drink and then blood drawn at 30–60 minute intervals for up to 3 hours to see how an individual's body is handling the glut of sugar. Normal result: Depends on how many grams of glucose are in the solution, which can vary.

Fasting blood sugar: This is a common test because it is easy to perform. After fasting overnight, blood is drawn in the early morning hours and tested to see if blood sugar is in the normal range.

Normal result: 70–99 milligrams per deciliter (mg/dL) or less than 5.5 mmol/L.

Two-hour postprandial test: This blood test is done 2 hours after the individual has eaten ('prandial' means meal).

Normal result: 70–145 mg/dL (less than 7.9 mmol/L).

Random blood sugar: A blood sugar test is performed regardless of when the last meal is eaten.

Normal result: 70–125 mg/dL (less than 7.0 mmol/L).

Hemoglobin A1C test: Glycated hemoglobin (A1C) test. This blood test indicates an individual's average blood sugar level for the past 2 to 3 months. It measures the percentage of blood sugar attached to hemoglobin, the oxygen-carrying protein in red blood cells. Therefore, this test gauges how high your blood sugar has been in recent months. Normal result for nondiabetics: 4–6%. Normal result for diabetics: 7% or lower (some groups suggest aiming for 6.5% or lower).

If a hemoglobin A1C test result is 8% or higher, it is a sign that blood sugar is not under control.

Management and Compliance

Oral antidiabetic drugs (OADs) are the first line of drug treatment. The progressive nature of type 2 diabetes usually requires a combination of 2 or more oral agents in the long-term, often as a prelude to insulin therapy. Insulin treatment is the cornerstone of diabetes management. It is the only means of achieving good glycemic control in insulin deficient patients with type 1 diabetes. Insulin is also used as an intermittent or permanent therapy in some patients with type 2 diabetes.

Medications can be used for individuals diagnosed with prediabetes, but who do not have full-fledged diabetes. Taking metformin and acarbose helps when diet and exercise are not providing adequate benefit but they are no substitute for the real thing. In clinical trials, exercise and dietary management were superior to both acarbose and metformin.

Adherence to medication, especially insulin is a key contributor to diabetes treatment outcome. Poor adherence results in worse glucose control and increased hospital admissions of patients due to diabetes complications. Factors like medication costs, regimen complexity, patient's emotional well-being, and patient's perceptions of medication side effects and medication-related intrusions on activities of daily living are associated with adherence to any diabetes medication.

Late Complication of Diabetes or Secondary Complication

Retinopathy, nephropathy, neuropathy, and atherosclerosis.

Retinopathy: It is characterized by retinal damage such as bleeding in retina. Due to this retinal damage or retinal detachment occurs from normal position which ultimately leads to cataract or glaucoma.

Diabetic nephropathy: In this renal capillaries become leaky; due to this protein appears in the filtrate or urine which is known as proteinurea, which leads to nephron syndrome. It may cause other kidney disorders such as renal atherosclerosis which leads to renal failure. Nephropathy occurs due to advanced glycation end product (AGE) accumulation. Glycation mainly occurs of collagen and other proteins. Initially, it is reversible, but later on become irreversible, but this deposits on renal capillaries.

Neuropathy: Defect in peripheral nervous system mainly involving nerves, and these become nonfunctional. Symptoms include disturbance in urinary bladder functioning, disturbance in bowel functioning.

Atherosclerosis: It occurs also due to advanced glycation end product (AGE) accumulation in blood vessels.

Burden of Diabetes-Related Complications in India

Both macrovascular and microvascular complications cause significant morbidity and mortality among diabetic subjects. The Chennai Urban Population Study (CUPS) and CURES provided valuable data from India on the complications related to diabetes. The prevalence of coronary artery disease was 21.4% among diabetic subjects compared to 9.1% in subjects with normal glucose tolerance. The prevalence of CAD in IGT subjects were 14.9% in the same study. It was also seen that the diabetic subjects had increased subclinical atherosclerosis as measured by intimal medial thickness (IMT) at every age point compared to subjects with normal glucose tolerance. A recent study showed that carotid intimal medial thickness increased with worsening grades of glucose tolerance as well as with increase in the number of components of metabolic syndrome. The prevalence of peripheral vascular disease (PVD) was 6.3% among diabetic subjects compared to 2.7% in nondiabetic subjects, and these figures are lower than the prevalence reported in Western populations. This is probably due to lower age at onset for diagnosis of type 2 diabetes in India. It is well-known that PVD is more common in older individuals. The CURES Eye study is the largest population-based data on the prevalence of diabetic retinopathy done in India. This study showed that the overall prevalence was 17.6%, which was lower when compared to the reports from the West. A recent population-based study reported that the prevalence of overt nephropathy was 2.2% in Indians while microalbuminuria was present in 26.9%. Glycated hemoglobin, duration of diabetes and systolic blood pressure were independently associated with diabetic nephropathy. Overall, Asian Indians appear to have a greater predilection for cardiovascular complications whereas the prevalence of microvascular complications appears to be lower than in Europeans.

Research Evidence Placing Individuals at Risk for Diabetes

According to Ramachandran A and Snehalatha C, Vijay V, Urbanization and associated lifestyle changes adversely affect the risk factors for diabetes unmasking the high genetic tendency existing in the population. Various epidemiological studies in Indians have shown that the increasing prevalence of diabetes could be attributed to a high genetic risk and lower risk thresholds for acquired risk factors such as age, obesity, abdominal adiposity and a high percentage of body fat. Diabetes occurs at a younger age in Indians compared to Whites. The risk of diabetes increases with a BMI of >23 kg/m and waist circumference of 85 cm for men and 80 cm for women in Asian Indians. For a given BMI, Asian Indians have higher central adiposity. There is also evidence of higher insulin resistance among Indians, and this is partly explained by higher body fat percentage. A large proportion of urban adults have the metabolic syndrome also which predisposes them to both diabetes and cardiovascular diseases. Recognition of these conditions and institution of early preventive measures are urgently needed.

In a paper by Ramachandran A, Das AK, Joshi SR et al. there is a need for novel therapeutic agents. Glucagon-like peptide-1 (GLP-1) is an incretin hormone secreted from the L cells in the lower gut. GLP-1 secretion is strongly correlated to gastric emptying rate, and GLP-1 secretion throughout the day is highly correlated to insulin release.

Byetta (exenatide) is the first in the incretin mimetic class (GLP-1 receptor agonists) that offers effective treatment for patients with type 2 diabetes. The dose is initially 5 µg subcutaneously twice daily and may be titrated to 10 µg subcutaneously twice daily to achieve the desired goal. Clinical trials have shown benefits by adding exenatide to metformin and SUs. The weight loss seen with exenatide is also an advantage over most of the current treatments. However, it is difficult to determine if nausea plays a role in weight loss. The concern for exenatide's use in type 2 diabetics is the reduction in gastric emptying. Also of interest is the preservation of the beta cells of the pancreas and the conversion of noninsulin-secreting cells to insulin-secreting cells in vitro. Studies are ongoing that will hopefully elucidate the true effect that exenatide has on the beta cells.

The NICE has updated the guidelines for the management of type 2 diabetes, which also gives guidance on use of exenatide. Though exenatide is not recommended for routine use in type 2 diabetes, it should be considered as an option in subjects with obesity who have HbA1c ≥7% with conventional oral agents or if another high-cost medication or insulin is recommended. Liraglutide is a once-daily human GLP-1 analog. Studies in animals and humans have demonstrated promising blood glucose–lowering effects as well as a favorable safety profile. In India, Victoza (liraglutide [rDNA origin] injection) is approved for 'use in type 2 diabetes.' Once-daily liraglutide was effective and well-tolerated when used as monotherapy or in combination with OADs in patients with type 2 diabetes, and is therefore a promising new treatment option for the management of type 2 diabetes. A double-blind, randomized, parallel group, placebo-controlled trial with an open-label comparator arm was conducted among 193 outpatients with type 2 diabetes. A once-daily dose of liraglutide provided efficacious glycemic control and was not associated with weight gain. Adverse events with the drug were mild and transient, and the risk of hypoglycemia was negligible. Another randomized, double-blind, parallel group, placebo-controlled trial showed that 8 weeks of 0.6 mg liraglutide treatment significantly improved glycemic control without weight gain in subjects with type 2 diabetes compared with those on placebo. No influence on 24 hour energy expenditure was detected. Adverse events were mainly mild and related to the gastrointestinal system. No episodes of hypoglycemia were observed. Subjects with a history of pancreatitis should not be given these agents.

Prevention strategies: Include 'health promotion' where the focus is active and healthy lifestyle and eating habits and 'primary prevention' which focuses on reduction of risk factors and promoting health at individual and community level.

Preventive Strategy through Patient Teaching – Emphasize Regular Monitoring and Early Detection

- Emphasize the importance of regular check-ups, especially to obese patients, even if there are no overly-avert symptoms of hyperglycemia.

- Educate parents on the reality of DM2 in childhood along with the importance of providing adequate nutrition to their children and scheduling annual health check-ups to identify early signs.

- When patients are discovered to fall within the prediabetic phase or become diagnosed with DM2, describe cellular function using terms and language that is appropriate to their level of understanding. As even someone who is highly educated in a non-medical discipline may not be familiar with the terminology, nurses and other medical professionals should not take for granted that patient and caregivers have understood. Once the patient obtains a basic understanding of the relationship between cells and glucose, the nurse can transition into a discussion as to why DM2 demands serious attention.

- Patients who are prescribed oral hypoglycemias may incorrectly assume that they do not have a serious progression of disease.

It is important to teach these patients that this is not always the case, and that failure to comply with prescribed regimens can lead to complications just as easily as for those individuals who used injectable insulin. Explain the importance of taking oral hypoglycemic as prescribed. Also, if the patient is using a sulfa agent, warn of the risks to hypoglycemia.

- Teach patient the importance of timely administration of medication so as to lower the risk of hypoglycemia and hyperglycemia.

- Teach to rotate the injection site within the same area in order to prevent lystrophy of the tissue and in order to promote consistent absorption; the abdomen offers the best absorption spot for insulin injections.

- Encourage the patient to invest in a glucometer that will meet their needs. An insulin starting kit is a good choice for patients with a new diagnosis of DM2 as it will contain the glucometer, test strips, disinfecting wipes, and lancets all in one package. Teach the patient the terminology relevant to insulin administration.

- Explain to patient the frequency of testing blood would depend upon their condition, but several checks are usually required throughout the day. This rate will increase if the patient is sick or under extreme stress as glucose levels tend to rise during these times.

- Teach the patient to call the health care provider when ill or encountered with other situations that impede hyperglycemic management.

- Teach the patient that certain medications can increase the need for insulin and may also mandate more frequent monitoring of glucose levels. Corticosteroids, ACE inhibitors, and beta-adrenergic blockers are just a few of the medications that are known to increase glucose values.

- While counseling patients on drug administration, there are several factors the nurse must take into consideration. a) Assess the patient's ability to comply with the prescribed regimen. b) Accurate dosing is essential for diabetic control and requires manual dexterity, cognitive awareness, and adequate vision to read labels. Patients with impaired sensory function may experience additional challenges in filling syringes from vials and administering injections accurately. Cognitive impairment makes administration even more challenging as such patients may lack the ability to plan meals and calculate dosing. The nurse must assess the patient's ability to perform such functions before determining the best approach to patient teaching.

Best Strategies for Preventing Diabetes are Practical Ways to Lower Your Risk

To prevent diabetes, the best one can do is to follow a healthy diet and a healthy lifestyle. Exercise and following a healthy diet are 50–50 in terms of importance in preventing diabetes and doing both provides the best benefit. If an individual is at risk for type 2 diabetes, there is nothing that can beat these two.

Firstly Family History

First identify family history of diabetes and one's risk for type 2 diabetes and being overweight. Being overweight can keep your body from making and using insulin properly. How overweight you are matters—higher the weight, the higher the risk.

To prevent diabetes, it is important for an individual to know his blood sugar levels. Studies have shown that treatment with modest lifestyle changes can often return blood sugar levels to normal and lower your risk for developing diabetes by at least 58%. An individual is more at risk for type 2 diabetes if:

- The individual has high blood pressure measuring 140/90 or higher, and BMI >25kg/m^2, waist circumference >90 cm in males and >85 cm in females.

- Has abnormal cholesterol levels with HDL (good) cholesterol at 35 or lower, or triglyceride levels at 250 or higher.

- Having heritage from the following countries: African American, American Indian, Asian American, Pacific Islander or Hispanic American heritage.

An individual should check oneself for blood glucose by ages 40–45 years if you fall into these categories. Even if you are younger, if you are overweight and have a family history, you must consider getting tested as incidences are increasing due to inactivity and obesity.

Secondly Exercise

Exercise not only helps you lose weight, but keep blood glucose, blood pressure, cholesterol and triglycerides at optimal levels. Even just moderate exercise of 30 minutes per day, 5 days a week can help.

Exercises May Include

Simple activities: Walking, using the stairs instead of elevators, moving around throughout the day.

Aerobic exercise: Brisk walking, swimming, bike riding, Strength training, Flexibility exercises.

Thirdly a Healthy Diet

The great thing about a healthy diet is that it is effective for controlling blood sugar (diabetes) cholesterol and blood pressure too. The quantity of food an individual eats is of key importance. Portion or serving of food should be controlled, which is very important, even if you are eating all the right foods. Some guidelines for a healthy preventive diet include:-

- Eating foods that are low in animal/saturated fats.
- Eating foods that are high in fiber.
- Avoid simple sugars.

- Get protein sources low in saturated fat like fish, chicken (not fried).
- Get vegetable protein that are also high in fiber like beans, and other varieties of mushrooms.
- Get dairy protein that is fat free like egg substitutes, skim and soya milk.
- If one can afford, the use of canola and olive oil in cooking; both have unsaturated fats.
- Healthy diet and exercise also work to prevent diabetes even among those who do not need to lose weight. For some who are at risk, and are at normal weight or only slightly overweight, weight loss is not a target per se, but the benefits in preventing diabetes.
- Medications for diabetes prevention: Take the oral antidiabetic drugs as prescribed by the treating physician.

Evidence-Based Strategies to Prevent Diabetes

Although the genes you inherit may influence the development of type 2 diabetes, they take a back seat to behavioral and lifestyle factors. Data from the Nurses' Health Study suggest that 90% of type 2 diabetes in women can be attributed to 5 such factors: i. excess weight, ii. lack of exercise, iii. a less-than-healthy diet, iv. smoking, and v. abstaining from alcohol, according to Hu FB, Manson JE, Stampfer MJ, et al.

Women in the low-risk group were 90% less likely to have developed diabetes than the rest of the women. Low-risk meant a healthy weight (BMI less than 25), a healthy diet, 30 minutes or more of exercise daily, no smoking, and having about 3 alcoholic drinks per week.

Similar factors are at work in men. Van Dam RM, et al. indicated that data from the Health Professionals Follow-up Study indicate that a 'Western' diet, combined with lack of physical activity and excess weight, dramatically increases the risk of type 2 diabetes in men.

Information from several clinical trials strongly supports the idea that type 2 diabetes is preventable. Knowler WC, et al. stated that diabetes prevention program examined the effect of weight loss and increased exercise on the development of type 2 diabetes among men and women with high blood sugar readings that had not yet crossed the line to diabetes. In the group assigned to weight loss and exercise, there were 58% fewer cases of diabetes after almost 3 years than in the group assigned to usual care. Knowler WC et al. in a later study stated even after the program to promote lifestyle changes ended, the benefits persisted: The risk of diabetes was reduced, albeit to a lesser degree, over 10 years. Similar results were seen in a Finnish study of weight loss, exercise, and dietary change, and in a Chinese study of exercise and dietary change **(Tuomilehto J et al., Lindstrom J et al., Pan XR et al., LiG et al.)**

Other Preventive Strategies

Weight Control

According Hu FB, Manson JE et al. being overweight increases the chances of developing type 2 diabetes 7 fold. Being obese makes you 20–40 times more likely to develop diabetes than someone with a healthy weight.

Get Moving—and Turn Off the Television

Findings from the Nurses' Health Study and Health Professionals Follow-up Study, conducted by Tanasescu M et al., Hu FB, Sigal RJ et al. suggest that walking briskly for a half hour every day reduces the risk of developing type 2 diabetes by 30%. More recently, Krishnan S et al. in the Black Women's Health Study, reported similar diabetes prevention benefits for brisk walking of more than 5 hours per week. This amount of exercise has a variety of other benefits as well. The more television people watch, the more likely they are to be overweight or obese, and this seems to explain part of the

TV viewing-diabetes link. The unhealthy diet patterns associated with TV watching may also explain some of this relationship.

Change Your Diet Pattern

Four dietary changes can have a big impact on the risk of type 2 diabetes other than alcohol and smoking:

- Choose whole grains and whole grain products over highly processed carbohydrates:

There is convincing evidence from a study conducted by Baliunas DO which stated that diets rich in whole grains protect against diabetes, whereas diets rich in refined carbohydrates lead to increased risk. In the Nurses' Health Studies I and II, for example, researchers looked at the whole grain consumption of more than 160,000 women whose health and dietary habits were followed for up to 18 years. De Munter JS et al. stated that women who averaged 2–3 servings of whole grains a day were 30% less likely to have developed type 2 diabetes than those who rarely ate whole grains. When the researchers combined these results with those of several other large studies, they found that eating an extra 2 servings of whole grains a day decreased the risk of type 2 diabetes by 21%.

De Munter JS et al. in their study stated whole grains do not contain a magical nutrient that fights diabetes and improves health. In China, for example where white rice is a staple, the Shanghai Women's Health Study found that women whose diets had the highest glycemic index had a 21% higher risk of developing type 2 diabetes, compared to women whose diets had the lowest glycemic index. **Krishnan S et al**. in 2007 reported similar findings in the Black Women's Health Study.

Skip the sugary drinks, and choose water, coffee, or tea instead: **Schulze MB et al**. in the Nurses' Health Study II, stated that women who drank one or more sugar-sweetened beverages per day had an

83% higher risk of type 2 diabetes, compared to women who drank less than one sugar-sweetened beverage per month. Combining the Nurses' Health Study results with those from 7 other studies found a similar link. What to drink in place of the sugary stuff? Water is an excellent choice. Coffee and tea are also good calorie-free substitutes. There is convincing evidence that coffee may help protect against diabetes; **(Huxley R et al. Van Dam RM et al. 2006)** emerging research suggests that tea may hold diabetes prevention benefits as well, but more research is needed.

Choose good fats instead of bad fats: The types of fats in your diet can also affect the development of diabetes. Good fats, such as the polyunsaturated fats found in liquid vegetable oils, nuts, and seeds can help ward off type 2 diabetes. **(Riserus U et al. 2009)** Trans-fats do just the opposite according to a study conducted by **Hu FB et al. and Mozaffarian D et al.;** trans-fats are found in packaged baked goods and fried foods in most fast food restaurants. Whereas according to **Kaushik M et al.** eating polyunsaturated fats from fish—also known as 'long chain omega 3' or 'marine omega 3' fats—does not protect against diabetes, even though there is much evidence that these marine omega 3 fats help prevent heart disease.

Limit red meat and avoid processed meat; choose nuts, whole grains, poultry, or fish instead: In a study conducted by **Pan A, Sun Q et al.** in 2011, the evidence was growing stronger that eating red meat (beef, pork, lamb) and processed red meat (bacon, hot dogs, deli meats) increases the risk of diabetes, even among people who consume only small amounts. The researchers looked at data from roughly 440,000 people, about 28,000 of whom developed diabetes during the course of the study. It increased the risk of type 2 diabetes by 20%.

The good news from this study: Swapping out red meat or processed red meat for a healthier protein source, such as nuts, low fat dairy, poultry, or fish, or for whole grains lowered diabetes risk by up to 35%.

If you smoke, try to quit: Willi C et al. in their study stated that smokers have roughly 50% more chance to develop diabetes than nonsmokers, and heavy smokers have an even higher risk.

Alcohol now and then may help: Hu FB et al., Joosten MM et al. concluded in their study that moderate amounts of alcohol, up to a drink a day for women, up to 2 drinks a day for men, increases the efficiency of insulin at getting glucose inside cells. And some studies indicate that moderate alcohol consumption decreases the risk of type 2 diabetes. **Baliunas DO et al.** stated in their study if you already drink alcohol, the key is to keep your consumption in the moderate range, as higher amounts of alcohol could increase diabetes risk. If you do not drink alcohol, there is no need to start—you can get the same benefits by losing weight, exercising more, and changing your eating patterns.

It can be concluded that the key to preventing can be boiled down to 5 words: Stay lean and stay active.

Preventive Strategies by the Government: There is a need for screening of people for diabetes or prediabetes which can help stop or slow the progression to diabetes. For those diagnosed with diabetes there is a need for cost-effective, accessible and comprehensive care. The alarming scenario led the government of India to start the national diabetes control program on pilot basis during the 7th Five Year Plan in 1987 in certain districts of Tamil Nadu, Jammu and Kashmir and Karnataka, but it could not be expanded further due to paucity of funds. Later in 1995–96 and 97–98 sums of 12 lakh and one core were allocated respectively.

Although India accounts for about 15% of the world's diabetes burden, India spends only 6.4% of worldwide spending on health care related to diabetes. There is a need for additional resource allocation for diabetes care, towards stronger prevention efforts, diagnostic infrastructure especially in rural areas, accessibility and affordability of treatment, and skilled health care workers, as recommended by the WHO Global Strategy. In January 2008 the Ministry of Health and Family welfare, Government of India launched the National Programme on Prevention and Control of Diabetes, Cardiovascular Disease, and Stroke (NPDCS), with an objective to prevent and control NCD, create awareness generation on lifestyle changes, early detection of NCDs and capacity building of health systems to tackle NCDs.

Preventive Strategies Adopted by Government Need to be Strengthen

As the major political barrier is the governments focus on economic growth and its role in transforming India into a developed nation, it has led to neglect of health related issues. It would strengthen health policies if in all policies made by government health becomes the focus. As communicable disease burden has reduced it should not get replaced by the burden of non-communicable disease.

Strengthening of government initiatives: Organization, institutions and NGO's at their level can organize awareness programs through public educational media, i.e., use of the National Channel Doordarshan and Radio to educate public about diabetes risk factors, preventive measures and complications in simple and clear messages in all major languages. At Bus stops and Railway stations the public address system can be used too.

Awareness can be created through rallies, folk arts, exhibitions at public places, campaigns, distribution of pamphlets, manuals, advertisements in magazines, newspaper, etc. None of these should be one time programs but should be ongoing.

Strengthening of preventive strategies should be focused at grass root level. Information on diabetes prevention in simple and understandable way should be communicated to school children and awareness created at PTA meetings regarding importance of early detection, risk factors and the importance of active healthy lifestyle and eating healthy foods.

Health care personnel can strengthen preventive strategies by displaying charts and posters in their clinics to create awareness on prevention of diabetes, healthy lifestyle and healthy food. They should encourage high risk group visiting their clinics to undergo assessment for diabetes.

Nursing Care: To be Planned Based on Individual Patient Need and Priority

1. Restore fluid/electrolyte and acid-base balance
2. Correct/reverse metabolic abnormalities
3. Identify/assist with management of underlying cause/disease process
4. Prevent complications
5. Provide information about disease process/prognosis, self-care, and treatment needs.

Discharge Goals

1. Homeostasis achieved
2. Causative/precipitating factors corrected/controlled
3. Complications prevented/minimized
4. Disease process/prognosis, self-care needs, and therapeutic regimen understood
5. Plan in place to meet needs after discharge.

Nurse Needs to Monitor and Interpret Diagnostic Test for Prevention of Complication

- **Serum glucose:** Increased 200–1000 mg/dL or more.
- **Serum acetone** (ketones) if strongly positive.

- **Fatty acids** that are lipids, triglycerides, and cholesterol level if elevated.

- **Serum osmolality** if level is altered elevated but usually less than 330 mOsm/L.

- **Glucagon:** Elevated level is associated.

- **Glycosylated hemoglobin (HbA1C):** A result greater than 8% represents average blood glucose of 200 mg/dL and signals a need for changes in treatment.

- **Serum insulin:** May be decreased/absent (type 1) or normal to high (type 2), indicating insulin insufficiency/improper utilization (endogenous/exogenous). Insulin resistance may develop secondary to formation of antibodies.

- **Electrolytes:** Sodium: May be normal, elevated, or decreased. Potassium: Normal or falsely elevated (cellular shifts), then markedly decreased. Phosphorus: Frequently decreased.

- **Arterial blood gases (ABGs):** Usually reflects low pH and decreased HCO3 (metabolic acidosis) with compensatory respiratory alkalosis.

- **CBC:** Hct may be elevated (dehydration); leukocytosis would suggest hemoconcentration, response to stress or infection.

- **BUN:** May be normal or elevated indicating dehydration/decreased renal perfusion).

- **Serum amylase:** May be elevated, indicating acute pancreatitis as cause of DKA.

- **Thyroid function tests:** Increased thyroid activity can increase blood glucose and insulin needs.

- **Urine:** Positive for glucose and ketones; specific gravity and osmolality may be elevated.

- **Cultures and sensitivities:** Possible UTI, respiratory or wound infections.

1. **Nursing Diagnosis: Risk for Infection**

Risk Factors May Include

- High glucose levels, decreased leukocyte function, alterations in circulation • Pre-existing respiratory infection, or UTI.

Desired Outcomes

Identify interventions to prevent/reduce risk of infection

Lifestyle changes to prevent development of infection/improve overall health.

Nursing interventions	Rationale
Observe for the signs of infection and inflammation: fever, flushed appearance, wound drainage, purulent sputum, and cloudy urine.	May have poor immunity and may also develop nosocomial infection. Patients with DM may be admitted with infection, which could have precipitated the ketoacidotic state.
Teach and promote good hand hygiene.	Reduces risk of cross-contamination.
Maintain asepsis during IV insertion, administration of medications, and providing wound or site care. Rotate IV sites as indicated.	Increased glucose in the blood creates an excellent medium for bacteria to thrive.
Provide catheter or perineal care. Teach female patients to clean from front to back after elimination.	Minimizes risk of UTI. Comatose patient may be at particular risk if urinary retention occurred before hospitalization. Note: Elderly female diabetic patients are especially prone to urinary tract and/or vaginal yeast infections.

Nursing interventions	Rationale
Provide meticulous skin care: gently massage bony areas, keep skin dry. Keep linens dry and wrinkle-free.	Peripheral circulation may be ineffective or impaired, placing the patient at increased risk for skin breakdown and infection.
Auscultate breath sounds.	Rhonchi may indicate accumulation of secretions possibly related to pneumonia or bronchitis. Crackles may result from pulmonary congestion or edema from rapid fluid replacement or heart failure.
Place in semi-Fowler's position.	Facilitates lung expansion; reduces risk of aspiration.
Reposition and encourage coughing or deep breathing if patient is alert and cooperative. Otherwise, suction airway using sterile technique as needed.	Aids in ventilating all lung areas and mobilizing secretions. Prevents stasis of secretions with increased risk of infection.
Provide tissues and trash bag in a convenient location for sputum and other secretions. Instruct patient in proper handling of secretions.	To minimize spread of infection.
Encourage and assist with oral hygiene.	Reduces risk of oral/gum disease.
Encourage adequate dietary and fluid intake (approximately 3000 mL/day if not contraindicated by cardiac or renal dysfunction), including 8 oz of cranberry juice per day as appropriate.	Decreases susceptibility to infection. Increased urinary flow prevents stasis and aids in maintaining urine pH/acidity, reducing bacteria growth and flushing organisms out of system. Note: Use of cranberry juice can help prevent bacteria from adhering to the bladder wall, reducing the risk of recurrent UTI.
Administer antibiotics as appropriate.	Early treatment may help prevent sepsis.

2. **Nursing diagnosis:** Risk for disturbed sensory perception.

Risk Factor

- Endogenous chemical alteration: glucose/insulin and/or electrolyte imbalance.

Desired Outcomes

- Maintain usual level of mentation
- Recognize and compensate for existing sensory impairments.

Nursing interventions	Rationale
Monitor vital signs and mental status.	To provide baseline from which to compare abnormal findings.
Call the patient by name, reorient as needed to place, person, and time. Give short explanations, speak slowly and enunciate clearly.	Decreases confusion and helps maintain contact with reality.
Schedule and cluster nursing time and interventions.	To provide uninterrupted rest periods and promote restful sleep, minimize fatigue and improve cognition.
Keep patient's routine as consistent as possible. Encourage participation in activities of daily living (ADLs) as able.	Helps keep patient in touch with reality and maintain orientation to the environment.
Protect patient from injury by avoiding or limiting the use of restraints as necessary when LOC is impaired. Place bed in low position and pad bed rails if patient is prone to seizures.	Disoriented patients are prone to injury, especially at night, and precautions need to be taken as indicated. Seizure precautions need to be taken as appropriate to prevent physical injury, aspiration, and falls.
Evaluate visual acuity as indicated.	Retinal edema or detachment, hemorrhage, presence of cataracts or temporary paralysis of extra ocular muscles may impair vision, requiring corrective therapy and/or supportive care.

Nursing interventions	Rationale
Observe and investigate reports of hyperesthesia, pain, or sensory loss in the feet or legs. Investigate and look for ulcers, reddened areas, pressure points, loss of pedal pulses.	Peripheral neuropathies may result in severe discomfort, lack of or distortion of tactile sensation, potentiating risk of dermal injury and impaired balance.
Provide bed cradle. Keep hands and feet warm, avoiding exposure to cool drafts and/or hot water or use of heating pad.	Reduces discomfort and potential for dermal injury.
Assist patient with ambulation or position changes.	Promotes patient safety, especially when sense of balance is affected.

3. **Nursing Diagnosis: Powerlessness.**

May Be Related To

- Long-term/progressive illness that is not curable
- Dependence on others.

Possibly Evidenced By

- Reluctance to express true feelings; expressions of having no control/influence over situation
- Apathy, withdrawal, anger
- Does not monitor progress, nonparticipation in care/decision making
- Depression over physical deterioration/complications despite patient cooperation with regimen.

Desired Outcomes

- Acknowledge feelings of helplessness
- Identify healthy ways to deal with feelings.

Nursing interventions	Rationale
Monitor laboratory values: blood glucose, serum osmolality, Hb/Hct, BUN/Cr.	Imbalances can impair mentation. Note: If fluid is replaced too quickly, excess water may enter brain cells and cause alteration in the level of consciousness (water intoxication).
Carry out prescribed regimen for correcting DKA as indicated.	Alteration in thought processes or potential for seizure activity is usually alleviated once hyperosmolar state is corrected.

Assist in planning own care and independently take responsibility for self-care activities.

Nursing interventions	Rationale
Encourage patient and/or significant others (SO) to express feelings about hospitalization and disease in general.	Identifies concerns and facilitates problem solving.
Acknowledge normality of feelings.	Recognition that reactions are normal can help patient problem-solve and seek help as needed. Diabetic control is a full-time job that serves as a constant reminder of both presence of disease and threat to patient's health.
Assess how patient has handled problems in the past. Identify locus of control.	Knowledge of individual's style helps determine needs for treatment goals. Patient whose locus of control is internal usually looks at ways to gain control over own treatment program. Patient who operates with an external locus of control wants to be cared for by others and may project blame for circumstances onto external factors.
Provide opportunity for SO to express concerns and discuss ways in which he or she can be helpful to patient.	Enhances sense of being involved and gives SO a chance to problem-solve solutions to help patient prevent recurrence.

Nursing interventions	Rationale
Ascertain expectations and/or goals of patient and SO.	Unrealistic expectations or pressure from others or self may result in feelings of frustration and loss of control. These can impair coping abilities.
Determine whether a change in relationship with SO has occurred.	Constant energy and thought required for diabetic control often shifts the focus of a relationship. Development of psychological concerns affecting self-concept may add further stress.
Encourage patient to make decisions related to care: ambulation, schedule for activities, and so forth.	Communicates to patient that some control can be exercised over care.
Support participation in self-care and give positive feedback for efforts.	Promotes feeling of control over situation.

4. **Nursing Diagnosis:** Imbalanced nutrition less than body requirements.

May Be Related To

- Insulin deficiency (decreased uptake and utilization of glucose by the tissues, resulting in increased protein/fat metabolism)
- Decreased oral intake: anorexia, nausea, gastric fullness, abdominal pain; altered consciousness
- Hypermetabolic state: release of stress hormones (e.g. epinephrine, cortisol, and growth hormone), infectious process.

Possibly Evidenced by

- Increased urinary output, dilute urine
- Reported inadequate food intake, lack of interest in food

- Recent weight loss; weakness, fatigue, poor muscle tone
- Diarrhea
- Increased ketones (end product of fat metabolism).

Desired Outcomes

- Ingest appropriate amounts of calories/nutrients
- Display usual energy level
- Demonstrate stabilized weight or gain towards usual/desired range with normal laboratory values.

Nursing interventions	Rationale
Weigh daily or as ordered.	Weighing serves as an assessment tool to determine the adequacy of nutritional intake.
Ascertain patient's dietary program and usual pattern then compare with recent intake.	Identifies deficits and deviations from therapeutic needs.
Auscultate bowel sounds. Note reports of abdominal pain, bloating, nausea, vomiting of undigested food. Maintain NPO status as indicated.	Hyperglycemia and fluid and electrolyte disturbances can decrease gastric motility and/or function (due to distention or ileus) affecting choice of interventions. Note: Chronic difficulties with decreased gastric emptying time and poor intestinal motility may suggest autonomic neuropathies affecting the GI tract and requiring symptomatic treatment.
Provide liquids containing nutrients and electrolytes as soon as patient can tolerate oral fluids then progress to a more solid food as tolerated.	Oral route is preferred when patient is alert and bowel function is restored.

Nursing interventions	Rationale
Identify food preferences, including ethnic and cultural needs.	If patient's food preferences can be incorporated into the meal plan, cooperation with dietary requirements may be facilitated after discharge.
Include SO in meal planning as indicated.	To promote sense of involvement and provide information to the SO to understand the nutritional needs of the patient. Various methods available or dietary planning include exchange list, point system, glycemic index, or preselected menus.
Observe for signs of hypoglycemia: changes in level of consciousness (LOC), cold and clammy skin, rapid pulse, hunger, irritability, anxiety, headache, lightheadedness, shakiness.	Hypoglycemia can occur once blood glucose level is reduced and carbohydrate metabolism resumes and insulin is being given. If the patient is comatose, hypoglycemia may occur without notable change in LOC. This potentially life-threatening emergency should be assessed and treated quickly per protocol.
Monitor by performing finger stick glucose testing.	Beside analysis of serum glucose is more accurate than monitoring urine sugar. Urine glucose is not sensitive enough to detect fluctuations in serum levels and can be affected by patient's individual renal threshold or the presence of urinary retention. (Normal levels for finger stick glucose testing may vary depending on how much the patient ate during their last meal. In general: 80–120 mg/dL (4.4–6.6 mmol/L) before meals or when waking up; 100–140 mg/dL (5.5–7.7 mmol/L) at bedtime.

Nursing interventions	Rationale
Administer regular insulin by intermittent or continuous IV method: IV bolus followed by a continuous drip via pump of approximately 5–10 U/hr so that glucose is reduced by 50 mg/dL/hr.	Regular insulin has a rapid onset and thus quickly helps move glucose into cells. The IV route is the initial route of choice because absorption from subcutaneous tissues may be erratic. Many believe the continuous method is the optimal way to facilitate transition to carbohydrate metabolism and reduce incidence of hypoglycemia.
Administer glucose solutions: dextrose and half-normal saline.	Glucose solutions may be added after insulin and fluids have brought the blood glucose to approximately 400 mg/dL. As carbohydrate metabolism approaches normal, care must be taken to avoid hypoglycemia.
Provide diet of approximately 60% carbohydrates, 20% proteins, 20% fats in designated number of meals and snacks.	Complex carbohydrates (apples, broccoli, dried beans, carrots, peas, and oats) decrease glucose levels/insulin needs, reduce serum cholesterol levels, and promote satiation. Food intake is scheduled according to specific insulin characteristics and individual patient response. A snack at bedtime of complex carbohydrates is especially important to prevent hypoglycemia during sleep and potential Somogyi response.
Administer other medications as indicated: metoclopramide (reglan); tetracycline.	May be useful in treating symptoms related to autonomic neuropathies affecting GI tract, thus enhancing oral intake and absorption of nutrients.

5. **Nursing Diagnosis:** Deficient fluid volume.

May Be Related To

- Osmotic diuresis (from hyperglycemia)
- Excessive gastric losses: Diarrhea, vomiting
- Restricted intake: Nausea, confusion.

Possibly Evidenced by

- Increased urinary output, dilute urine
- Weakness; thirst; sudden weight loss
- Dry skin/mucous membranes, poor skin turgor
- Hypotension, tachycardia, delayed capillary refill.

Desired Outcomes

- Demonstrate adequate hydration as evidenced by stable vital signs, palpable peripheral pulses, good skin turgor and capillary refill, individually appropriate urinary output, and electrolyte levels within normal range.

Nursing interventions	Rationale
Assess patient's history related to duration or intensity of symptoms such as vomiting, excessive urination.	Assists in estimation of total volume depletion. Symptoms may have been present for varying amounts of time (hours to days). Presence of infectious process results in fever and hypermetabolic state, increasing insensible fluid losses.
Monitor vital signs	
Orthostatic BP changes.	Hypovolemia may be manifested by hypotension and tachycardia. Estimates of severity of hypovolemia may be made when patient's systolic BP drops more than 10 mmHg from a recumbent to a sitting then a standing position.
Respiratory pattern: Kussmaul's respirations, acetone breath.	Lungs remove carbonic acid through respirations, producing a compensatory respiratory alkalosis for ketoacidosis. Acetone breath is due to breakdown of acetoacetic acid and should diminish as ketosis is corrected. Correction of hyperglycemia and acidosis will cause the respiratory rate and pattern to approach normal.
Respiratory rate and quality, use of accessory muscles, periods of apnea, and appearance of cyanosis.	In contrast, increased work of breathing, shallow, rapid respirations, and presence of cyanosis may indicate respiratory fatigue and/or that patient is losing ability to compensate for acidosis.
Temperature, skin color, moisture, and turgor.	Although fever, chills, and diaphoresis are common with infectious process, fever with flushed, dry skin and decreased skin turgor may reflect dehydration.
Assess peripheral pulses, capillary refill, and mucous membranes.	Indicators of level of hydration, adequacy of circulating volume.

Nursing interventions	Rationale
Monitor intake and output. Monitor urine specific gravity.	Provides ongoing estimate of volume replacement needs, kidney function, and effectiveness of therapy.
Weigh daily.	Provides the best assessment of current fluid status and adequacy of fluid replacement.
Maintain fluid intake of at least 2500 mL/day within cardiac tolerance when oral intake is resumed.	Maintains hydration and circulating volume.
Promote comfortable environment. Cover patient with light sheets.	Avoids overheating, which could promote further fluid loss.
Investigate changes in mental state and LOC.	Changes in mental state can be due to abnormally high or low glucose, electrolyte abnormalities, acidosis, decreased cerebral perfusion, or developing hypoxia. Regardless of the cause, impaired consciousness can predispose patient to aspiration.
Insert and maintain indwelling urinary catheter.	Provides for accurate ongoing measurement of urinary output, especially if autonomic neuropathies result in neurogenic bladder. May be removed when patient is stable to reduce risk of infection.

6. **Nursing diagnosis:** Fatigue.

May Be Related To

- Decreased metabolic energy production
- Altered body chemistry: Insufficient insulin
- Increased energy demands: Hypermetabolic state/infection

Possibly Evidenced by

- Overwhelming lack of energy, inability to maintain usual routines, decreased performance, accident-prone
- Impaired ability to concentrate, listlessness, not interested in surroundings

Desired Outcomes

- Verbalize increase in energy level
- Display improved ability to participate in desired activities

Nursing interventions	Rationale
Discuss with patient the need for activity. Plan schedule with patient and identify activities that lead to fatigue.	Education may provide motivation to increase activity level even though patient may feel too weak initially.
Alternate activity with periods of rest and uninterrupted sleep.	To prevent excessive fatigue.
Monitor pulse, respiratory rate, and BP before and after activity.	Indicates physiological levels of tolerance.
Discuss ways of conserving energy while bathing, transferring, and so on.	Patient will be able to accomplish more with a decreased expenditure of energy.
Increase patient participation in ADLs as tolerated.	Increases confidence level, self-esteem and tolerance level.

Other Possible Nursing Care

Knowledge deficit: Regarding disease process/treatment and individual care needs—may be related to unfamiliarity with information, misinterpretation, possibly evidenced by requests for information, statements of concern, inadequate follow-through of instructions, and development of preventable complications.

Risk for risk-prone behavior: Risk factors may include all-encompassing changes in lifestyle, self-concept requiring lifelong adherence to therapeutic regimen, and internal/altered locus of control.

Risk for unstable blood glucose: Risk factors include lack of adherence to diabetes management, medication management, inadequate blood glucose monitoring, physical activity level, failure of lifestyle modification, stress, and rapid growth periods.

Key Points

Diabetes is becoming the most common non-communicable disease adding to the economic burden, with increased shift from traditional measures, industrialization and focus on economic growth. Individuals in the rural area have adapted to motorized ways of farming putting them at risk for diabetes, while in the urban area affordability has brought changes in lifestyle and stress. Along with genetic factors and environment factors, these changes have placed Indians at high risk for diabetes. Though government machinery are in place the general public needs to adapt to healthy lifestyle, and create awareness and adopt preventive strategies for diabetes so as to bring the alarming number down.

Bibliography

1. A Ramachandran, AK Das, SR Joshi, CS Yajnik, S Shah, KM PrasannaKumar, Current Status of Diabetes in India and Need for Novel Therapeutic Agents, JAPI, June 2010, 58: 7-9.

2. Abate N, Chandalia M. Ethnicity and type 2 diabetes: focus on Asian Indians. Journal of Diabetes Complications 2001; 15: 320-7. 40. Joshi R. Metabolic syndrome – Emerging clusters of the Indian phenotype. Journal of Association of Physicians India 2003; 51: 445-6.

3. Alder AI, Shaw EJ, Stokes T, Ruiz F: Newer agents for blood glucose control in type 2 diabetes: Summary of NICE guidance. British Medical Journal, 2009; 338.

4. AlEssa H, Bupathiraju S, Malik V, Wedick N, Campos H, Rosner B, Willett W, Hu FB. Carbohydrate quality measured using multiple quality metrics is negatively associated with type 2 diabetes. Circulation, 2015; 1–31: A: 20.

5. Amit Vaibhav, OP Singh, Anil KR Tripathi: Present scenario of Diabetes Mellitus and its Treatment Possibilities, Asian Journal of Modern and Ayurvedic Medical Science, ISSN 2279–0772

6. Anjana RM et al. Prevalence of diabetes and prediabetes (impaired fasting glucose and/or impaired glucose tolerance) in urban and rural India: phase I results of the Indian Council of Medical Research-INDIA diabetes (ICMR-INDIAB) study. Diabetologia. 2011 Dec; 54(12): 3022–7. doi: 10.1007/s00125-011-2291-5. Epub 2011 Sep 30.

7. Baliunas DO, Taylor BJ, Irving H, et al. Alcohol as a risk factor for type 2 diabetes: A systematic review and meta-analysis. Diabetes Care. 2009; 32: 2123–32.

8. De Munter JS, Hu FB, Spiegelman D, Franz M, Van Dam RM. Whole grain, bran, and germ intake and risk of type 2 diabetes: a prospective cohort study and systematic review. PLoS Medicine, 2007; 4: e261.

9. De Munter JS, Liu S, Gao Y-T, et al. Prospective Study of Dietary Carbohydrates, Glycemic Index, Glycemic Load, and Incidence of Type 2 Diabetes Mellitus in Middle-aged Chinese Women. Archive of Internal Medicine, 2007; 167: 2310–2316.

10. Deepa R, Sandeep S, Mohan V. Abdominal obesity, visceral fat and type 2 diabetes – "Asian Indian phenotype". In: Mohan V, Rao GHR, editors. Type 2 diabetes in South Asians: Epidemiology, risk factors and prevention. New Delhi: Jaypee Brothers Medical Publishers (P) Ltd; 2006 p. 138–52.

11. Djousse L, Biggs ML, Mukamal KJ, Siscovick DS. Alcohol consumption and type 2 diabetes among older adults: the Cardiovascular Health Study. Obesity (Sliver Spring), 2007; 15: 1758–65.

12. Harder H, Nielsen L, Tu DT, Astrup A. The effect of liraglutide, a long-acting glucagon-like peptide 1 derivative, on glycemic control, body composition, and 24-h energy expenditure in patients with type 2 diabetes, Diabetes Care 2004; 27: 1915–21.

13. Holst JJ. On the physiology of GIP and GLP-1, Hormone Metabolic Research, 2004; 36: 747–54.

14. Hu FB, Manson JE, Stampfer MJ, et al. Diet, lifestyle, and the risk of type 2 diabetes mellitus in women, North England Journal of Medicine, 2001; 345: 790–7.

15. Hu FB, Sigal RJ, Rich-Edwards JW, et al. Walking compared with vigorous physical activity and risk of type 2 diabetes in women: a prospective study, JAMA, 1999; 282: 1433–9

16. Huffman MD et al. Incidence of cardiovascular risk factors in an Indian urban cohort, results from the New Delhi birth cohort. Journal of American College of Cardiology. 2011 April 26; 57(17): 1765–74. doi: 10.1016/j.jacc.2010.09.083.

17. *Huxley R, Lee CM, Barzi F, et al. Coffee, decaffeinated coffee, and tea consumption in relation to incident type 2 diabetes mellitus: a systematic review with meta-analysis.* Archive of Internal.

18. *Joosten MM, Grobbee DE, van der AD, Verschuren WM, Hendriks HF, Beulens JW. Combined effect of alcohol consumption and lifestyle behaviors on risk of type 2 diabetes. American Journal of Clinical Nutrition, 2010. Apr 21 Epub ahead of print.*

19. *Kaushik M, Mozaffarian D, Spiegelman D, Manson JE, Willett WC, Hu FB. Long-chain omega-3 fatty acids, fish intake, and the risk of type 2 diabetes mellitus. American Journal of Clinical Nutrition, 2009; 90: 613–20.*

20. Knowler WC, Barrett-Connor E, Fowler SE, et al. Reduction in the incidence of type 2 diabetes with lifestyle intervention or metformin, North England Journal of Medicine, 2002; 346: 393–403.

21. Knowler WC, Fowler SE, Hamman RF, et al. 10-year follow-up of diabetes incidence and weight loss in the Diabetes Prevention Program Outcomes Study, Lancet, 2009; 374: 1677–86.

22. Kostecka M, Eating habits of preschool children and the risk of obesity, insulin resistance and metabolic syndrome in adults. Pakistan Journal of Medical Science, 2014 Nov-Dec.; 30(6): 1299–303.doi: 10.12669/pjms.306.5792.

23. *Krishnan S, Rosenberg L, Palmer JR. Physical activity and television watching in relation to risk of type 2 diabetes: the Black Women's Health Study, American Journal of Epidemiology, 2009; 169: 428–34.*

24. *Krishnan S, Rosenberg L, Singer M, et al. Glycemic Index, Glycemic Load, and Cereal Fiber Intake and Risk of Type 2 Diabetes in US Black Women. Archive of Internal Medicine, 2007; 167: 2304–2309.*

25. Kumar A, Goel MK, Jain RB, Khanna P, Chaudhary V. India towards diabetes control: Key issues. Australasia Medical Journal. 2013; 6(10): 524–31.

26. Li G, Zhang P, Wang J, et al. The long-term effect of lifestyle interventions to prevent diabetes in the China Da Qing Diabetes Prevention Study: a 20-year follow-up study, Lancet 2008; 371: 1783–9.

27. Lindstrom J, Ilanne-Parikka P, Peltonen M, et al. Sustained reduction in the incidence of type 2 diabetes by lifestyle intervention: follow-up of the Finnish Diabetes Prevention Study, Lancet, 2006; 368: 1673–9.

28. Madsbad S, Schmitz O, Ranstam J, Jakobsen G, Matthews DR., Improved glycemic control with no weight increase in patients with type 2 diabetes after once-daily treatment with the long-acting glucagon-like peptide 1 analog liraglutide

(NN2211): A 12-week, double-blind, randomized, controlled trial, Diabetes Care, 2004;27: 1335–42.

29. McKeigue PM, Shah B, Marmot MG. Relation of central obesity and insulin resistance with high diabetes prevalence and cardiovascular risk in South Asians. Lancet 1991; 337: 382–6.

30. Medicine, *2009; 169: 2053–63.*

31. Melton LJ, Macken KM, Palumbo PJ, Elveback LR. Incidence and prevalence of clinical.

32. Misra A, Khurana L. The Metabolic syndrome in South Asians: epidemiology, determinants and prevention, Metabolic syndrome and related disorders, 2009 Dec. 7(6): 497–514.

33. Misra A, Vikram NK. Insulin resistance syndrome (metabolic syndrome) and obesity in Asian Indians: evidence and implications. Nutrition, Los Angeles County, California, 2004 May; 20(5): 482–91.

34. Mohan V, Gokulakrishnan K, Sandeep S, Srivastava BK, Ravikumar R, Deepa R. Intimal media thickness, glucose intolerance and metabolic syndrome in Asian Indians – the Chennai Urban Rural Epidemiology Study (CURES – 22). Diabetes Medicine 2006; 23: 845–50.

35. Mohan V, Pradeepa R. Epidemiology of diabetes in different regions of India, Health Administrator 2009; 22: 1–18.

36. Mohan V, Shanthirani CS, Deepa M, Deepa R, Unnikrishnan RI, Datta M. Mortality rates due to diabetes in a selected urban South Indian population – the Chennai Urban Population Study (CUPS). Journal of Association of Physicians India 2006; 54: 113–7. 37.

37. Mohan V, Sharp PS, Cloke HR, Burrin JM, Schumer B, Kohner EM. Serum immunoreactive insulin responses to a glucose load in Asian Indian and European Type 2 (noninsulin-dependent) diabetic patients and control subjects, Diabetologia 1986; 29: 235–7.

38. *Mozaffarian D, Katan MB, Ascherio A, Stampfer MJ, Willett WC. Trans fatty acids and cardiovascular disease, North England Journal of Medicine, 2006; 354: 1601–13.*

39. *Pan A, Sun Q, Bernstein AM, et al. Red meat consumption and risk of type 2 diabetes: 3 cohorts of US adults and an updated meta-analysis American Journal of Clinical Nutrition., 2011 Aug 10. [Epub ahead of print]*

40. Pan XR, Li GW, Hu YH, et al. Effects of diet and exercise in preventing NIDDM in people with impaired glucose tolerance. The Da Qing IGT and Diabetes Study, Diabetes Care, 1997; 20: 537–44.

41. Peripheral vascular disease in a population-based cohort of diabetic patients. Diabetes Care 1980; 3: 650–4. 34.

42. Premalatha G, Shanthirani S, Deepa R, Markovitz J, Mohan V. Prevalence and risk factors of peripheral vascular disease in a selected South Indian population: the Chennai Urban Population Study. Diabetes Care 2000; 23: 1295–300. 228 Indian Journal of Medical Research, March 2007 33.

43. Ramachandran A, Snehalatha C, & Vijay V, Low-risk threshold for acquiring diabetogenic factors in Asian Indians, Diabetes Research and Clinical Practice;2004 Sept.65(3): 189–95.

44. Ramachandran A, Snehalatha C, Current Scenario of diabetes in India, Journal of Diabetes, 2009 March1(1): 18–28, doi: 10.1111/j.1753-0407.2008.00004.xEpub 2008 dec17.

45. Ramachandran A, Snehalatha C, Viswanathan V, Viswanatha M, Haffner SM. Risk of non-insulin-dependent diabetes mellitus conferred by obesity and central adiposity in different ethnic groups: a comparative analysis between Asian Indians, Mexican Americans and Whites. Diabetes Research and Clinical Practices 1997; 36: 121–5.

46. Ranjit UI, Rema M, Pradeepa R, Deepa M, Shanthirani CS, Deepa R, et al. Prevalence and risk factors of diabetic nephropathy in an urban Indian population – The Chennai Urban Rural Epidemiology Study (CURES) (in press).

47. Rema M, Premkumar S, Anitha B, Deepa R, Pradeepa R, Mohan V. Prevalence of diabetic retinopathy in urban India: the Chennai Urban Rural Epidemiology Study (CURES) eye study, I. Investigative Ophthalmology Visual Science 2005; 46: 2328-33. 35.

48. *Riserus U, Willett WC, Hu FB. Dietary fats and prevention of type 2 diabetes, Prog Lipid Research, 2009; 48: 44–51.*

49. SA Kaveeshwar, Jon Cornwall, 'The current state of diabetes mellitus in India,' Australia Medical Journal.2014: 7(1): 45–48. (online 2014 Jan31.doi: 10.4066/AMJ.2013.1979)

50. *Schulze MB, Manson JE, Ludwig DS, et al. Sugar-sweetened beverages, weight gain, and incidence of type 2 diabetes in young and middle-aged women. JAMA, 2004; 292: 927–34.*

51. Tanasescu M, Leitzmann MF, Rimm EB, Hu FB. Physical activity in relation to cardiovascular disease and total mortality among men with type 2 diabetes. Circulation 2003.

52. Tuomilehto J, Lindstrom J, Eriksson JG, et al. Prevention of type 2 diabetes mellitus by changes in lifestyle among subjects with impaired glucose tolerance, North England Journal of Medicine, 2001; 344: 1343–50.

53. V Mohan, S Sandeep, R Deepa, B Shah & C Varghese. Epidemiology of Type 2 diabetes: Indian scenario, Office of the World Health Organization Representative to India, New Delhi, India, January 10, 2007

54. Van Dam RM, Rimm EB, Willett WC, Stampfer MJ, Hu FB. Dietary patterns and risk for type 2 diabetes mellitus in U.S. men, Annual Internal Medicine, 2002; 136: 201–9.

55. *Van Dam RM, Willett WC, Manson JE, Hu FB. Coffee, caffeine, and risk of type 2 diabetes: a prospective cohort study in younger and middle-aged U.S. women. Diabetes Care. 2006; 29: 398–403.*

56. Whiting Dr., Guariguata L, Weil C, Shawj. IDF Diabetes atlas: Global estimates of the prevalence of diabetes for 2011 and 2030. Diabetes Research Clinical Practice. 2011; 94: 311–21.

57. WHO Expert Consultation. Appropriate BMI for Asian populations and its implications for policy and intervention strategies. Lancet. 2004 Jan 10; 363(9403): 157–63.

58. Wild S, Roglic G, Green A, Sicree R, King H. Global prevalence of diabetes-estimates for the year 2000 and projections for 2030. Diabetes Care. 2004; 27(3): 1047–53.

59. Willi C, Bodenmann P, Ghali WA, Faris PD, Cornuz J. Active Smoking and the Risk of Type 2 Diabetes: A Systematic Review and Meta-analysis. JAMA, 2007; 298: 2654–2664.

60. Yajnik CS, Fall CH, Vaidya U, et al. Fetal growth and glucose and insulin metabolism I 4 year old Indian children, Diabetes medicine 1995;12: 330–336.

61. Yajnik CS. Early life origins of insulin resistance and type 2 diabetes in India and other Asian countries. International Nutrition 2004; 134: 205–210.

62. Zimmet P, The burden of type 2 diabetes: Are we doing enough? Diabetes Metabolism, 2003; 29: 6S9–6S18.

Chapter V (E)

Preventive Strategies for Osteoporosis

Dr. Nancy Fernandes

Introduction

India is a vast tropical country that receives ample sunlight throughout the year and hence it is hard to believe that vitamin D deficiency is common across all ages and sexes in India as one reviews existing literature. There is widespread prevalence of varying degrees (50–90%) of vitamin D deficiency with low dietary calcium intake in Indian population according to various studies published earlier according to **Harinarayan CV, Joshi SR (2009)**. Apart from low dietary intake, people suffering from hepatic, renal, dermatological disorders, alcoholics and inflammatory rheumatological conditions also have vitamin D deficiency.

Osteoporosis is one among the 5 non-communicable diseases of aging; its treatment cost is more expensive than treating diabetes, hyperlipidemia, hypertension or heart disease. Osteoporosis is a common disorder of bone metabolism in which the mass of bone is decreased. Mineral and protein matrix components are reduced, resulting in structural deterioration of bone tissue. Without prevention or treatment, osteoporosis can progress without pain or a symptom until a bone breaks, that is fracture occurs. Fractures from osteoporosis commonly occur in the hip, spine, ribs, and wrist.

Meaning of Osteoporosis

Osteoporosis means porous bone. Osteoporosis is a bone disease in which the bone loss occurs, as a result the bones become weak and are more likely to break.

Magnitude of Osteoporosis

Reduction in bone density occurs in approximately in one-fourth of all elderly persons, most frequently in women between the ages of 50–70 years 50% of premenopausal women and 30%–60% of men with osteoporosis develop secondary osteoporosis resulting in further bone loss. In India, it is estimated that 60 million adults have osteoporosis with nearly 2.3 million added annually. 25% of women over 60 years of age develop vertebral fracture due to osteoporosis; approximately 30% of hip fractures and 20% of vertebral fractures in men are attributed to osteoporosis. According to WHO in Figure 5E.1, out of 8 Indian males suffer from osteoporosis, 1 out of 3 Indian females suffer from osteoporosis making India one of the largest affected countries in the world. Expert groups pegged in 2003, the number of osteoporosis patients at approximately 26 million with the numbers projected to increase to 36 million in 2013. A significantly large proportion of south Indian men had osteoporosis and vitamin D deficiency was concluded in study conducted by **Sahana Shetty, et al.**

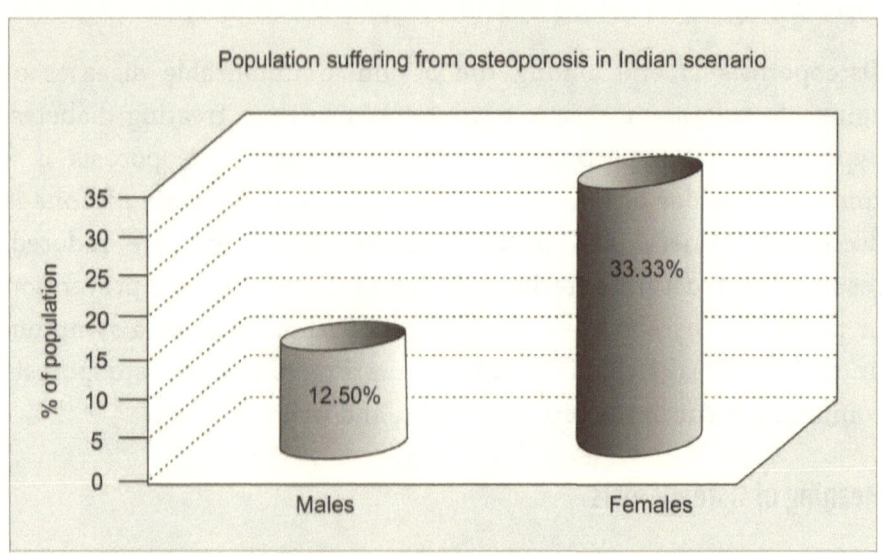

Fig. No. 5(e) 1: *Indian scenario of osteoporosis as given by WHO*

Magnitude of Osteoporosis in the Indian Scenario

In a study conducted by **Neelam Aggarwal et al. in 2011,** the prevalence of low bone mineral density (BMD) was found in more than half of this population (53%). The mean age in group I (normal BMD) was found to be 50.56 ± 5.74 years as compared to 52.50 ± 5.94 in group II with low BMD (P=0.02). The 2 groups were similar with respect to parity, education, socio-economic status, family history of osteoporosis, hormone replacement therapy, and thyroid disorders. 46.8% of the women in group I and 33% of the women in group II had low physical activity and there was no statistically significant difference in sunlight exposure between the groups. Parity or the number of children and type of menopause was not seen to have much association with low BMD in our study. Lack of exercise and low calcium diet were significantly associated with low BMD. Multiple logistic regression analysis showed that age, exercise, menopause, and low calcium diet acted as significant predictors of low bone density. Whereas Ranu Patni concludes in her study that the BMD of Indian females was 1.5–2 standard deviations (SDs) lower than that of the reference Western population in all the comparative age groups, **Mitra et al**. in her study concludes that genetic variations at estrogen receptor alpha (ER alpha) gene locus, perhaps, are associated with BMD in Indian women and may influence some determinant of bone metabolism resulting in accelerated bone loss with age.

Rama Vidya states that a large community-based, 4 center study (Hyderabad, Lucknow, Mumbai, and New Delhi), reported by the Indian Council of Medical Research (ICMR), has determined the peak bone mineral density (PBMD) values at the hip, lumbar spine, and forearm in healthy Indian men and women aged 20–29 years. (n = 404 men, n = 404 women). The mean BMD values in women were 0.901 ± 0.111, 0.538 ± 0.044, and 0.954 ± 0.095 at the hip, forearm, and spine. The ICMR study has proposed the cut-off values for diagnosing osteoporosis in women as 0.624, 0.428, and 0.717 g/cm^2.

Risk Factors Contributing to Osteoporosis

In spite of the adequate sunlight in India vitamin D a fat-soluble is dependent on number of factors like latitude, atmospheric pollution, clothing, skin pigmentation and duration of time of exposure to sunlight. Bones may seem like hard and lifeless structures, but they are in fact living tissue. Old bone is constantly broken down and remodeled that is through a process called bony resorption by our bodies, while new bone is simultaneously deposited. When bone is broken down faster than it is deposited, low bone mass that is a condition called osteopenia and osteoporosis can occur.

Osteoporosis can occur at any age. However, it is more common in people older than 50 years of age, and the older a person is, the greater the risk is of osteoporosis. This is because during childhood and teenage years, new bone is generally added faster than old bone is removed. This is the time when a diet rich in calcium, phosphate, and vitamin D is important. As a result, bones become larger, heavier, and denser.

Maximum bone density and strength is reached by 20–25 years of age. The density and strength of the bones is fairly stable between 25–45 years of age. A slight loss of bone density begins to occur after age of 30 years because bone slowly begins to break down through a process called resorption, this process is faster than new bone formation. For women, bone loss is fastest in the first few years after menopause, but it continues gradually into the postmenopausal years. As bone density loss occurs, osteoporosis can develop. This process is slower by 10 years in men.

Cause of Vitamin D Deficiency in India can be attributed to several factors:

- Changing food fads and food habits contribute to low dietary calcium and vitamin D intake.

- High fiber diet containing phosphates and phytates which can deplete vitamin D stores and increase calcium requirement (Khadilkar AV, 2010).

- Genetic factors like having increased 25(OH) D-24 – hydroxylase which degrades 25(OH) D to inactive metabolites (Awumey EM et al. 1998).

- It has been shown that increment in serum 25(OH) D in response to treatment depends on the heritability of vitamin D binding protein (Fu L, Yun F et al. 2009).

- With modernization, the number of hours spent indoor has increased thereby preventing adequate sun exposure. This is particularly true in the urban Indians.

- Increased pollution can hamper the ultraviolet rays to adequately synthesize vitamin D in the skin (Babu US et al. 2010).

- Cultural and traditional habits prevalent in certain religions like 'Burka' and the 'pardah' system in Muslims are well-known.

- Repeated and unplanned, unspaced pregnancies in dietary deficient patients can aggravate vitamin D deficiency in the mother and the fetus.

- At Risk Population

- Certain risk factors are associated with developing osteoporosis. Many individuals with osteoporosis have several risk factors, but some individuals with osteoporosis have none.

- Individuals who may be at risk of not getting enough vitamin D include:

- People who are housebound or particularly frail.

- People with a poor diet.

- People who keep covered up in sunlight because they wear total sun block or adhere to a certain dress code (wear burka).
- Women who are pregnant or breastfeeding.

Some risk factors cannot be changed. These include the following:

Sex: Women are more likely to develop osteoporosis than men, due to deficit estrogen level especially in postmenopausal women. However, men are also at risk and constitute 20% of the patient population with osteoporosis.

Age: The older a person is, the greater the risk of osteoporosis.

Physical build: People who are small and have thin bones are at greater risk than those who weigh less than 127 pounds.

Race: White and Asian women are at the highest risk.

Family and personal history: If a person's parents had/have osteoporosis, he or she may be at risk, history of fracture on the maternal side of the family, and a personal history of any kind of bone fracture as an adult (after age of 50 years). Some risk factors can be modified. These include the following:

Levels of sex hormones: Low estrogen in women, particularly after menopause, and hypogonadism (small gonads) in male, low or testosterone deficiency in men are associated with osteoporosis. Those with catabolic hormone excess, e.g. Cushing disease.

Diet: Diets low in calcium, phosphate, and vitamin D are risk factors.

Use of medications: Certain types of medications can damage bone and lead to what is termed as 'secondary osteoporosis' Glucocorticoids/corticosteroids, which are medications prescribed for a wide range of diseases, including arthritis, asthma, Crohn's disease, lupus, and other diseases, can cause osteoporosis.

Medication Associated with Osteoporosis

- Anticoagulants (heparin)
- Anticonvulsants (some)
- Cyclosporine A and tacrolimus
- Cancer chemotherapy drugs
- Glucocorticoids (and adrenocorticotropic hormone [ACTH])
- Gonadotropin-releasing hormone agonists
- Lithium
- Methotrexate
- Proton pump inhibitors
- Selective serotonin reuptake inhibitors (SSRIs)
- Thyroxine.
- Others include

Individuals having anorexia nervosa, prolonged immobilization, inactive lifestyle, especially weight-bearing exercise, cigarette smoking, and excessive intake of alcohol.

Clinical Features

In many people, low bone mass, i.e. osteopenia and osteoporosis occur without any symptoms. In people with osteoporosis, a simple everyday movement, such as picking up a grocery bag, can cause a sudden onset of back pain and that can be the first symptom. As the involved bone tissue loses its density and tensile strength increasing risk of fracture, even slight trauma may fracture the brittle osteoporotic bone. See fig 5E.2 to 4 depicting normal bone structure and change due to osteoporosis. As osteoporosis progresses over a period of time, the bony building blocks of the spine (vertebrae) can begin to collapse. Collapsed vertebrae may be felt as severe back pain or cause a loss of height or spinal deformities. When the spinal vertebrae collapse in the upper back, it can lead to a hump of curvature (Dowager's hump). The most common bones broken in osteoporosis are the hip, spine, wrist, and ribs, although any bone in the body can be affected by osteoporosis and can break. In others walking may become difficult and painful as their knee joint may wear off.

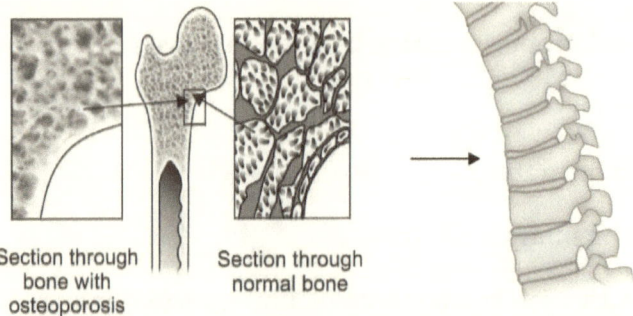

Fig. No. 5(e) 2: *Image on the left shows decreased bone.* **Fig. No. 5(e) 3:** *Arrow indicates vertebral fractures density in osteoporosis. The image on the right shows normal bone density*

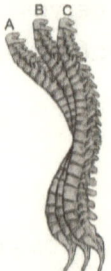

Fig. No. 5(e) 4: *A to C: A. Normal spine, B. Moderately osteoporotic spine, C. Severely osteoporotic spine*

Diagnosis in Osteoporosis

Unfortunately, many people do not know they have osteoporosis until they develop a fracture or experience pain. By that time, bones are already weak. However, osteoporosis can be prevented or delayed by early detection and treatment. Early diagnosis becomes the second most important step for individuals at risk of developing osteoporosis and associated spine fractures.

A bone density test is also termed as bone mineral test or BMD test is the gold standard diagnostic procedure to detect osteoporosis. Bone density test measures the solidness of bone in various sites of the body, such as the hip, spine, and wrist. These tests are quick taking less than 15 minutes, painless, and non-invasive and are extremely helpful in screening for and making a diagnosis of osteoporosis. A bone density test can detect osteoporosis before a fracture occurs and can predict the chances of having a fracture in the future.

According to National Osteoporosis Foundation and the US 'Preventive task force' a bone density is recommended in the following situations: women above 65 years, postmenopausal women under age of 65 years with multiple risk factors, cases undecided about hormone replacement therapy, long-term on oral steroids and individuals with hyperparathyroidism.

DEXA Scan or DXA Scan

A dual energy X-ray absorptiometry scan of BMD can determine the rate of bone loss or track bone density change over time and/or be used to monitor the effects of treatment. It will indicate whether the person has normal bone density, low bone mass or osteoporosis. The test is performed by passing low energy X-rays through a bone most of the lower spine and hips.

Blood Test

In individuals with osteoporosis, serum calcium levels, phosphate and vitamin D levels will be low.

A combination of results of the dexa bone density test, history and physical examination and other necessary examination and diagnostic test will provide the facts to accurately diagnose:

The presence of osteopenia, i.e., loss of bone density, a precursor to osteoporosis.

Indicated if osteoporosis is a primary or secondary problem, this is essential as line of treatment will differ.

To focus the treatment on out beating the condition by providing personalized treatment to slow bone loss or rebuild bone density to help avoid an osteoporosis-related fracture.

Disease Burden

Burden of non-communicable diseases are increasing in all the developing countries and India is experiencing an epidemiological transition, reflecting the burden of non-communicable disease due to lifestyle change. Osteoporosis-related fractures are inflicting a major economic loss on health care systems. Worldwide, osteoporosis-fractures contributes 0.83% to the global burden of non-communicable disease and 1.75% global burden in Europe, hip fractures account for 0.82 million DALY's in women, account for 41% of global burden of osteoporosis (Johnell, 2006). Osteoporosis-fractures are amounting to 1% of the DALY's among non-communicable diseases in the world (WHO scientific group, 2004). Worldwide health expenditure on osteoporosis is rising more than the general inflation rate in all countries according to Cummings, whereas according to NHA there is no data available on health costs of osteoporosis, but India is spending 0.4% of total health budget on the non-communicable disease. According to the report of International Osteoporosis Foundation (IOF) the estimated annual direct cost of treating osteoporosis fracture of people in the workplace in USA, Canada and Europe alone is approximately USD 48 billion while they forecast the world wide cost burden of osteoporosis to increase by 2050 to USD131.5 billion. Studies have indicated that once an individual suffers first vertebral fracture, there is a five-fold increase in the risk of developing a new fracture within a month, and this too adds to the burden of osteoporosis.

Strategies to Prevent Osteoporosis

The FAO/WHO Expert Consultation states that in most locations of the world between 42° N and 42°S latitude there is abundant sunshine. This is responsible for physiological production of vitamin D endogenously in the skin from 7-dehydrocholesterol present in the subcutaneous fat. 30 minutes of exposure of the skin over the arms and face to sunlight, without application of sunscreen, preferably between 10 am to 2 pm (as maximum ultraviolet B rays are transmitted during this time) daily is adequate to avoid vitamin D deficiency.

Your genes are responsible for determining your height and the strength of your skeleton, but lifestyle factors such as diet and exercise influence how healthy your bones are. Hence preventive strategies play a major role in reducing the incidences of osteoporosis. Once you are identified as at risk for osteoporosis, the biggest challenge for the individual is behavioral changes such as stopping smoking altogether, radically changing a diet to include adequate calcium and vitamin D intake, and starting a regular exercise program. While the changes in a patient's behavior are often difficult to undertake, they are definitely worth it when one considers the negative consequences of sustaining an osteoporosis-related fracture.

Steps to Strengthen Osteoporosis Prevention Strategies

The first step in preventing osteoporosis and associated spine fractures is to determine whether an individual is at risk or high risk for developing this bone condition.

Different physical characteristics and lifestyle choices can contribute to osteoporosis in both men and women.

Osteoporosis can be prevented by reaching the peak bone mass (maximum bone density and strength) during the childhood and teenage years and by continuing to build more bone as one gets older, particularly after the age of 30 years.

Maintaining adequate level of calcium and vitamin D by adequate consumption of milk or eating milk products, doing physical activity and exercise, avoiding smoking and excessive alcohol intake. They may be administered calcitonin which inhibits bone resorption.

Monitoring administered medication such as glucocorticoids prescribed for a wide range of diseases, including arthritis, asthma, Crohn's disease, lupus, and other diseases of the lungs, kidneys, and liver which can lead to a loss of bone density. If an individual needs to take glucocorticoids then prophylactic steps to prevent osteoporosis should be taken.

Antiepileptics such as asphenytoin—Dilantin and barbiturates, gonadotropin-releasing hormone (GnRH) analogs used in treatment of endometriosis, excessive consumption of antacids containing aluminum, thyroid hormone therapy, and even cancer medications are known to cause loss of bone mass. Then calcium and vitamin D supplementation should be advised to prevent loss of bone mass and prevent osteoporosis.

Postmenopausal women may be treated with cyclic estrogen.

Calcium Intake

The recommended amounts of calcium for adults are as follows:

- For premenopausal women 25–50 year-old and postmenopausal women on estrogen replacement therapy: 1,000–1,200 mL of calcium per day. 1,500 mL of calcium per day is recommended for pregnant or lactating women.
- For postmenopausal women less than age of 65 years not on estrogen replacement therapy: 1,500 mL of calcium per day.
- For men ages 25–65 years: 1,000 mL of calcium per day.
- For all people (women and men) over age of 65 years: 1,500 mL of calcium per day.

Vitamin D Intake

The recommended amounts of vitamin D for adults are as follows:

- For people over 50 years and postmenopausal women: 400–800 IU of vitamin D per day. For people over 65 or 70 years, at least 600 IU is usually recommended.

- For people 25–50-year-old and premenopausal women: 400 IU of vitamin D per day.

Regular Weight-Bearing Exercise

The importance of exercise in the fight against osteoporosis cannot be underestimated. Changing to a healthier diet can have little effect on bone mass when not combined with regular exercise. Starting the right kind of exercise in combination with other preventive measures like appropriate calcium intake, can help build bone mass especially in high risk fracture sites like the wrist, hip and spine. Manske S et al., states that best exercise outcome is dependent on strain magnitude (how much impact the exercise has on the bones and muscles), strain rate (how often maximum vs. minimum strain is applied), and strain frequency (how often strain occurs in a given amount of time).

Putting Stress on the Bones Fights Fractures

The key here is weight-bearing exercise—which means exercise one performs while on their feet that works the bones and muscles against gravity. Popular forms of weight-bearing exercise include:

- Walking
- Jogging
- Stair climbing
- Dancing

- Hiking
- Volleyball
- Tennis
- Certain types of weight lifting/resistance exercises (e.g. squats).

The particular form of exercise will depend on the person's overall physical health, the extent of bone loss, and whether the person already regularly engages in physical activity. It is recommended that individuals speak with their physician about the appropriate types of exercise to include in their osteoporosis treatment plan, especially people who have been sedentary most of their adult life or who are already diagnosed with low bone mass (termed osteopenia) or osteoporosis.

Certain movements, like those that require twisting of the spine or bending forward from the waist (like sit-ups or toe touches), and most high-impact exercise, can put certain people at risk for fracture and should be avoided.

Recommendations on frequency of exercise needed to increase bone density vary. Depending on one's diagnosis and doctor-recommend activity restrictions, typical exercise routines that are recommended may range from:

- 20–30 minutes of aerobic exercise 3–4 times weekly to 30 minutes of moderate physical activity every day plus strength training 2–3 times per week.

Many patients benefit from working with an exercise specialist trained in exercise; physiology, physical education, physical therapy, or a similar specialty to learn the proper progression of exercise, how to stretch and strengthen muscles safely, and how to correct poor posture habits. This is particularly true for those with relatively advanced osteoporosis (who are most at risk for a fracture) and those who are starting a new exercise program. The exercise specialist should be familiar with the special needs of people with osteoporosis.

Habits: Smoking, Alcohol Abuse

These are 2 lifestyle habits, considered diseases in certain cases, which are important to eliminate especially for those suffering from osteoporosis.

Smoking

In any amounts has a detrimental effect on bone density. Alcohol intake of greater than 3 ounces per day (or about 2–3 typical drinks) has been shown to increase bone loss. If one considers that studies have shown that people who smoke are more likely to drink than nonsmokers and that people who drink are more likely to smoke than nondrinkers, it is no surprise that stopping either activity (or both) can be particularly difficult. Patients with either of these problems are advised to address these factors as part of their osteoporosis and fracture prevention plan and seek appropriate medical treatment as necessary.

Smoking and Osteoporosis

Smoking impacts a person at risk for developing osteoporosis in several ways. In studies, smoking has been shown to:

- Reduce blood supply to the bones
- Slow the production of bone-forming cells
- Impair the absorption of calcium
- Reduce the protective effect of estrogen replacement therapy

Because those who smoke have weakened bones, they are more likely to experience exercise-related injuries, such as fractures or sprains. When individuals do sustain a fracture, it would takes longer to heal.

If surgical intervention is needed, recovery period would prolong and increase the risk of complications.

While it is very difficult for many individuals to quit smoking, for a person at risk for osteoporosis, quitting smoking is definitely worth the effort as it will greatly reduce the risk of sustaining a fracture.

Excessive Alcohol and Osteoporosis

The effect of moderate alcohol use on bone health is unclear, and some studies suggest moderate alcohol intake (usually defined as up to one drink per day for women and up to 2 drinks per day for men) is beneficial. However, the damaging effects of heavy alcohol use are fairly consistently supported.

Although alcohol's damaging effects on bone are most striking in people who drink heavily during adolescence and young adulthood, research has shown that elderly women (between the ages of 67 and 90 years) who consumed an average of more than 3 ounces of alcohol per day (the equivalent of 6 typical alcoholic drinks) had greater bone loss than women who had minimal alcohol intake (Hannan et al., 2000).

Nutrition

An individual should take a healthy diet with enough calcium and vitamin D which helps make bones strong (Table 5E.1). Many people get less than half the calcium they need. Good sources of calcium are: Low fat milk, yogurt, cheese, leafy green vegetables, dried fruits, and tofu, and foods fortified with calcium such as orange juice, cereals, and breads.

Vitamin D can be found in eggs, milk and oily fish. However, most vitamin D is made in the skin in response to sunlight. Short exposure to sunlight without wearing sunscreen (10 minutes twice a day) throughout the summer should provide an individual with enough vitamin D for the whole year.

Table 5(e) 1: Recommended calcium and vitamin D intakes

Life-stage group	Calcium mg/day	Vitamin D (IU/day)
Infants 0–6 months	200	400
Infants 6–12 months	260	400
1–3-year-old	700	600
4–8-year-old	1,000	600
9–13-year-old	1,300	600
14–18-year-old	1,300	600
19–30-year-old	1,000	600
31–50-year-old	1,000	600
51–70-year-old males	1,000	600
51–70-year-old females	1,200	600
>70-year-old	1,200	800
14–18-year-old, pregnant/lactating	1,300	600
19–50-year-old, pregnant/lactating	1,000	600

Definitions: mg = milligrams; IU = International Units

Source: Food and Nutrition Board, Institute of Medicine, National Academy of Sciences, 2010.

Preventive Strategies for Individuals at Risk for Fall

Men and women with osteoporosis need to take care not to fall down. Some reasons why falls occur are: Poor vision, poor balance, diseases that affect gait, medicine, such as sleeping pills.

Some Tips to Help Prevent Outdoor Falls are:

- Use a cane or walker.
- Wear rubber-soled shoes to prevent slipping.
- Walk on grass when sidewalks are slippery.

Some Ways to Help Prevent Indoor Falls are:

- Keep rooms free of clutter, especially on floors.
- Use plastic or carpet runners on slippery floors.
- Wear low-heeled shoes that provide good support.
- Do not walk in socks, stockings, or slippers.
- Be sure carpets and area rugs have skid-proof backs or are fixed to the floor.
- Be sure stairs are well lit and have rails on both sides.
- Put grab bars on bathroom walls near tub, shower, and toilet.
- Use a rubber bath mat.
- Keep a flashlight next to your bed.
- Use a sturdy step stool with a handrail and wide steps.
- Add more lights in rooms ensure floor is well lit.
- Buy a cordless phone to keep with you so that you do not have to rush to the phone when it rings and so that you can call for help if you fall.

Treatment in Osteoporosis

The treatment can be classified into 2, curative and preventive. Osteoporosis treatment includes both lifestyle changes and medications. Treatment programs focus on nutrition, exercise, and safety issues to prevent falls that may result in broken bones. There are articles which indicate herbals like Dandelion Tea, Red Clover, Black Cohosh 20 or 40 mg twice daily, handful of sesame seeds had every morning, may also help osteoporosis but there is no research evidence, hence should be taken with caution.

Medication may be prescribed to slow or stop bone loss, increase bone density, and reduce fracture risk. There are oral medications available in the market. One well-known medication used to treat osteoporosis, alendronate (e.g. Fosamax), helps strengthen bones by encouraging mineral deposition in the vertebral bodies. This in turn can lower the risk of compression fractures. Fosamax is taken orally and it can be very irritating to the esophagus, so it should be taken with water and the patient should avoid lying down for 30 minutes after taking the drug to keep it from refluxing back into the esophagus.

Calcitonin (e.g. Miacalcin), a hormone that improves bone strength by favoring the bone-forming cells and inhibiting the bone-destroying cells. This medication serves to lower the risk of vertebral fractures, and has the added benefit of reducing low back pain in those who already have had a compression fracture. Miacalcin is administered by a nasal spray once a day.

The most important component of any osteoporosis treatment plan is regular monitoring and follow-up to ensure that the treatment plan is working effectively and make adjustments as necessary. The most important thing required in the treatment of 'Osteoporosis' is the restoring of bone architecture and only a drug with anabolic actions. This role is achieved by 'Teriparatide.' It acts directly through receptors on osteoblasts and stimulates the osteoprogenitor cells, leading to activated bone formation. It reactivates bone lining cells and improves matrix synthesis.

The most important component of any osteoporosis treatment plan is regular monitoring and follow-up to ensure that the treatment plan is working effectively and make adjustments as necessary.

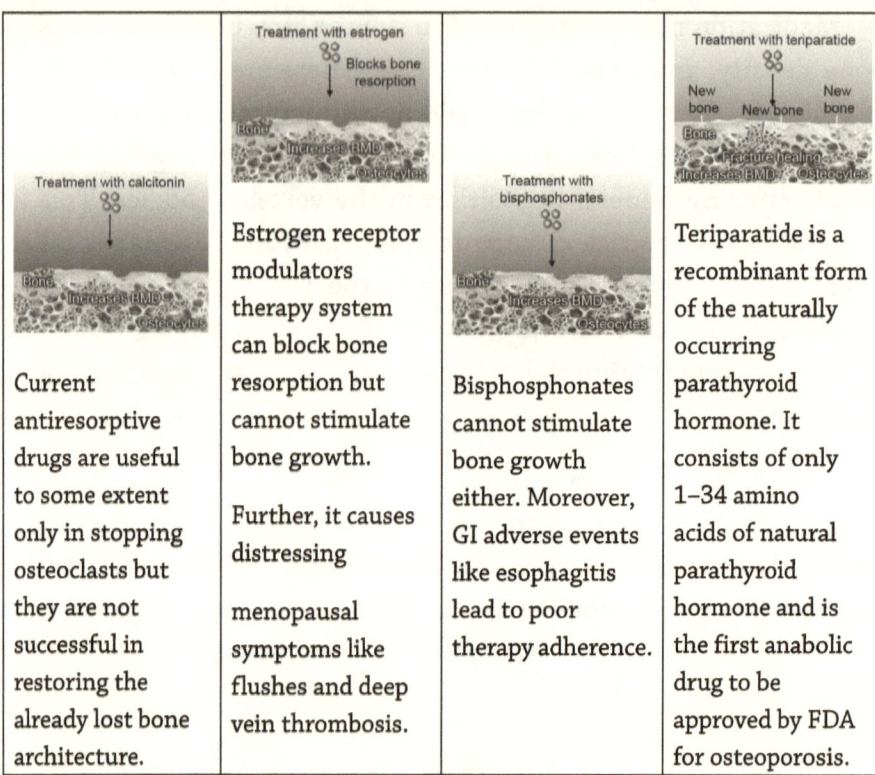

Fig. No. 5(e) 5: *Treatment in osteoporosis*

Complications of osteoporosis: The major complication of osteoporosis is fracture of bone including non-union and delayed union. It also causes disability by severely weakened bones.

Depending on which bones fracture and how they fracture, there can be further complications. For example, if a spinal vertebra in the low back has collapsed by a compression fracture, this can cause bone to directly press against nervous tissue of the spinal cord, causing severe pain and loss of function of the lower extremities. Collapse of vertebrae in the thoracic vertebrae can cause difficulty in breathing.

The preventive strategy to be adopted by individuals at risk is to strength their back muscles through back strengthening exercise to prevent spine fracture under supervision of physiotherapist, and to be physically active throughout life span.

Research-based Evidence Related to Preventive Strategies in Osteoporosis

In a study conducted by Delaney MF, 'Strategies for the prevention and treatment of osteoporosis during early menopause,' it is stated that during the perimenopause, both the quantity and quality of bone decline rapidly, resulting in a dramatic increase in the risk of fracture in postmenopausal women. Although many factors are known to be associated with osteoporotic fractures, measures to identify and treat women at risk are underused in clinical practice.

Consequently, osteoporosis is frequently not detected until a fracture occurs. Identification of postmenopausal women at high risk of fracture therefore is a priority and is especially important for women in early postmenopause, who can benefit from early intervention to maintain or to increase bone mass and, thus, reduce the risk of fracture. Most authorities recommend risk factor assessment for all postmenopausal women, followed by BMD measurements for women at highest risk (i.e. all women aged > or = 65 years, postmenopausal women aged <65 years with > or =1 additional risk factors for osteoporosis, and postmenopausal women with fragility fractures). All postmenopausal women can benefit from non-pharmacologic interventions to reduce the risk of fracture, including a balanced diet with adequate intake of calcium and vitamin D, regular exercise, measures to prevent falls or to minimize their impact, smoking cessation, and moderation of alcohol intake.

Several pharmacologic agents, including the bisphosphonates (e.g. alendronate, risedronate, and ibandronate) and the selective estrogen receptor modulator, raloxifene, have been shown to increase bone mass, to reduce fracture risk, and to have acceptable side effect profiles. Women who have discontinued hormone therapy are in particular need of monitoring for fracture risk, in the light of the accelerated bone loss and increased risk of fracture that occurs after withdrawal of estrogen treatment.

Yet another study was published in the journal of obstetrics and gynecology a systematic review of literature by **Khan A, Fortier M et al.,** the objective of which was to provide guidelines for health care providers on prevention, diagnosis and clinical management of postmenopausal osteoporosis. This study once again emphasized on the strategies for identification and evaluating high risk individuals using BMD and bone turnover markers for assessing diagnosis and response to management. The study also made recommendations regarding nutrition, physical activity, and selection of pharmacologic therapy to prevent and manage osteoporosis.

Reid IR, concluded calcium supplementation does not completely arrest postmenopausal bone loss but slows the rate of decline by 30–50%. Published data are inconsistent. In general, hormone replacement therapy and the potent bisphosphonates produce greater effects on bone density and there is a greater consistency among the results. Controlled trials of exercise interventions in postmenopausal women show that exercise can positively influence bone density by a few percent.

Masi L, Bilezikian JP, in the paper, 'Osteoporosis: new hope for the future,' reviewed established work and newer approaches to osteoporosis, and also emphasize identification of women with osteoporosis well before they begin to suffer some of its devastating consequences. The paper states that one of the most important approaches to therapy is prevention. Measures of importance relate to the establishment of peak bone mass in young adulthood. Along with issues of lifestyle, adequate calcium intake looms large as one of the important nutritional features of a program designed to establish peak bone mass. Calcium is also important later on in life to prevent bone loss and to help restore bone that might have been lost due to osteoporosis, with respect to vitamin D stores. The factors leading to this deficiency include routine avoidance of sun, which is a major source of vitamin D, avoidance of milk, which is fortified with vitamin D, and physiological factors that make it more difficult for an older individual to activate vitamin D and to respond to it.

Thus, along with adequate calcium, it is important that vitamin D stores are adequate. If vitamin D stores are inadequate or if they are marginal, a supplement regimen is usually advisable. Another helpful preventive measure is an exercise program. It is also important to minimize the likelihood of falling because hip fractures do not generally occur among those who do not fall. Attention to factors that may predispose an individual to fall, such as her balance, eyesight, stairs, and bathtubs that are difficult to get into and out of, are all items that need attention. The controversy surrounding hormone replacement therapy in postmenopausal women continues to be active. On the other hand, there is no question that estrogen replacement therapy in the menopausal years is a highly effective means to prevent bone loss. In its absence, women experience a 5 -to 8-year period of accelerated bone loss beyond what would be expected to occur as a function of age alone. Estrogen essentially prevents this bone loss, and it continues to be prevented for as long as estrogens are taken.

N de Jong, MJ Chin, A Paw, et al. studied, 'Dietary supplements and physical exercise affecting bone and body composition in frail persons.' The objective of the study was to determine the effect of enriched foods and all-around physical exercise on bone and body composition in frail elderly persons. A 17-week randomized, controlled intervention trial, following a 2 × 2 factorial design (1) enriched foods, (2) exercise, (3) both, or (4) neither, was performed in 143 frail elderly persons (aged 78.6 +/− 5.6 years). Foods were enriched with multiple micronutrients; exercises focused on skill training, including strength, endurance, coordination, and flexibility. Main outcome parameters were bone and body composition. The findings indicated exercise preserved lean mass (mean difference between exercisers and non-exercisers: 0.5 kg +/− 1.2 kg; $P < .02$). Groups receiving enriched food had slightly increased BMD (+0.4%), bone mass (+0.6%), and bone calcium (+0.6%) compared with groups receiving non-enriched foods, in whom small decreases of 0.1%, 0.2%, and 0.4%, respectively, were found. These groups differed in BMD (0.006 +/−0.020 g/cm^2; $P = .08$), Total bone mass (19 +/− g; $P = .04$), and bone calcium (8 +/− 21 g; $P = .03$). Thus it was concluded that foods containing a physiologic dose of micronutrients slightly increased bone density, mass, and calcium, whereas moderately intense exercise preserved lean body mass in frail elderly persons.

Kulak and Bilezikian stated in their paper, 'Osteoporosis: preventive strategies,' that in the United States alone, osteoporosis affects over 20 million women. The cost of treating the complications of osteoporosis exceeds 10 billion dollars. Half of those who sustain a hip fracture never return to their former lifestyle. In addition, there is a major increase in mortality within the first year of a hip fracture. These facts dictate an urgent need to address issues relevant to the prevention of osteoporosis. Only by preventing bone loss will it be possible to meet the challenge of dealing effectively with this major public health problem. There are 3 major components of an effective preventive strategy.

The first is to ensure that optimal peak bone mass is achieved during childhood, adolescence and early adulthood. Although much of peak bone mass is determined by genetic influence, there are other factors of importance over which one has control. These include adequate dietary calcium intake, good nutrition, exercise and hormone sufficiency. The second aspect to prevention is maintaining bone mass that has been acquired. Bone maintenance requires adequate calcium intake and exercise as well as avoiding tobacco and excessive alcohol. Certain diseases (i.e. hyperthyroidism) and medications (i.e. steroids, anticonvulsants) will tend to erode the repositories of bone at any time in life. The third aspect to prevention is counteracting the process of age related bone loss that occurs after 40–45 years of age. In women, the menopause markedly accelerates bone loss. Measures to ensure that bone loss is minimized during the middle years and beyond include adequate nutrition (vitamin D and calcium) and hormone sufficiency. For women, hormone replacement therapy is a gold standard of therapy because it arrests bone loss associated with the menopause. For women who cannot or will not take estrogen, newer, effective approaches, such as estrogen analogs and the non-hormonal bisphosphonates, are available. With this three-phased approach, requiring constant attention to bone health over one's entire life, the risk of developing osteoporosis and its complications can be minimized.

Need to Strengthen National Program

A report by **Divya Ramamurti,** in 'The Hindu' online edition on 18th Feb, 2005. 'Awareness on osteoporosis needs to be raised' quotes Rohini Handa, Secretary General of Osteoporosis Society of India, that in India osteoporosis is yet not taken seriously, as every fracture a person sustains after 50 years is attributed to old age instead of osteoporosis.

Therefore two-pronged approach is required in India. A public health approach which emphasizes nutrition, exercise and sunlight exposure beginning in childhood, so as to achieve a better peak bone mass, and a clinical based approach which allows greater accessibility and affordability of DXA scanning as well as widespread use of appropriate pharmacologic therapy through inclusion in government programs or reimbursement policies.

The Indian Society of Bone Mineral Research (ISBMR) stated in their study that public awareness in urban areas is due to the media. Literature indicates government of India does not recognize osteoporosis as a major health problem. However ISBMR and some other societies like Arthritis Foundation of India are involved in conducting public awareness programs for prevention of osteoporosis. ISBMR regularly programs on television, radio, newspaper and leading magazines. But there still exists a need for awareness on a macro level to disseminate information on osteoporosis.

As there is evidence of the risk factors causing osteoporosis from a younger age when peak bone mass needs to develop, educating on prevention of osteoporosis should be target in school and colleges.

Strengthening the Health System

In India, there is no data available on health costs of osteoporosis. In India, government is spending 4.6% of its GDP on health. Total public health expenditure is 20.3%, private expenditure is 77.4% and the external support is 2.3% (NHA of India). India is spending 0.4% of total health budget on the non-communicable disease **(NHA of India, 2001–2002)**.

There is a need for national campaigns to encourage increasing BMD through behavioral modification, change in lifestyle, physical activity and consumption of calcium rich foods.

There is need to sensitize and increase awareness regarding osteoporosis in the public about the prevention and its future consequences of osteoporosis and gain their involvement in reducing the incidences of fracture due to osteoporosis.

Have more diagnostic centers in the both rural and urban areas at cost-effective rates.

Development of Infrastructure to Deal with Osteoporosis

There is a need to allocate funds and human resource to develop the infrastructure to support the prevention and control of osteoporosis. There is a need to shift from medical information to programmed approach towards self-care management at government and private institutions.

Strengthening of Training Programs

There is a need to train health personnel as well as registered medical practitioners in early identification and management of osteoporosis and its consequences.

Physician education program in orthopedics to focus on osteoporosis. Structured government programs to provide education at national level training of osteoporosis and inclusion of it in undergraduate programs.

The primary health care teams need to promote early case identification of high risk individuals and refer them to referral centers for management. There is also a need for community-based screening strategies for especially rural poor and lower socio-economic section of society.

Strengthening of preventive measures through researches to develop BMD standard from Indian perspectives, developing pragmatic, effective strategies to overcome vitamin D insufficiency.

Public Awareness to Strengthen Prevention of Osteoporosis

Government agencies/Ministry of health to take up bone health program as a priority; initiate a media campaign to spread awareness about lifestyle issues across the country; implement strategies to correct vitamin D nutrition, including fortification of milk and food.

The National Rural Health Mission started in 2005 does not include osteoporosis in its list of non-communicable diseases. It includes national program for prevention and control of cancer, diabetes, cardiovascular disease and stroke although they are yet to be addressed. Hence government and advocacy of health care official could encourage including osteoporosis in the nation health plan. School health programs to ensure children receive vitamin D and calcium fortified food in all government added schools. Canteen of institutions can at their level provide calcium rich food.

Health checkup for all new recruits should include assessment of non-communicable disease, especially osteoporosis, as it often gets excluded due to the cost of DXA or bone mineral assessment. The government should provide machinery for assessment or subsidize the cost for procurement so that bone mineral scan can become affordable to all.

There is a need for strengthening primary prevention by increasing awareness, lifestyle modification and screening and making secondary prevention affordable as treatment need to be cost-effective compared to late diagnosis and treatment of fractures. Referral system needs to be strengthened as are the secondary and tertiary level of health care.

Key Points

There is conclusive evidence to indicate that with individual efforts to change lifestyle, half of the chronic diseases that caused disability and death could be prevented. Earlier diagnosis and prevention of fractures should decrease the medical, social and economic burdens of this disease.

It is nearly impossible for anyone to satisfy vitamin D needs through diet. It requires a 3 pronged attack, sun exposure, supplements and food. Health care practitioners can be instrumental in educating their patients about the fact that, with intelligent dietary and lifestyle choices, osteoporosis is largely preventable for most people.

WHO has emphasized that reduction in non-communicable disease can be through preventive measure like keeping healthy behavior, which includes healthy diet, maintaining normal weight and being physically active throughout life span. An important aspect of osteoporosis preventive strategies is improving knowledge at rural and urban areas to adapt healthy living, early detection of osteoporosis and confirmatory test of all fracture patients to rule out osteoporosis-related fracture.

References

1. Awumey EM, Mitra DA, Hollis BW et al. Vitamin D metabolism is altered in Asian Indians in the southern United States: a clinical research center study. J Clin Endocrinol Metab 1998; 83: 169–73.

2. Babu US, Calvo MS. Modern India and the vitamin D dilemma: evidence for the need of a national food fortification program. Molecular Nutrition and Food Research. 2010; 54: 1134–47.

3. Boning up on Osteoporosis. India Times, 2004 http://health.indiatimes.com/article show/329953 cms.

4. Brown JP, Josse RG. Clinical practice guidelines for the diagnosis and management of osteoporosis in Canada. Canadian Medical Association Journal. 2002; 12: 167 (10 Suppl): S1–34.

5. Castelo-Branco C. Management of osteoporosis: an overview, drugs aging. 1998; 12: 25–32.

6. Chapurlat R, Delmas PD. Therapeutic strategies for osteoporosis. Annales de Medecine Interne (Paris). 2000; 151(6): 471–6.

7. Cranney A, Horsley T, O'Donnell S, Weiler H et al. Effectiveness and safety of Vitamin D in relation to bone density, Evidence report/technology assessment (Full Rep.). 2007; (158): 1–235.

8. Cummings SR, Melton LJ. Epidemiology and outcomes of osteoporotic fracture. Lancet, 2002, 3rd edition, 359: 1761–7.

9. Delaney MF. Strategies for the prevention and treatment of osteoporosis during early postmenopause Am J Obst and Gyne. Feb. 2006; 194(2 Supplement): S12–23.

10. Dietary Supplement Fact Sheet: Vitamin D. Referenced in National Institutes of Health, Office of Dietary Supplements. http://ods.od.nih.gov/factsheets/VitaminD-HealthProfessional/#h10.

11. Food and Nutrition Board, Institute of Medicine, National Academy of Sciences, 2010.

12. Fu L, Yun F, Oczak M, et al. Common genetic variants of the vitamin D binding protein (DBP) predict differences in response of serum 25-hydroxyvitamin D[25(OH)] to vitamin D supplementation. Clinical Biochemistry. 2009; 42: 1174–7.

13. Harinarayan CV, Joshi SR. Vitamin D status in India—its implications and remedial measures. J Assoc Physicians India. 2009; 57: 40–8.

14. Hudson T, N. D; Osteoporosis: Strategies for prevention and management. 2006, Oct.17.

15. Institute of Medicine, Food and Nutrition Board. Dietary Reference Intakes: Calcium, Phosphorus, Magnesium, Vitamin D and Fluoride. National Academy Press, Washington DC, 1999.

16. Intas Pharmaceuticals Ltd. terifrac.com/osteoporosis_prevelence.htm.

17. International Osteoporosis Foundation (2002) Osteoporosis in the Workplace: The social, economic and human costs of osteoporosis on employees, employers and governments.

18. Khadilkar AV. Vitamin D deficiency in Indian adolescents. Indian Pediatr. 2010; 47: 756–7.

19. Khan A, Fortier M et al. Osteoporosis in menopause J Obsta, Canada: JOGC. 2014; 36(9): 839–43.

20. Klippel J H et al. Primer on the Rheumatic Diseases. New York: Springer, 2008.

21. Kulak CA Bilezikian JP. Osteoporosis: preventive strategies. Int J FertilWomens Med. March-April 1998; 43(2): 56–64.

22. Levis S, Theodore G. Summary of AHRQ's comparative effectiveness review of treatment to prevent fractures in men and women with low bone density or osteoporosis: update of the 2007 report. J Manag Care Pharm. 2012; 18 (4Suppl. B): S1–15; S13.

23. Londhey V (Ed). Vitamin D Deficiency: Indian Scenario, JAPI, 2011, Nov. Vol. 59, New Delhi: ICMR: Published by Director

General; 2010. Population-based reference standards of Peak Bone Mineral Density of Indian males and females—an ICMR multi-center task force study; 1–24.

24. Manske S, Lorincz C, Zernicke R. Bone health: part 2, physical activity. Sports Health. 2009; 1(4): 341-6.

25. MasiL, Bilezikian JP. Osteoporosis: new hope for the future. Int J Fertil Womens Med. 1997; July-Aug.; 42(4): 245–54.

26. Mitra S, Desai M, Khatkhatav MI. Association of estrogen receptor alpha gene polymorphisms with BMD in postmenopausal Indian women. Molecular Genetics and Metabolism, 2006; 87(1): 80–7.

27. National health account of India 2001–2002, Ministry of health, Government of India, WHO India [online] (http://www.who.int/nha/NHA_ India _NHA_2001-02.pdf.).

28. National Osteoporosis Foundation. Physician's guide to prevention and treatment of postmenopausal osteoporosis. Washington DC, USA: 2003.

29. N de Jong, MJ Chin, A Paw, LC de Groot, G J Hiddin K & WA Van Staveren,'Dietary supplements and physical exercise affecting bone and body composition in frail persons.' Am J Public Health, June 2000; 90(6): 947–54.

30. Ontario Health Technology Assessment series, Clinical Utility of Vitamin D testing: an evidence-based analysis. 2010; 10(2): 1–93. Epub 2010 Feb 1.

31. Osteoporosis Society of India, Action Plan Osteoporosis: Consensus statement of an expert group. New Delhi, 2003.

32. Patni R. Normal BMD values for Indian females aged 20–80 years. J Midlife Health. 2010; 1: 70-3.

33. Population-based reference standards of Peak Bone Mineral Density of Indian males and females – an ICMR multi-center task force study; ICMR: Published by Director General; New Delhi: 2010; 1–24.

34. Rao H, Rao N, Sharma LR. A clinical study of bone mineral density using heel ultra-densitometer in Southern Maharashtra. Indian J Orthop. 2003; 37: 9.

35. Reid IR. Therapy of osteoporosis: calcium, vit. D and exercise. Am J Med Sci; 1996; 312(6): 278–86.

36. Report of Joint FAO/WHO Expert Consultation on vitamin and mineral requirement in human nutrition: Bangkok 1998. Second Edition FAO Rome, 2004. Available at http://whqlibdoc.who.int/publications/2004/9241546123.pdf.

37. Sharma S, Khandewal S. Effective risk assessment tool for osteoporosis in Indian menopausal female. J Midlife Health. 2010; (2): 79–85.

38. Shetty S, Kapoor N, Naik D et al. Osteoporosis in Healthy South Indian Males and the Influence of Life Style Factors and Vitamin D Status on Bone Mineral Density. J Osteoporosis, Vol. 2014(2014), Article ID 723238, http;//dx.doi.org/10.1155/2021/723238.

39. The NIH Osteoporosis and Related Bone Diseases, National Resource Center, 'Secondary Osteoporosis.' Vol: 4, no. 1, December 2001.

40. Vaidya R, Shah R. Bone mineral density and reference standards for Indian women. J Midlife Health. 2010; 1(2): 55.

Chapter V (F)

Preventive Strategies for Alzheimer's Disease

Dr. T. Sivabalan

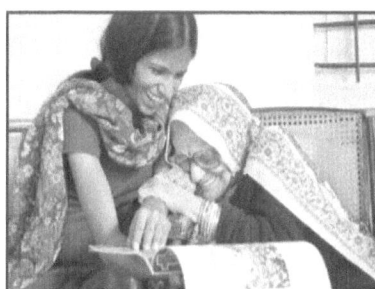 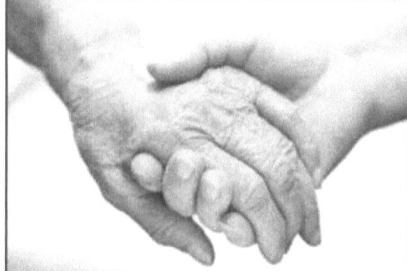

Introduction

More than a century ago, in 1906, a German physician, Alois Alzheimer, first described the disease which has come to be known as the Alzheimer's disease. It's a type of dementia that progressively affects the memory, thinking, mobility and communication, etc. The increase in the older population and increased life expectancy in our country has led to a growing incidence of age related diseases such as dementia, and interestingly advancement of the disease cannot be halted.

National Institute on Aging highlighted that worldwide the Alzheimer's is one of the leading causes of dementia, which affects more than half of the individuals suffering from dementia. Alzheimer's disease is an aging (above 60 years) related brain disorder which progressively affects the memory, cognition, thinking skills and behavioral abilities such as ability to carry out simple tasks. Later an Alzheimer's patient may have difficulties in carrying out daily life and activities.

Epidemiology

Among elderly population the Alzheimer disease is a major public health concern in the world. It is estimated that by the year 2050, people aged above 60 years will account for 22% of the world's population and four-fifths of such people will be living in Asian countries. The number of people suffering from Alzheimer's disease has been estimated to be around 24 million across all nations in the world.

Aging and its related changes are a global phenomenon, and India's experience is not exceptional where the rapid demographic transition along with fast-paced social restructuring is in place. Among the general population, soon there will be a sharp inclination of number of elderly people in the country. In the year 2001, India was home to more than 75 million elderly, who constitute 7.5% of the population, while this number is expected to grow dramatically in the forthcoming years.

The Dementia India report – 2010, highlighted that there is a marked variation in the rate of demographic aging within India which ranges from 4% to 11%. The regions with elderly population above 8% include Himachal Pradesh (9%), Punjab (9%), Tamil Nadu (8.8%), Maharashtra (8.7%), and Orissa, Goa and Pondicherry which had (8.3%) of elderly respectively. Alzheimer's and Dementia remain a largely hidden problem in India, mainly in the parts where poverty and illiteracy levels are high. There is a great demand for support, care and services for the elderly affected with Alzheimer's/Dementia; meeting the needs of the elderly is a more urgent and challenging task before all, including health care professionals.

> **'Being proactive is a vital step on the journey toward successful ageing'**

Changes in the Brain

In Alzheimer's disease, brain damage appears before the occurrence of problems in memory and cognitive functions. During this phase (preclinical) Alzheimer's disease persons do not have any manifestations; however changes in the brain remain constant and progressive in nature. The brain changes will be abnormal deposition of proteins forming amyloid plaques and tau tangles throughout the brain. Presence of amyloid plaques in the healthy neurons stops their functioning, and develops loose connections with other neurons, followed by the cells dying. Commonly the initial damage takes place in the hippocampus (essential for memory). As damage progresses, increased numbers of neurons die, followed by other parts of the brain also being affected, and brain begins to shrink. Finally most part of the brain gets affected and this leads to memory, cognition and behavioral problems.

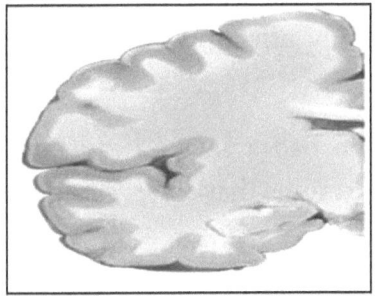 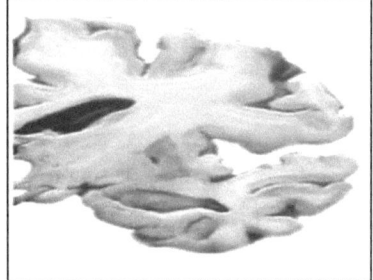

Fig. No. 5(f) 1: *Healthy brain*   *Alzheimer's brain*

Risk Factors

Alzheimer's is a complex, progressive and chronic non-communicable disease of the aging population. There are varieties of factors which influence the person's chance of developing the disease. The common risk factors are age, genetics, environment, and lifestyle factors. As mentioned earlier, the Alzheimer's causes progressive changes in the brain tissues for years before the occurrence of first symptoms.

Age: Aging factor is the most influential and prime risk factor for development of Alzheimer's disease. Individuals above 65 years of age have double the risk in every 5 years of life, and further, it is very much common beyond 80 years of age.

Genetics: Genetic materials (genes) play an important role in the development (early or late onset) of Alzheimer's disease. The individuals of early age group (30–50 years) have onset of Alzheimer's known as early onset Alzheimer's. It is associated with family history, and caused by the mutations in amyloid precursor protein (APP) or presenilins 1 and 2 genes. Mutations in these genes lead to production of beta amyloid 42 which causes death of neurons. Late onset Alzheimer's disease is a common type and individuals in the aging population (above 60 years) commonly suffer from this. Mutations in Apolipoprotein E (APOE) increase (3 to 15 times) the risk of Alzheimer's disease, affecting around 30% of the population while 5% of people are affected with early onset of Alzheimer's.

Gender: Alzheimer's disease commonly affects women more than men 1.

History of head injury: People who had a severe head injury or suffered with repeated head injury/trauma have a greater risk of developing Alzheimer's disease.

Lifestyle factors: Variety of evidence reveals that the risk factors responsible for developing heart disease are also likely to increase the chances of development of Alzheimer's disease. The common risk factors are: lack of exercise/obesity, smoking, high blood pressure, high blood cholesterol, elevated homocysteine levels, uncontrolled diabetes and a diet lacking in fruits and vegetables.

Down syndrome: People with Down syndrome can experience premature aging, due to which they're at a higher risk for age related health problems like Alzheimer disease.

Vitamin deficiencies: The elevated amount of amino acid homocysteine and deficiency of vitamin B12 and folate are linked with brain shrinkage and increased risk of Alzheimer's disease.

Aluminum toxicity: The chronic exposure to aluminum (neurotoxin) causes the brain cell degenerative changes and leads to Alzheimer's disease, dementia and brain damage.

Electromagnetic radiation: Electromagnetic radiation is associated with accelerating aging which enhances the cell death, and leads to Alzheimer's disease and cancer.

Box No: 1 Warning Signs of Alzheimer's Disease

- Memory loss
- Difficulty performing familiar tasks
- Problems with language
- Disorientation to time and place
- Poor or decreased judgment
- Problems with abstract thinking
- Misplacing things
- Changes in mood or behavior
- Changes in personality
- Loss of initiative

(The Alzheimer's Association, 2009)

Scientific Evidence: 01

A systematic review of incident rates for dementia and Alzheimer's disease among aging population showed that the incidence of Alzheimer's increased with aging. It was noticed that around 64% of persons with 90 years of age exhibited Alzheimer's disease. Alongside, female gender, smoking, head injury and low levels of education significantly increased the risk of Alzheimer's[2].

Scientific Evidence: 02

A study on prevalence and risk factors of dementia among urban aging population in Kerala, India, found that the prevalence of dementia was 34/1000 population. The common type was Alzheimer's disease (54%) followed by vascular dementia (39%), and 7% were due to infection, tumor and trauma. It was noticed that, family history of dementia was associated with Alzheimer's disease and hypertension was associated with vascular dementia. Study highlights that multiple factors are involved in the development of Alzheimer's disease[3].

Scientific Evidence: 03

A community based longitudinal study on association of head injury and the occurrence of Alzheimer's disease was done. It was observed that the history of head injury with loss of consciousness was associated with early onset of dementia due to Alzheimer's disease. The risk of Alzheimer's was increased in individuals who had head injury with loss of consciousness for more than 5 minutes. The study concluded that head injury is a risk factor for Alzheimer's disease[4].

Diagnosis

Alzheimer's disease is diagnosed by utilizing the following techniques/tests like: a) health history (on overall health, past medical history, ability to carry out the activity of daily living (ADL), changes in personality and behavior, etc.) b) physical (clinical) examination to assess mental status, memory, problem solving ability, attention, counting, and language skills c) blood investigations for hemoglobin, electrolytes, vitamin B12 and d) imaging tests for brain (Computed Tomography (CT) scan, Magnetic Resonance Imaging (MRI) scan and Positron Emission Tomography (PET) scan) to identify the brain changes.

> **'Most people living with Alzheimer's are not aware of their diagnosis'**

Treatment

Alzheimer's is a chronic, progressive and complex disease, where a single drug or therapy may not cure the disease. However, the treatment approaches focus on helping the people to maintain optimal mental function, manage/correct behavioral symptoms, and slow or delay the symptoms of disease. National Institute on Aging – Alzheimer's disease Education and Referral center, USA, reported that several medications are approved by the Food and Drug Administration (FDA) to treat symptoms of Alzheimer's. Donepezil, Rivastigmine and Galantamine are commonly used to treat the mild to moderate Alzheimer's, whereas Memantine is used to treat moderate to severe Alzheimer's. These drugs improve the health status by regulation of neurotransmitters, which are the brain chemicals that transmit messages between the neurons.

Alongside it helps to maintain thinking, memory and communication skills, and helps with behavioral problems; however, these drugs will not change the underlying disease process.

> **'Patience is the key to management of Alzheimer's disease'**

Table No. 5(f) 1: Common symptoms experienced by people with alzheimer's disease – World Alzheimer's Report: 2009

Early stage	Middle stage	Late stage
The early stage is often overlooked. Relatives and friends see it as 'old age,' just a normal part of aging process. Because the onset of disease is gradual, it is difficult to be sure exactly when it begins.	As the disease progresses, limitations become clearer and more restricting. Become very forgetful, especially of recent events and people's names.	The last stage is one of nearly total dependence and inactivity. Memory disturbances are very serious and the physical side of the disease becomes more obvious.

Early stage	Middle stage	Late stage
Become forgetful, especially regarding things that just happened. May have some difficulty with communication, like difficulty in finding words. Become lost in familiar places. Lose track of the time, including time of day, month, year, and season. Have difficulty in making decisions and handling personal finances. Have difficulty carrying out complex household tasks. Mood and behavior: may become less active/ motivated and lose interest in activities and hobbies. may show mood changes, including depression or anxiety. may react unusually angrily or aggressively on occasions.	Have difficulty in comprehending time, date, place and events; may become lost at home as well as in the community. Have increasing difficulty with communication (speech and comprehension). Unable to successfully prepare food, cook, clean or shop. Unable to live alone safely without considerable support. Behavior changes may include wandering, repeated questioning, calling out, clinging, disturbed sleeping, hallucinations (seeing or hearing things which are not there). May display inappropriate behavior in the home or in the community (disinhibition or aggression).	Usually unaware of time and place. Have difficulty in understanding what is happening around them. Unable to recognize relatives, friends and familiar objects. Unable to eat without assistance, may have difficulty in swallowing. Increasing need for assisted self – care (bathing and toileting). May have bladder and bowel incontinence Change in mobility (unable to walk or be confined to a wheelchair or bed). Behavior changes may escalate and include aggression towards carer, nonverbal agitation (kicking, hitting, screaming or moaning). Unable to find his/her way around in the home.

General Management of Alzheimer's Disease

Creating a safe and Supportive environment

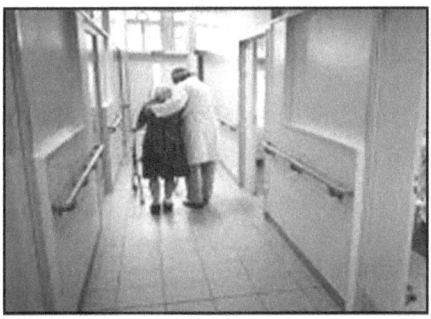

Fig. No. 5(f) 2: *Safe environment*

Adapting the living situation to the needs of a person with Alzheimer's is an important component of the treatment plan. For Alzheimer's patients, establishing and strengthening routine habits and minimizing memory demanding tasks makes life easier.

The following steps may be followed to support a person's sense of well-being and ability to do activities:

- Create a calm and quiet soothing environment, and try to modify the environment to reduce the potential stressors.

- Always keep keys, wallets, mobile phones and other valuables in the same place at home, so they don't become lost.

- Develop the habit of carrying a mobile phone (along with important numbers) at all locations (so that people can track the location via phone).

- Make sure that the regular appointments are on the same day at the same time as much as possible.

- Use a calendar or white board in the home to track daily schedules. Build the habit of checking off completed items, so that the person can be sure that they were completed.

- Remove excess furniture; install side rails or hand rails on stairways as well as in bathroom/washrooms.

- Ensure that shoes and slippers are comfortable and provide good traction.
- Reduce the number of mirrors, because people with Alzheimer's may find images in mirrors confusing or frightening.
- Request the treating physician to simplify the drugs regimen to once a day (OD) dose.

Preventive Strategies

Though the exact reason for development of Alzheimer's disease is not completely known to the medical fraternity, there are numerous preventive strategies available to manage the problems/symptoms in a comprehensive manner. Prevention is crucial for stopping the alarming spread of this disease. Delaying the onset of the disease could reduce the total number of cases by 50%. The following are the preventive strategies helpful to reduce the occurrence and the impact of Alzheimer's disease.

> **'Stay mentally Active and Healthy'**

I. Exercise Therapy

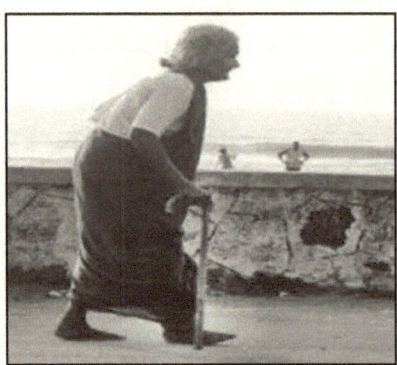

Fig. No. 5(f) 3: *Walking as Physical therapy*

Regular exercise is an important part of everybody's wellness plan – and those with Alzheimer's are no exception. Exercise therapy triggers a change in the way the amyloid precursor protein is metabolized, thus it slows down the onset of Alzheimer's disease. Activities such as a daily 30 minutes' walk and activities like gardening, housekeeping, taking the stairs and walking with pet animals are encouraged, which help in preventing the Alzheimer's disease.

Table No. 5(f) 2: Recommended physical therapy for Alzheimer's disease

Early stage	Middle stage	Late stage
Walking	Walking	Walking
Aerobic exercises	Flexibility exercises	Gardening
Stretching exercises	Breathing and relaxation exercises	Coordination activities
Cycling		Exercises to maintain range of motion
Breathing and relaxation exercises	Stretching and strengthening exercises	Balance exercises
Recreational activities	Range of motion exercises	Recreational activities
Swimming	Balance training	Activities mimicking
Cognitive therapy including education	Cognitive stimulation therapy	Activities of daily living
		Cognitive stimulation therapy

Source: **Kaur J, Garnawat D, Bhatia MS and Sachdev M. Rehabilitation in Alzheimer's disease – Psycho physiotherapy. Delhi psychiatric journal, 2013; 16 (1): 166 – 715**

The scientific evidences highlight that the exercise program resulted in significant improvement in cortical connectivity and activation, and improved cognitive functional brain network connectivity[6]. Alongside, the exercises improved the production of neurotrophic factors, increased cerebral blood flow, increased neurogenesis, enhanced neural survival, mobilization of gene expression impacting neuronal plasticity, increased growth factors in hippocampus and decreased risk of cerebrovascular diseases[7,8].

> **'Reading is to the mind, what exercise is to the body'**

II. Mental Exercises

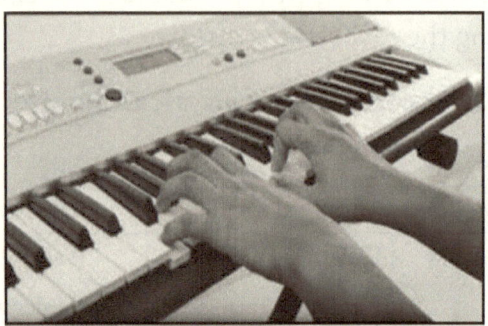

Fig. No. 5(f) 4: *Mental exercises*

An active brain (i.e., engage the brain in any kind of mental activities) may reduce the risk of Alzheimer's disease.

Following are the recommended exercises for sharpening the mental skills.

Play music: Learn to play any of the musical instruments or listen to music

Take a cooking class: Cooking uses a number of senses (smell, touch, sight and taste) which involve different parts of the brain

Learn a new language: The listening and hearing stimulates brain and keeps the brain cells active. The rich vocabulary is linked with reduced risk for cognitive decline

Improve the hand eye abilities: Perform a new hobby that involves fine motor skills such as knitting, drawing, painting or assembling a puzzle, etc.

Start doing new sports: Start doing athletic exercises that utilize the brain and body such as yoga, golf or tennis, etc.

Sensible use of leisure times: Use the leisure hours in reading newspapers, doing maths, visiting museums and playing puzzle games, etc.

The scientific literatures highlighted that there is a strong correlation between more/frequent social activities with better cognitive function. Studies on impact of activities like listening to music, reading books/newspapers, engaging with puzzle games and visiting museums shows that the risk of developing Alzheimer's disease was 47% lower for those who did the activities most often than for those who did not do such activities, or did them less frequently.

National Institute on Aging highlighted that the theories on role of mental exercises on Alzheimer's disease are: a) these activities helps in protecting the 'cognitive reserve' thus the brain has ability to operate effectively even if it is damaged or disrupted, and b) these activities help the brain to become more adaptable in mental functions, thus it can compensate for declines in other functions of the brain.

III. Nutrition

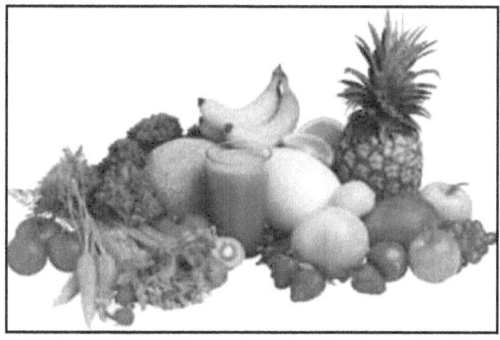

Fig. No. 5(f) 5: *Nutrition*

Individuals with Alzheimer's may forget to eat, lose interest in preparing meals or eat, and do not eat a healthy combination of foods. They may also forget to drink enough, which may lead to dehydration and constipation.

Maintain healthy balanced diet by using whole grains, fruits and vegetables, fish, nuts, olive oil, blueberries and strawberries, etc.

Consume more of vitamin B 12 rich foods such as green leafy vegetables, beans, peas, poultry, eggs, milk, cheese, yogurt, fish and red meat, etc. Try to consume vitamin B12 – 2.4 microgram (mcg), Folate – 400 mcg and vitamin C – 90 mcg daily. These vitamins help in maintaining healthy nerve cells and RBCs, and are important for the optimal brain function.

Include vitamin C rich food items like broccoli, citrus fruits, strawberries, sweet peppers and tomatoes, etc. The antioxidant vitamins such as vitamin C and E protect the brain against damage caused by the free radicals and other metabolic waste products. The neuron is sensitive to the damage caused by free radicals which is believed to cause development of Alzheimer's disease.

IV. Stop Smoking

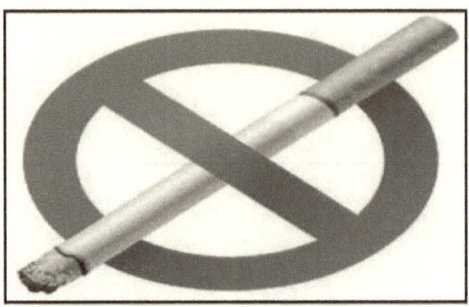

Fig. No. 5(f) 6: *Stop smoking*

World Health Organization report on Tobacco use and Dementia 2014 highlights that smokers have 45% higher risk of developing dementia than nonsmokers, and 14% of all Alzheimer's cases worldwide can potentially be attributed to smoking. Smoking (tobacco consumption) increases the risk of Alzheimer's disease and dementia. Further smoking inhibits the absorption of nutrients like vitamin C which leads to vitamin deficiency. To avoid all these impacts stop smoking; other measures to stop smoking are: a) think positive b) change the diet and drink c) be prepared for nicotine withdrawal symptoms d) make a plan to quit smoking e) seek help and support from family and health care professionals.

V. Screening for Blood Pressure, Cholesterol and Diabetes Mellitus

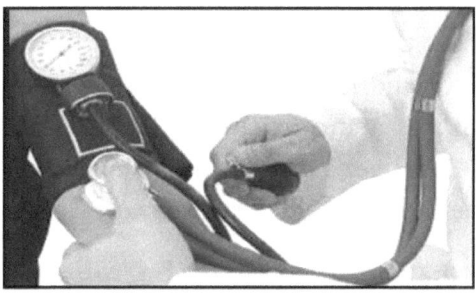

Fig. No. 5(f) 7: *Screening for Blood Pressure*

Regular screening helps to understand the current health status and intimates the need to take corrective actions via health care. The appropriate management for high blood pressure (BP), high cholesterol and other vascular risk factors may help to minimize the risk of Alzheimer's disease. Clinical trials reported that patients who were treated for high BP, high cholesterol, heart disease and diabetes had less progression of memory and thinking impairment and were less likely to develop dementia[9]. Individuals who are above 45 years of age need to undergo regular screening of blood pressure, cholesterol and blood sugar assessment to identify the risk of developing hypertension, diabetes and vascular diseases, thereby preventive measures may be initiated to prevent the Alzheimer's disease.

VI. Avoid Aluminum Toxicity

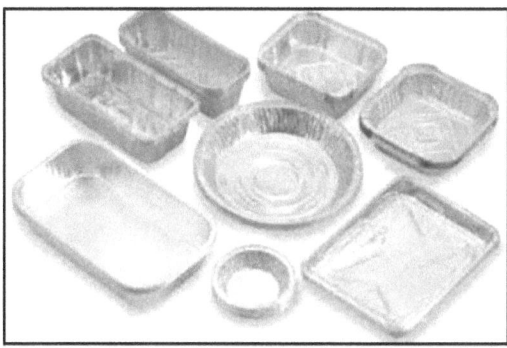

Fig. No. 5(f) 8: *Avoid Aluminium*

The longevity of exposure to aluminum causes brain cell degeneration which leads to Alzheimer's disease and brain damages. The growing evidence emphasizes that aluminum is a neurotoxin which could cause cognitive deficiency and Alzheimer's disease. The oligomerization of β amyloid protein and neurotoxicity in the molecular mechanism for development of Alzheimer's disease, and the aluminum play a crucial role as cross linker in β amyloid oligomerization.

The following measures need to be followed to avoid the aluminum toxicity:

- Eat completely cleaned foods.
- Avoid use of aluminum foils for cooking and covering the cooked foods.
- Avoid using aluminum or non-stick cookware, and prepare the food items with stainless steel, copper or iron cookware.
- Avoid eating the canned (aluminum cans) foods such as soups, vegetables, sauces, etc.
- Filter the water before drinking, and avoid processed foods and foods sprayed with pesticides.
- Minimize the use of skin care products and cosmetics and use natural cosmetics and organic skin care products.
- Perform regular exercises which increase the perspiration and sweating to eliminate the metals from the body.

VII. Minimize the Electromagnetic Radiation Exposure

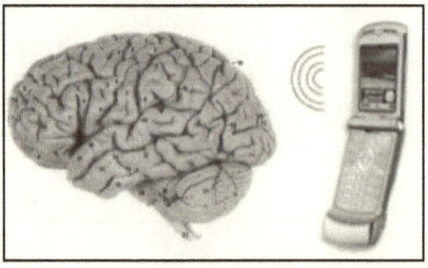

Fig. No. 5(f) 9: *Electromagnetic radiation*

Electromagnetic radiation is associated with accelerating aging which enhances increased cellular necrosis which leads to Alzheimer's disease and dementia.

- Avoid areas of wireless networking.
- Refrain from or minimize using cellular phones and cordless phones.
- Place the head of the bed on a wall that is opposite to an electric panel, electric meter, refrigerator, freezer, television, computer, air conditioner or any other electronic device that produces electromagnetic radiation during sleeping hours.
- Never sleep in a bed with an electric heating pad, electric blanket, or waterbed heater plugged in to a wall outlet.
- If cordless devices must be used, recharge them at night and locate the charging units away from bedrooms.
- Use flat screen LCD model computers that produce low level electromagnetic radiation.

VIII. Reduce the Risk of Head Injury

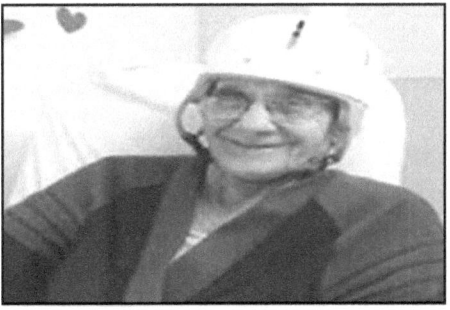

Fig. No. 5(f) 10: *Preventing head injury*

Individuals who had a severe head injury or repeated head trauma appear to have a greater risk of developing Alzheimer's disease and brain damages. Research has shown that the moderate to severe traumatic brain injury had increased risk of developing Alzheimer's disease and dementia years after head injury. Alongside, studies have reported that a head injury patient has 2 times greater risk of developing Alzheimer's disease than someone with no history of head injury.

Follow the general safety guidelines to minimize the risk of head injury like:

- Avoid alcohol or drug use while driving
- Always wear seat belts while driving a motor vehicle
- Wear helmets while driving motorcycle/bikes and while playing contact sports like skiing, skating or riding a horse, etc.
- Install side rails/hand rails in bathrooms/wash rooms and both sides of staircases
- Keep the stairs and floors clear of clutter
- Improve the lighting in the home and nearby vicinity
- Get regular vision check-ups

IX. Lifestyle Changes to Prevent Cardiovascular Disease

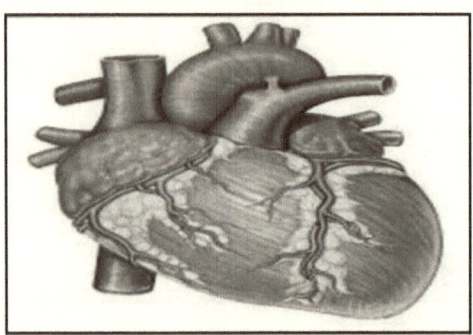

Fig. No. 5(f) 11: *Cardiovascular diseases*

Healthy lifestyle changes can lower the risk of cardiovascular diseases thereby reducing the chance of developing Alzheimer's disease. The occurrence of cardiovascular diseases can be reduced up to 80% by practicing healthy lifestyle modifications[10]. The scientific evidences have demonstrated that the healthy life style factors can prevent or slow the process of development of Alzheimer's disease and other age related cognitive disorders. The healthy lifestyle changes are: 1) eat healthy diet, 2) be physically active, 3) maintain healthy body weight, 4) stop smoking and 5) manage stress.

X. Lower the Homocysteine Level

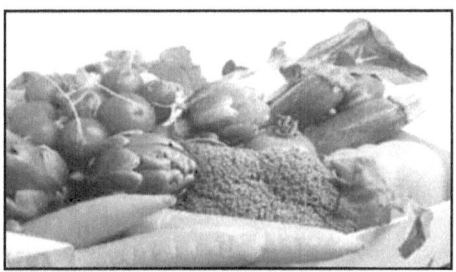

Fig. No. 5(f) 12: *Foods rich in Homocysteine*

It's an amino acid that builds the protein, and higher the level of homocysteine, higher is the risk factor for Alzheimer's disease and cognitive impairment. There is a strong association between hyperhomocysteinaemia and development of Alzheimer's disease. The possibility of occurrence of Alzheimer's disease can be minimized up to 75% by lowering the homocysteine concentrations[11].

Foods rich in folate and vitamin B12 have been shown to lower the homocysteine levels. The active form of folate – L methylfolate may improve up to 700% higher than synthetic folic acid; therefore it is more effective in lowering the homocysteine levels[12]. Thus the food which is rich in these vitamins is recommended daily. Such food items are: spinach, broccoli, green leafy vegetables, cauliflower, beetroots, potatoes, fortified cereals, fish, red meat, poultry, eggs, etc. Regular consumption of these food items minimizes the homocysteine level; thereby it reduces the risk of Alzheimer's disease.

'Alzheimer's disease: With awareness, there is hope'

Scientific Evidence: 04

Study on comparing the effect of a functional task exercise program to a cognitive training program in older adults (>60 years) with mild cognitive impairment. The duration of exercise programs was 10 weeks, and the outcome measures were carried out on 6 months follow up. The results showed that between the groups the functional task exercise group showed significant differences in general cognitive functions, memory, executive function, functional status and everyday problem solving ability. The improvements were sustained over time at 6 month follow up. The trial affirms that the functional tasks exercise program is feasible, cost effective for improving cognitive functions and functional status of older adults with mild cognitive impairment[13].

Scientific Evidence: 05

Effects of physical activity on cognitive impairment were studied as a five year follow up study among 4,615 individuals. It was observed that high levels of physical activity are associated with a 42% reduction in the risk of cognitive impairments in the future, suggesting that increased physical activity improves brain health. Similarly, high levels of physical activity were associated with a 50% reduction in Alzheimer's risk and a 37% reduced risk of dementia from any other cause. At the population level, it was observed that more than 1 in 7 cases of Alzheimer's disease could be prevented if everyone who is currently inactive were to become physically active at a level consistent with current activity recommendations. It is evident that physical activity is associated with a reduced risk of cognitive impairment[14, 15].

Scientific Evidence: 06

Engaging with more mentally stimulating activities such as reading, learning new language, playing music, crosswords, puzzles, etc. throughout life is associated with better cognitive function, reduced cognitive decline and a reduced risk of developing dementia. Systematic reviews have shown that those who achieve higher level of education, have more mentally demanding occupations or participate in higher numbers of mentally stimulating leisure activities have around a 50% lower risk of developing dementia[16].

Scientific Evidence: 07

A case control study was done on benefits of a cognitive rehabilitation program (play, assertive training, relaxation techniques, use of memory aids, memory training and motor exercises) in patients (n=28) with mild cognitive impairment. After 4 weeks of intervention results showed significant improvements on activities of daily living, mood, verbal and nonverbal episodic memory. Study demonstrates that patients with cognitive impairment benefit from a cognitive rehabilitation program with regard to activities of daily living, mood, and memory performance[17].

Scientific Evidence: 08

A prospective study was conducted from 1993 to 2000 on 815 elderly to examine whether fish consumption and intake of n-3 fatty acids protect against Alzheimer's disease. Results showed that a total of 131 elderly developed Alzheimer's disease. Elderly who had fish once per week or more had 60% less risk of Alzheimer's disease compared with those who rarely or never ate fish. Alongside, the intake of n-3 polyunsaturated fatty acids was associated with reduced risk of Alzheimer's disease. Results of the study recommend that the dietary intake of n-3 fatty acids and weekly consumption of fish reduce the risk of Alzheimer's disease[18].

Individual Preventive Measures

The preventive strategies adopted at individual level, enables people to have better control over the various determinants of health and thereby improve their health status, well-being and Quality of Life (QOL). It is accomplished by specific protective measures carried out by the people.

a) Consume more omega-3 fatty acids.

It was found that the use of diet rich in omega-3 fatty acids might help to protect the brain against cognitive decline and Alzheimer's disease. It helps to reduce the levels of an unhealthy protein associated with Alzheimer's disease[19]. The omega-3s are rich in foods such as fish and nuts. Along with these, eating well balanced diet, and more plants and fewer animal products are recommended. However avoid unhealthy saturated fats such as dairy foods, meat and butter, etc.

b) Follow good practices to have healthy heart.

The risk factors for hypertension and heart disease are also the risk factors for Alzheimer's disease. Making lifestyle modifications to prevent these diseases may help to prevent another (Alzheimer's). The risk factors include: a) a sedentary lifestyle b) history of smoking c) consumption of unhealthy diet d) high blood pressure e) high cholesterol and f) poorly controlled diabetes.

c) Keep the brain active and life socialized.

It is important to stay healthy throughout life in relation to mental and social aspects. The mental and social stimulation through engaging in activities throughout life reduces the risk of Alzheimer's disease. The following are the activities which help to keep the brain more active and healthy: a) a mentally stimulating job that keeps you interested and active b) advanced education, such as college degrees and extended learning classes c) having friends and engaging in social activities and d) participating in mentally challenging activities such as reading, doing puzzles, video games or playing memory games, etc.

d) Consult the physician for medicine use.

Non-Steroidal Anti-Inflammatory Drugs (NSAIDs) such as Advil and Statin (used to treat high cholesterol and lower the risk of Alzheimer's disease) help to reduce the chance of developing Alzheimer's disease. Try to use these drugs along with multivitamin supplements every day.

e) Use of memory aids.

In day-to-day life, memory aids helps the people who have mild Alzheimer's. A calendar, plan of daily activity, anecdotes on simple safety measures and written directions on use of common household items are the helpful memory aids.

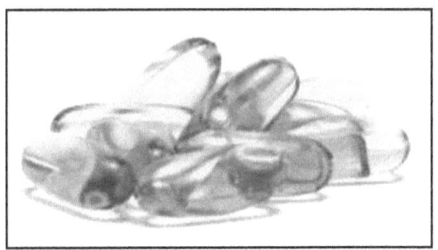

Omega3 fatty acid foods

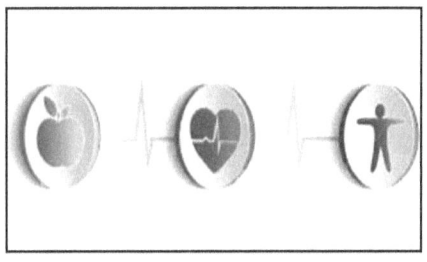

Healthy practices for heart

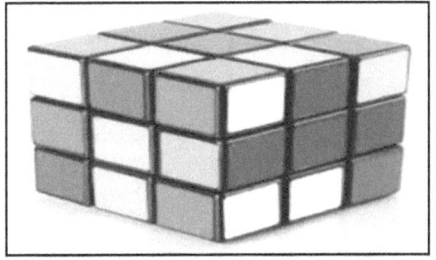

Mentally challenging activity

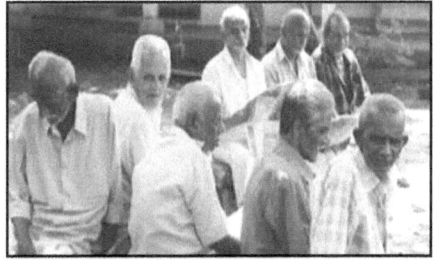

Elderly group (friends)

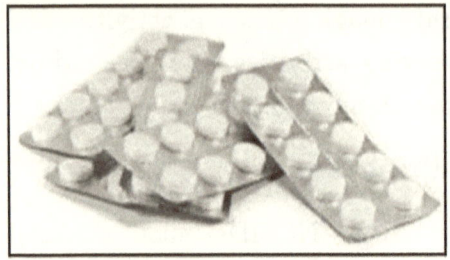 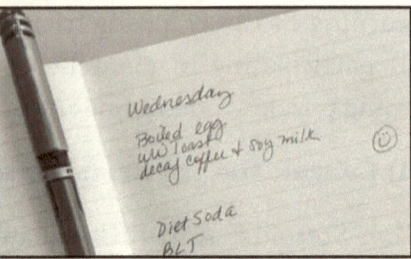

Use of medicines   Use of daily plan/notes

Fig. No. 5(f) 13: *Memory aids*

'Memories matter; fight against Alzheimer's'

Role of Family Members

As there are no cures for Alzheimer's disease, the family and society support is vital and has great significance. As the number of cases is expected to rise drastically the family members are the main care givers and patients need constant support. Most people who have Alzheimer's disease are cared for at home by family members, care givers and home nurses. However, people with mild Alzheimer's disease are involved in planning and organizing the home care activities.

The following are the roles and responsibilities of family members for the prevention and care of Alzheimer's disease person.

I. Home Care

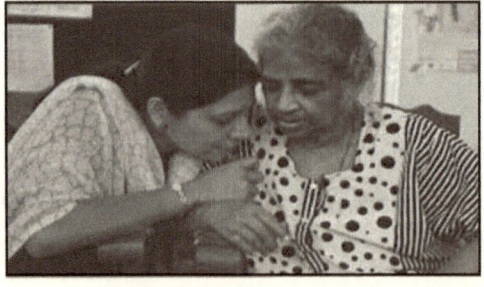

Fig. No. 5(f) 14: *Home care*

- Make sure that the home is safe
- Communicate clearly and loudly (short, simple and familiar words)
- Maintain eye to eye contact and use touch for reassurance and support
- Advice the person to eat well balanced diet with more fruits and vegetables
- Use familiar objects such as chair, vessels or other objects and label the rooms and objects
- Keep routines for daily activities such as meals, baths, hobbies, etc.
- Reinforce and support the person's efforts to remain independent, even if the tasks take more time or aren't done correctly.

II. Managing Behavior

Sleeplessness, wondering, agitation, anxiety and aggression are the common behavioral problems of Alzheimer's disease person. The care giver/family members must identify the triggers for Alzheimer's aggression, and try to follow the below mentioned measures for managing the behavior problems[20].

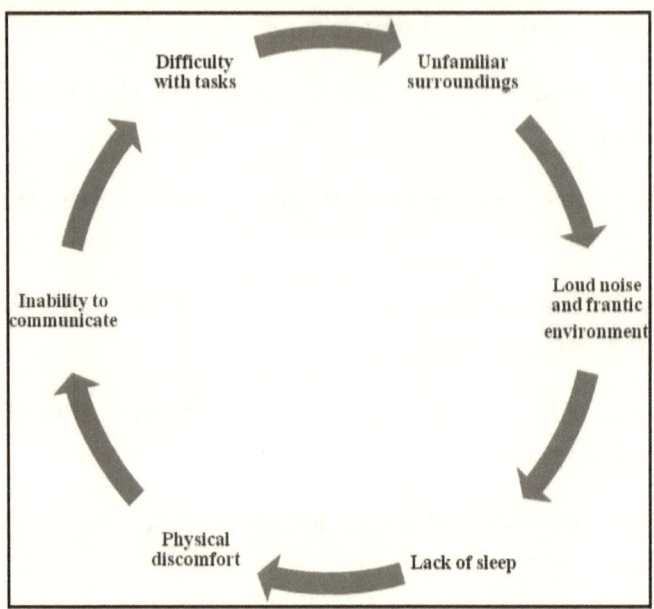

Fig. No. 5(f) 15: *Causes/triggers of aggressive behavior in Alzheimer's disease*

The measures to overcome the behavioral problems of Alzheimer's disease are:

- Be positive and reassuring, and speak with a quiet, soothing voice.

- Repeat the questions or re-explain earlier discussions many times. Don't be aggressive and be patient.

- Keep distractions to a minimum level, try to keep noise level low, and develop simple routines for bathing, dressing, eating and other routine activities.

- Identify and remove or avoid any source of agitation such as pictures, objects, music, TV shows, etc. (which disturbs the person).

- In case of wandering, lock outside doors, and use alarms and other devices to alert caregiver and others when the person wanders outdoors or into unsafe areas.

- Provide a safe place for wandering, such as an enclosed yard or garden.
- Notify neighbors and others of Alzheimer's disease person's tendency to wander and provide your phone/mobile number for help and assistance, in case of missing or emergency.
- Do not confront the person or don't try to discuss the angry behavior; and instead distract the person to a more pleasurable topic or activity.
- Try to get help from others.

> **'Follow 3Rs – Repeat, Reassure and Redirect'**

III. Managing Sleep Problems

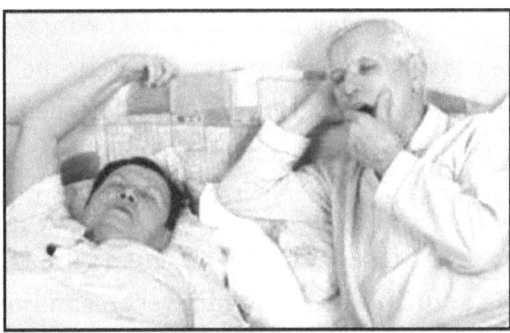

Fig. No. 5(f)16: *Sleep problems*

The normal sleep wake cycle is often affected with brain disorders; similarly Alzheimer's disease patients may exhibit wakefulness, disorientation, confusion, and insecurity at night time.

To overcome these sleep problems try to follow the below mentioned measures:

- Improve the sleep hygiene: Provide a comfortable bed, try to minimize the noise and light, and play smooth music to help them to fall asleep.

- Keep a regular sleep schedule: Always be consistent with the timing of sleeping and keep the nighttime routine the same. Provide bath and warm milk before the bed time.

- Keep a night lamp on: Individuals suffering from dementia imagine things in the dark and become upset. Keeping the night lamp on and keeping a pet may also help soothe the patient and allow them to sleep.

- Place a commode next to the bed: Always keep the bedside commode in the bedroom for nighttime urination. Walking to the washroom in the middle of the night (sleeping hours) may wake up the person too much, and then he can't get back to sleep.

- Increase physical activity: It is recommended that the physical activity during the day time needs to be increased, thereby it helps the person to feel more tired at bedtime and go to sleep. However if the person feels very much fatigued during day time try to provide short naps during the day (keep in mind that too much day time sleep may increase the insomnia).

- Limit the tea/coffee: Limit the patient's caffeine intake such as tea, coffee, and other carbonated beverages and junk foods during the day.

- Encourage exercise: Encourage him to perform some kind of physical activities before the bed time which enhances the induction of sleep.

IV. Managing Depression

In Alzheimer's disease, apathy, lack of motivation and depression are the commonly reported problems. The patient may sit alone for a long period of time staring blankly, further he may have anger, irritability, and frequent crying spells, which suggest the presence of depression. **The following are the simple and comprehensive tips which can help you to manage the depression and other related symptoms.**

- Acknowledge the person's feelings and grieving, etc.
- Always try to engage the person in his favorite activities.
- Encourage the person to remember the pleasant past memories/events.
- Play music with a strong tempo, and encourage the person to clap and involve in it.
- Use simple humor, such as a book of jokes or TV comedies to lighten things up for both patient and caregiver.
- Visit to health care professional if the person shows manifestation of depression.
- Involve the person in elderly care program that engages the person in appropriate activities.

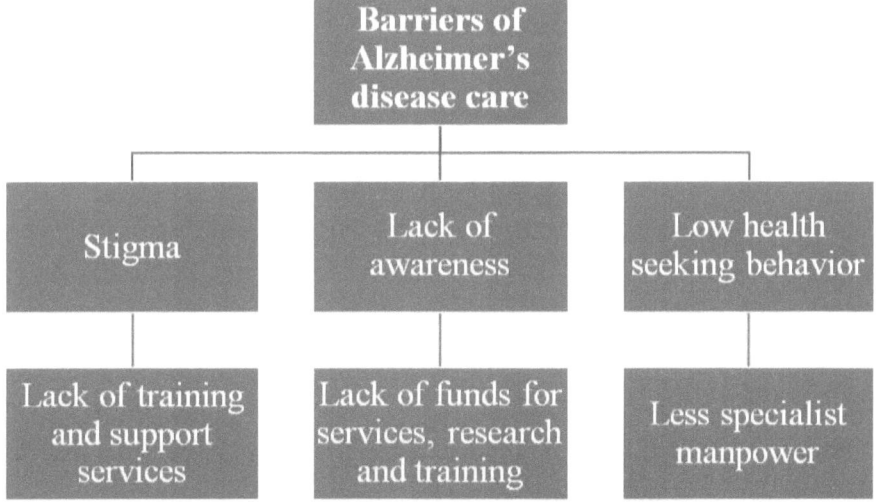

Fig. No. 5(f) 17: *Barriers of Alzheimer's disease care*
Source: Dementia India Report 2010

'Say NO to Alzheimer's disease; it's time to take it down'

Tips to prevent Alzheimer's disease risk:

- Exercise regularly
- Eat a healthy balanced diet rich in fruits and vegetables
- Engage in social and intellectually stimulating activities
- Control diabetes
- Lower the high blood pressure level
- Lower high blood cholesterol level
- Maintain a healthy body weight (BMI)
- Stop smoking
- Get treatment for depression

Conclusion

The biological phenomenon of aging process is universal, aging and health have a variety of socio cultural determinants. In 2012, World Health Organization has declared dementia a public health priority. Due to the aging of the world population the number of patients with Alzheimer disease will rise significantly. Currently India has huge burden of people with Alzheimer's and dementia. If no treatment is available, this will be a major health issue with enormous financial burdens to health care systems. Thus, there is an urgent need for both early recognition, diagnoses with specific markers as well as appropriate treatment, and effective therapies to be undertaken at different stages of the disease.

Though specific treatment is not readily available for Alzheimer's disease, the disease severity and its impact can be controlled effectively by following a variety of preventive strategies as mentioned above. The prevention and control of Alzheimer's disease enhances the individual's well-being, health, Quality of Life (QOL), Activities of Daily Living (ADL), survival and cost of care, etc. The family members and care givers play a pivotal role in managing the disease at home and health care settings. It was widely acknowledged that the family is the primary support for elderly people with Alzheimer's disease.

Key Points

- Alzheimer's disease is a chronic, progressive and irreversible brain disorder of the elderly.

- It commonly affects memory, thinking, cognition and ability to carry out activities.

- The incidence rate increases substantially with age, and affects 50% of persons over the age of 85.

- The cause of Alzheimer's disease is unknown, however accumulation of protein called amyloid in the brain is suspected to play a role.

- Along with aging factor, genetic factors, diabetes, hypertension and others also contribute significantly for occurrence of Alzheimer's.

- The impact of Alzheimer's disease or dementia on the individual, family and society will increase exponentially in terms of the burden, disablement and costs of care.

- The common warning signs of Alzheimer's disease are: memory loss, difficulty in performing familiar tasks, problems with language, disorientation to time and place, poor or decreased judgment, problems with abstract thinking, misplacing things, changes in mood or behavior, changes in personality, and loss of initiative.

- Alzheimer's disease is diagnosed when: 1) a person has sufficient cognitive decline to meet criteria for dementia 2) the clinical course is consistent with that of Alzheimer's disease 3) no other brain diseases or other processes are better explanations for the dementia.

- The management of Alzheimer's disease consists of medication based and non – medication based treatments. Families are the main carers and they need support and training.

- Family members/caregivers play a significant role in managing and prevention of Alzheimer's disease and its symptoms.

- Create more awareness on Alzheimer's disease among the general public and health care professionals.

- Along with existing evidence, there is a need of more epidemiological and clinical research in treatment and prevention of Alzheimer's disease.

- Awareness, quality education and training, research and strong political will are the central causes to achieve the goal, i.e., commitment to Alzheimer's disease care.

References

1. Canadian study of Health and Aging Working Group. Canadian Study of Health and Aging: study methods and prevalence of dementia. Can Med Assoc J, 1994; 150: 899–913.

2. Launer LJ, Anderson K, Dewey ME, Letenneur L, Ott A, Amaducci LA et al. Rates and risk factors for dementia and Alzheimer's disease. Results from EURODEM pooled analysis. Neurology, 1999; 52: 78–84.

3. Shaji S, Bose S and Varghese A. Prevalence of dementia in an urban population in Kerala, India, British Journal of Psychiatry, 2005; 186: 136–140.

4. Schofield PW, Tang M, Marder K, Bell K, Dooneief G, Chun M et al. Alzheimer's disease after remote head injury: an incidence study. J Neurol Neurosurg Psychiatry, 1997; 62: 119–124.

5. Kaur J, Garnawat D, Bhatia MS and Sachdev M. Rehabilitation in Alzheimer's disease – Psycho physiotherapy. Delhi psychiatric journal, 2013; 16 (1): 166–71.

6. Geda YE. Physical exercise as a preventive or disease modifying treatment of dementia and brain aging. Mayo clinic Proc, 2011; 86 (9): 876–84.

7. Geda YE, Robert RO and Knopman. Physical exercise and mild cognitive impairment – A population based study. Arch Neural, 2010; 67 (1): 80–86.

8. Pandav RS and Blit JV. Exercise level and cognitive decline. Alzheimer's disease Assoc Disord, 2004; 18: 57–64.

9. Yan – Jiang Wang. Vascular risk factors promote conversion from mild cognitive impairment to Alzheimer's disease. Neurology, 2011; 76 (17): 1485–1491.

10. Buttar SH, Timao Li and Ravi N. Prevention of cardiovascular diseases: Role of exercise, dietary interventions, obesity and smoking cessation. Exp Clin Cardiol, 2010; 10 (4): 229–249.

11. Morris MS. Homocysteine and Alzheimer's disease. Lancet Neurol. 2003; 2 (7): 425–28.

12. Heijer M, Brouwer IA, Bos GM, Blom HJ, Vander Put NM, Spaans AP, Thomas CS et al. Vitamin supplementation reduces blood homocysteine levels: A controlled trial. Arterioscler Thromb Vasc Biol, 1998; 18 (3): 356–61.

13. Law LF, Barnett F, Yau MK, Gray MA. Effects of functional tasks exercise on older adults with cognitive impairment at risk of Alzheimer's disease: a randomized controlled trial. Age and Ageing, 2014: 1–8.

14. Balsamo S, Willardson JM, Frederico S, Prestes J, Balsamo DC, Dahan CNet al. Effectiveness of exercise on cognitive impairment and Alzheimer's disease. International journal of general medicine, 2013; 6: 387–91.

15. The Role of Physical Activity in the Prevention and Management of Alzheimer's disease – Implications for Ontario. Ontario Brain Institute, 1–18.

16. Scarmeas N, Levy G, Tang MX, Manly J and Stern Y. Influence of leisure activity on the incidence of Alzheimer's disease. Neurology, 2001; 57: 2236–2242.

17. Kurz A, Pohl C, Ramsenthaler M and Sorg C. Cognitive rehabilitation in patients with mild cognitive impairment. Int J Geriatr Psychiatry, 2009; 24 (2): 163–68.

18. Morris MC, Evans DA, Bienias JL, Tangney CC, Bennett DA, Wilson RS et al. Consumption of fish and n-3 fatty acids and risk of incidence of Alzheimer's disease. Arch Neurol, 2003; 60(7): 940–46.

19. Sifferlin A. Study: Eating Omega-3s may help reduce Alzheimer's risk. Alzheimer's disease, 2012, available at http://healthland.time.com/2012/05/03/eating-omega-3s-may-help-reduce-alzheimers-risk/retrieved on 20.02.2016.

20. Xiao – Ling Li, Nan Hu, Shan Tan, Tai Yu and Lan Tan. Behavioral and psychological symptoms in Alzheimer's disease. Bio Med Research International, 2014; 1–10.

Chapter V (G)

Preventive Strategies for Mental Health Disorder

Dr. K Lalitha & R Rajalakshmi

Introduction

The consideration of individuals with mental and psychological issue is a developing general health concern. These disorders profoundly have common and high passionate toll on people, families and society. The health care delivery system is trying to improve the health of society but due to the low resources, it is difficult to achieve completely. Counteractive preventive action of emotional instability and the advancement of psychological well-being prosperity may imply a decent utilization of existing assets. From the time mental hygiene development started in the twentieth century, numerous thoughts have been created on conceivable methodologies to forestall behavioral problems and mental disorders in kids and grown-ups. It is perceived that mental and neurological disorders, including Alzheimer's illness is a huge reason for morbidity and worldwide non-communicable disease burden, for which there should be some necessary preventive actions.

Epidemiology

World Health Organization found that globally more than 450 million individuals experience the ill effects of mental health problems. Right now mental and behavioral disorders represent around 12% of the worldwide burden of illnesses. This is likely to increase to 15% by 2020. Significant extents of mental disorders originate from poor and moderate economic countries. There are lacunae in psychiatric epidemiology due to under reporting, stigma, absence of satisfactory financing and trained labor and low priority of mental health in the health policy.

Table No. 5(g) 1: Mental Illness Statistics

S.no	Mental illness	Millions/Total population
1	All Mental disorders	80 m
2	Chronic mental illness(CMDs)	60 m
3	Child/Adolescent disorders	20 m
4	Mood Disorders	18 m
5	Alcoholism	10 m
6	Epilepsy	0.5 m
7	Schizophrenia	0.2 m
8	Geriatric disorders	0.3 m
9	Mental retardation	0.1 m

Source: Mental Illness Statistics in India National Mental Health Program: 2015 Projections by Ministry of Health and Family Welfare, Govt. of India

Mental Illness

The American Psychiatric Association (APA 2000) defines a mental disorder as "a clinically significant behavioral or psychological syndrome or pattern that occurs in an individual and is associated with present distress or disability or with a significantly increased risk of death, pain, disability, or an important loss of freedom." General criteria to determine mental disorders include disappointment to have one's attributes, capacities, and achievements, ineffective relationship with others, disappointment with one's place on the world, insufficient adapting to life occasions, and absence of self-improvement. Moreover, the individual's conduct must not be socially anticipated or authorized (APA, 2000).

Risk Factors of Mental Illness

Common Social, Environmental and Economic Risk Factors

- Easy access to some drugs and liquor in living area
- Feeling of loneliness in the individual life
- Absence of education, transport, lodging because of the low financial status
- Facing frequent problems in the neighborhood
- Peer dismissal because of numerous reasons
- Poor social circumstances in the living range
- Poverty and inadequate nutrition in the regular life
- Racial shamefulness and sexual differences in the work place and society.
- Stress due to continuous urbanization and industrialization in the country
- Increased violence and wrongdoing and terrorism in the society.
- Problem related to unemployment in the youths and stress in the work place.

Individual Risk Variables

- Scholastic difficulties and poor academic performance
- Taking care of chronically ill patients
- Abused and neglected person
- Persons suffering from sleep deprivation
- Continuous suffering from pain
- Pregnancy in young age

- ➤ Abused children, adolescents and senior citizens
- ➤ Lack of emotional maturity
- ➤ Over usage of substances
- ➤ Introduction to hostility, brutality and injury
- ➤ Disorganized family
- ➤ Feeling lonely for a long time
- ➤ Living in low socio-economic background
- ➤ Suffering from chronic illness
- ➤ Parental dysfunctional behavior
- ➤ Parental substance misuse
- ➤ Perinatal psychological issues
- ➤ Any kind of loss in the life and unpleasant life occasions
- ➤ Poor work abilities and propensities
- ➤ Physical disabilities or physically challenged
- ➤ Incompetence in social skills

Chronological Classification of Etiological Factors

- ➤ **Predisposing factors** These are the factors which will make the person vulnerable to develop the mental illness, for example, genetic endowment, operative childhood period, eternal deprivation and broken families.

- ➤ **Precipitating factors** – These will occur just before the onset of illness such as loss of job, financial difficulties, death of loved one and natural disaster, etc.

- ➤ **Perpetuating factors** – These factors will prolong the illness after the onset also, e.g. low self-esteem, continued family issues and chronic physical illness.

Diagnostic Evaluations

The psychiatric illness will be identified through the general physical examination along with neurological examination and mental status, mini mental status examination. Further, hospital laboratory will be utilized for diagnostic procedures. Indicative lists of laboratory investigations are as follows:

Laboratory Investigations

- Hb, TLC, DLC, Platelet count
- Bleeding Time, Clotting time
- Fasting/PP blood sugar
- Lipid profile
- Serum electrolytes
- Liver Function Test
- Kidney Function Test
- Thyroid function test
- HIV testing
- VDRL
- Urine routine & Urine Sugar
- Drug level estimation
- Genetic and endocrine examination

Radiological Investigation

With the new methods, other than old or conventional modalities, it has been possible to not only anatomically visualize but also functionally evaluate the tissues or organs. Chest X-ray, Ultrasound,

Magneto encephalography, Positron Emission Tomography/CT and Electromagnetic imaging are the added radiological investigations to rule out brain pathology for mental disorders. Current advanced MRI modalities that can be used in addition to routine examinations include high resolution imaging (3Tesla), functional magnetic resonance imaging(f-MRI), perfusion MRI (p-MRI), diffusion-weighted imaging (DWI), diffusion tensor imaging(DTI), and magnetic resonance spectroscopy (MRS). It is aimed to review the functional or micro anatomical structure or metabolite changes in brain and imaging of the psychiatric disorders.

Psychological Tests

In order to assess the psychiatric symptoms, levels of stress, personality traits, cognitive functioning and psychodynamics, psychological tests are carried out.

Following are some psychological tests done in the mental health arena.

- Anxiety self-rating scale
- **Beck's** anxiety scale
- **Beck's** depression scale
- Binet Kamat test of intelligence
- Bhatia battery of intelligence
- Clinical global impression
- Child behavior checklist
- **Cattel's** 16 factor personality inventory
- CAGE questionnaire
- Extra pyramidal symptom rating scale

- Eysenck personality inventory
- Global assessment of functioning scale
- Hamilton anxiety scale
- Hamilton depression scale
- Insight and treatment attitude questionnaire
- Manic state rating scale
- Marital satisfaction inventory
- Nurses observation for inpatient evaluation (NOSIE)
- NIMHANS neuropsychological battery of lobe dysfunction
- Positive and negative symptom scale for schizophrenia
- Psychiatric symptom check list
- Rorschach inkblot test
- Wechsler intelligence scale for children
- Suicide intent scale
- Social adjustment scale
- Thematic apperception scale
- Wechsler adult intelligence scale
- Yale brown obsessive compulsive scale

Signs and Symptoms of Mental Illness Organic Mental Disorders

Delirium

Persons suffering from Delirium have disturbances in consciousness and cognition, disorientation, problems in reviewing particularly the memory and time, created over a brief time frame. It is characterized by the following features

   a. Easily diverted
   b. Difficulty in concentration
   c. Perceptual disturbances (visual and auditory)
   d. Decreased level of consciousness
   e. Difficulty in speech
   f. Fearful and anxious

Dementia

It is a dynamic, steady, and lasting subjective disability which prompts numerous permanent intellectual shortages; basically memory debilitation happens. It includes no less than one of the accompanying:

- Aphasia (disintegration of speech or dialect capacity)
- Apraxia (hindered capacity to execute motor activities)
- Agnosia (powerlessness to name or perceive objects)
- Echolalia (repeating the heard words) and Palilalia (repeating words or sounds again and again)

Substance Abuse Disorder

Substance misuse is a maladaptive use of liquor or medications. It might prompt dependence, tolerance, and withdrawal state in person. Regularly utilized psychotropic substances are liquor, opioid, cannabis, cocaine, amphetamines, Hallucinogens, tranquilizers and hypnotics such as barbiturates, unstable solvents, nicotine and stimulants, for example, caffeine. A man with this issue will proceed with the substance use in spite of destructive impacts to health, way of life or partners.

Some of the common signs and symptoms of various substance abuse disorders.

Alcohol Abuse

Malaise, mood swing, poor personal hygiene, tendency to blame others, maladaptive behavior, psychosomatic changes, inapt sexual and aggressive behaviors, impaired judgment, slurred speech, incoordination, insecure step or walk, disabled consideration and memory.

Sometimes patients may have the simple withdrawal symptoms to delirium tremens when they stop the alcohol. It is characterized by mild tremors, nausea, vomiting, weakness, irritability, insomnia and anxiety, to vivid hallucination, sever psychomotor agitation, dehydration, rise of blood pressure, papillary dilatation, hyperthermia, cardio vascular collapse and death. Alcohol induced amnestic disorder will occur due to prolonged use of alcohol which leads to vitamin B deficiency followed by **Wernicke's** syndrome (peripheral neuropathy) and **Korsakoff's** syndrome with gross memory loss and poor attention. Prolonged usage of the alcohol further induces in human beings psychiatric illness such as psychosis and neurosis and sexual disorders.

Other Substance Use Disorders

Opioids, cannabis, Cocaine, Amphetamine, Lysergic acid diethylamide, Barbiturates, Inhalent or volatile solvents are considered to be some other substances used by people.

Opioid Use Disorders

People who have acute intoxication of opioid may show the following features

- ➢ Respiratory depression
- ➢ Hypotension

- ➢ Subnormal temperature
- ➢ Pinpoint pupils.

Cannabis Use Disorder

- ➢ Alteration in psychomotor activity
- ➢ Flashback
- ➢ Lacrimation
- ➢ Dry mouth

Cocaine Use Disorder

Acute intoxication from cocaine leads to papillary dilatation sweating, hypertension, tachycardia and hypomania.

Amphetamine Use Disorder

Acute intoxication from Amphetamine leads to hyperpyrexia, panic, paranoid hallucination, papillary dilatation, sweating, hypertension, tachycardia and hypomania.

LSD Use Disorder

LSD use disorder is characterized by depersonalization, derealization, illusion, paranoid ideation.

Barbiturate Use Disorder

Abusing of barbiturates leads to reduction of memory, slurred speech and liability of mood.

Inhalants or Volatile Solvent Use Disorder

Using of inhalant or solvent by human being results in slurring of speech, belligerence, excitement and euphoria as some of the neurological disturbances.

Schizophrenia

Schizophrenia is diagnosed as a psychotic disorder. As indicated by the WHO classification, a few types of schizophrenia and manifestations can be distinctive relying upon which type a person has, for example, disturbance in thought process, perception and affect. A person having schizophrenia may have decline in social and occupational functions.

Types of Schizophrenia and its Symptoms

Paranoid Schizophrenia

- Detachment
- Suspiciousness
- Hostility and delusions
- Anxiety and anger
- Fearfulness
- Aggression
- Hearing unusual sounds or voices

Disorganized Schizophrenia

- Intense social withdrawal
- Confused speech or unusual and unwanted behaviors
- Flat or improper affect
- Stereotyped practices
- Excessive facial expression
- Maladjustment with daily activities

Catatonic Schizophrenia

- Stupor
- Waxy flexibility
- Major psychomotor reduction
- Reduction in usual mobility
- Automatic obedience
- Stereotyped or repetitive behavior
- Repetition of heard words (Echolalia)
- Excessive purposeless motor actions

Undifferentiated Schizophrenia

Undifferentiated schizophrenia is another sort of schizophrenia. It may not fulfill the criteria of previously said types of schizophrenia

- Delusions and perceptual disturbance (visual or auditory)
- Jumbled speech
- Disorganized or Catatonic behavior
- Complete flattening of the mood
- Withdrawal behavior from the society

Residual Schizophrenia

Residual schizophrenia has the criteria of significant past history of schizophrenia, along with severe decline in social interaction and role functions.

Some Common Disturbances of Schizophrenia

- Alteration in visual or auditory perceptions
- Repetition of words, phrases or expressions

- Absence of verbal communications
- Patient will derive some meaningless words
- Believing that someone else is taking away the thoughts
- Patients believe that others can hear their thinking or thoughts
- Persistent thought that others are inserting the thoughts inside the brain.

Unusual Motor Activities

Akathisia: Displaying motor apprehension and solid trembling; the patient can't sit or lie in the same place.

Dyskinesia: Reduction in the physical movement.

Mood Disorders

This is a state of mental illness, in which patients have lot of mood variations, which may influence the physical, mental and social working of a person. Classifications of mood disorders are Unipolar Depression, Bipolar Mania Depression, and Period of normal mood.

Unipolar Disorder: This is a kind of depression and its signs and symptoms are as below:

- Changes in sleep pattern (too much or too little)
- Unable to concentrate and take decisions
- Loss of self-esteem (hopelessness, helplessness)
- Sad mood or lack of interest in life for 2 or more weeks
- Change in appetite (increase or decrease)
- Suicidal Ideation

Bipolar Disorder

This is a condition in which cyclic mood changes will take place. A person may experience manic episodes, periods of profound depression, and times of normal behavior in between. This occurs equally in both the genders.

Clinical Course of Mania

Episode of unusual, grandiose, or agitated mood lasting at least one week with 3 or more of the following symptoms:

- Decreased need for sleep
- Irritability towards others
- Inflated self-esteem
- Pressured speech
- Flight of ideas
- More activities with increased energy
- Distractibility

Anxiety Disorders

Anxiety disorders are sometimes related with depression, eating disorders, and frequent hospitalization. They are also linked to genetic, social, and environmental factors. Persons with anxiety disorders may have a risk of developing the habit of drinking alcohol and other substance use disorders. Some of the common physiological and psychological symptoms of anxiety disorders are given below:

Physiological Responses

- Increased respiration rate and pulse rate due to increased level of adrenaline secretion
- Pupils will be dilated for better vision
- Flight or fight responses may occur
- Blood vessels will be constricted in peripheral circulation, which leads to skin being cool and pale
- Increased level of arterial blood pressure leading to increased heart rate
- Increased level of glycogenolysis process to raise free glucose for energy

Psychological Responses

- Behavioral changes
- Thought disturbances
- Agitation
- Increased motor activity

Panic Disorders

Described as repetitive, sudden panic attacks take place after a month of constant concern or stress over having another attack. One episode of panic attack may last 15–30 minutes in which a patient encounters fast, exceptional, raising tension, inconvenience and physiological and psychological discomfort.

Phobias

An illogical, intense, persistent fear of a specific object or social situation that causes extreme

Distress and interferes with having a normal life. Phobic disorders can be divided into 3 types as follows:

- ☐ Social Phobia, in which strong persisting fear of an interpersonal situation like embarrassment may occur
- ☐ Specific Phobias, in which patient may have fear towards closed space (Claustrophobia), Fear of height (Acrophobia), Fear of marriage (Gamatophobia), etc.
- ☐ Agoraphobia, in which a person will have fear while being alone in a public place

Obsessive Compulsive Disorder (OCD)

Obsessive compulsive disorder is portrayed by repeated interfering unnecessary thoughts that appear to be difficult to control, connected to ritualized conduct or behavior.

Obsessive thoughts: Recurrent considerations, thoughts, perceptions, or wrong driving forces that irritate a man's life; has no power over them.

Compulsive behavior: Behaviors or customs like washing the hands, forgetting about it over and again, praying constantly, which are aimed at pushing out the obsessive thoughts and lessening tension.

Post-Traumatic Stress Disorder

Post-traumatic Stress Disorder is caused by encountering a compelling traumatic occurrence, for example, a robbery or mischance; yet PTSD additionally may happen when a man has been "in relationship with an interpersonal stressor" over a timeframe.

Side effects of PTSD happen inside 3 months or more after the injury. PTSD is portrayed by outrage, anger, and blame, detachment from others, weeping and not having any desire to discuss the unpleasant occasion, bad dreams, etc. and manifests in physiological side effects (GI trouble) such as being irritable and having insomnia. Later they may mishandle substance.

Somatoform Disorders

Somatization implies transference of mental thoughts and states into physical reactions. Somatoform disorders are portrayed as the nearness of physical manifestations that recommend a therapeutic condition without obvious natural premise to account completely for them.

The 3 focal elements of somatoform issue are as per the following

- Repeated physical problems recommend significant therapeutic illness, however there are no supportable findings.
- Emotional factors and clashes appear to be critical in the beginning, become worse, and maintain the symptoms.
- Warning sign or improved well-being concerns are not under the patient's present cognizant control.

The 5 Particular Somatoform Issues Are as Detailed Below

1. **Somatization Disorder:** Characterized by various physical reactions. It starts by 30 years of age, reaches out more than quite a while, and has aches and GI, sexual, and pseudo neurologic problems.

2. **Conversion Disorder:** Involves unexplained, generally sudden shortfalls in sensory or motor activities.

3. **Pain disorder:** Pain disorder is the essential physical manifestation which is for the most part unrelieved by analgesics and significantly influenced by mental elements regarding onset, seriousness, intensification, and support.

4. **Hypochondriasis:** Preoccupation with the apprehension that one has a genuine infection (illness conviction) or will get a genuine ailment (sickness fear).

5. **Body dysmorphic disorder:** Preoccupation with an envisioned or misrepresented imperfection in individual appearance; for example, supposing one's nose is too vast or teeth are slanted and ugly.

Eating Disorders

The identifying element of eating disorders is found frequently with the adolescent age group. There will be persistent worry and embarrassment about weight gain, hence patients may not follow proper and regular dietary pattern in order to maintain or to reduce the weight.

Anorexia Nervosa

An existence undermining dietary problem described by the patient's refusal or failure to keep up a negligibly ordinary body weight, extreme apprehension of putting on weight or getting to be fat, altogether irritated view of the shape or size of the body, and undaunted powerlessness or refusal to recognize the reality of the issue or even that one exists. The defining symptoms are:

- ☐ Lose weight basically through eating less, fasting, or exorbitantly working out.
- ☐ Not eating enough nourishment and supplements to renew cells.

- ☐ Has experienced amenorrhea for no less than 3 sequential cycles.
- ☐ Paleness in the eyes and all over body.
- ☐ Decreased level of blood pressure, temperature and pulse rate.
- ☐ Elevated level of blood urea and nitrogen.
- ☐ Decreased level of protein in the body.
- ☐ Frequent experience of difficulty in passing stool due to hardness and pain.
- ☐ Inability to tolerate the coldness.

Bulimia Nervosa

Bulimia is commonly analyzed in the age group of late adolescents with the characteristics of eating more or binge eating, and following that evacuating inappropriately through purging by using laxatives, diuretics, enemas and emetics, in order to reduce the energy absorption in the body and to reduce the weight.

Sexual Disorders

Sexual issues are any sort of issues earlier to, while performing, or after the sexual contact. It might be physiological or psychological in nature. Sexual dysfunction disorder can be portrayed as a debilitation or unsettling influence in any of the periods of the sexual reaction cycle. These include not being interested in having sex with partner, no arousal or enjoyment or having genital pain during coitus. Some other problems are gender identity disorder with psychological feelings characterized by persistent discomfort with one's own sexual identity, paraphilias, repetitive or preferred sexual fantasies or behaviors that involve preference for use of a nonhuman object, or repetitive sexual activity with humans involving real or simulated suffering, or repetitive sexual activity with non-consenting partners. (APA 2000)

Personality Disorders

Personality disorders are characterized as a grid of persevering attributes and dispositions of a person that decide a man's change in accordance with nature.

Table No. 5(g) 2: Types of Personality

Type of Personality	Symptoms
Paranoid	Doubtfulness and non-trusting behavior
Schizoid	Detached social behavior
Schizotypal	Magical thinking, social isolation and perceptual distortion.
Antisocial	Lack of concern for others, violation of laws and rights of others, aggressive behaviors
Borderline	Unstable emotional relationship, suicidal threats
Histrionic	Attention seeking and Dramatic
Narcissistic	No feeling of empathy, continuous need of attention.
Dependent	Unable to take decisions and clinging
Avoidant	Low self-esteem, fearful of rejection
Obsessive compulsive	Follows ordering and arranging, unable to relax, over concerned with laws and rules and regulations.
Passive aggressive	Stubborn, not responding to the demand

Child and Adolescent Disorders

Psychiatric disorders in children are not recognized as effectively because of negligence and carelessness. Child and adolescent disorders are briefed here for understanding.

Mental Retardation

Significant subnormal general impairment of intellectual functioning is noted with marked reduction of adaptive behaviors during the developmental period. In youngsters mental retardation is categorized based on their intelligence quotient. There are 4 sorts of mental retardation. They are mild, moderate, severe and profound.

- Mild mental retardation: IQ 50–70
- Moderate mental retardation: IQ 35–50
- Severe mental retardation: IQ 20–35
- Profound mental retardation: IQ under 20

Common Signs and Symptoms of Mental Retardations

- Developmental delay in milestones, impaired intellectual function, poor schooling performance, difficultly in performing self-care and daily activities, reduction of psychomotor activities, communication and language problems.

Disorder

Children with autistic disorder may have difficulty in communication; usually children with autism disorder have restricted repetitive stereotyped behavior and make peculiar sounds or shout in order to express their feelings. Most commonly found in boys; recognized no later than 3 years old.

Signs and Manifestations

- Children with autistic disorder have poor eye to eye contact
- Changes in facial experience
- Lack of experience during communication
- Child will not maintain relation with guardians or companions, lack of delightfulness, clear nonattendance of disposition and passionate effect, can't be occupied with play
- Repetitive behaviors, for example, hand-fluttering, body bending, or head slamming

Attention Deficit Disorder

Attention deficit hyperactive disorder is portrayed by absentmindedness, hyperactivity, and rashness during any kind of activity. It is frequently analyzed when a child begins schooling. There are 3 sorts, first is predominantly inattentive, second is predominantly hyperactive – impulsive, and third is combination of both. Children with first type normally have poor attention and lack of interest to do the task, are easily distracted, may forget easily also. A hyperactive – impulsive type child will not sit in a place, will be very restless, cannot remain in the same place, and will frequently disturb others. In kids, this issue is frequently unnoticed.

Conduct Disorder

The Conduct Disorder is frequently noticed in children and adolescents, with maladaptive behaviors which may violate rules and regulation and rights of others. This behavior is learned from peers, family members or social surroundings. "It is characterized by persevering withdrawn conduct in kids and youths that fundamentally weakens their capacity to work in social, scholarly, or word related zone."

Clinical Manifestations

- Aggression to individuals and creatures.
- Destructive behaviors like destroying others' property.
- Dishonesty and robbery from inside of the family and outside of the family.
- Having the behavior of violating rules and regulation.
- Altered self-esteem and lack of realization in life.
- Inability to tolerate the frustrations.
- Early onset of sexual conduct, liquor and substance misuse, smoking, risk-taking behavior.

- Antisocial behavior and poor scholastic performance.
- Committing more crimes even after getting punishment.

Oppositional Defiant Disorder

Repetitive negativistic behavior, rebellious, insubordinate, and unfriendly conduct towards higher authorities that persists for no less than 6 months," ODD is characterized by losing temper, contending, disobedience, irritating others, accusing others, being furious, angry, resentful or malicious. It comprises of a continuing example of uncooperative, rebellious, and antagonistic conduct towards power figures without major reserved infringement. A specific level of oppositional conduct is regular in youngsters in immaturity. Oppositional disobedient turmoil is analyzed just when practices are more incessant and extraordinary than in unaffected associates and cause brokenness in social, scholastic, or work circumstances.

Elimination Disorder

Encopresis: It is characterized by repeated passing of fecal matter in inappropriate places like clothes and places other than toilet.

Enuresis: Repeated voiding of urine during the day or night into clothes or bed by a child, not less than 5 years old.

Common Treatment

Pharmacological Treatment

Antipsychotic Drugs

- Known as narcoleptics, such drugs are used to treat the symptoms of psychosis, such as the delusions and the hallucinations seen in schizophrenia, schizoaffective disorder, and the manic phase of bipolar disorder.
- Antipsychotics work by blocking receptors of the neurotransmitter, dopamine.

- Dopamine receptors are classified into subcategories (D1, D2, D3, D4, and D5), and D2, D3, and D4 have been associated with mental illness.

- The typical antipsychotic drugs are potent antagonists (blockers) of D2, D3, and D4. This makes them effective in treating target symptoms but also produces many extra pyramidal side effects because of the blocking of the D2 receptors.

- Newer, atypical antipsychotic drugs such as clozapine (Clozaril) are relatively weak blockers of D2, which may account for the lower incidence of extra pyramidal side effects.

- The newer antipsychotics also inhibit the reuptake of serotonin, increasing their effectiveness in treating the depressive aspects of schizophrenia.

Table No. 5(g) 3: List of Antipsychotics

Typical Antipsychotics	Usual Dosage(mg/day)
Chlorpromazine	50–1200
Thioridazine	150–800
Trifluoperazine	5–40
Thiothixine	5–60
Fluphenazine	☐ Oral: 2–20 ☐ Intramuscular: 12.5–250mg
Haloperidol	☐ Oral: 2–60 ☐ Intramuscular: 5–30 ☐ Depot: 50–250mg repeated 4 weeks once
Atypical Antipsychotics	
Clozapine	300–900
Resperidone	2–8
Olanzapine	10–20
Qutiapine	150–800
Aripiprazole	10–60

Problems Associated with Antipsychotics

Extrapyramidal reactions

(EPS) are the real symptoms of antipsychotic medications. They incorporate severe dystonia (increased muscular tone and involuntary movements), pseudo Parkinsonism, and akathisia (urge to move about). Blockage of the D2 receptors in the midbrain area of the brain stem is the cause for advancement of EPS. Some of the other problems during the EPS are:

Contorted head and neck (**Torticollis**) – Snugness of the whole body with head back and a curved neck (**Opisthotonus**), eyes moved in a bolted position (**Oculogyric emergency**)

Prompt treatment with anticholinergic medications as per rule brings quick alleviation.

Pseudo Parkinsonism or medication impelled Parkinsonism frequently occurs along with EPS. The symptoms include stiff, stooped posture, mask like face, shuffling festinating gait, drooling, tremor, brady cardia. Treatment of these manifestations can incorporate including an anticholinergic specialist or amantadine, which is a dopamine agonist that improves transmission of dopamine hindered by the antipsychotic drug.

Neuroleptic Malignant Disorder

(NMS) is a conceivably deadly eccentric response to an antipsychotic. Death rates have been accounted for at 10% to 20%. Manifestations of Neuroleptic malignant disorder incorporate unbending nature, high fever, autonomic instability, for example, unstable blood pressure, diaphoresis, and pallor, delirium, altered level of enzymes and electrolytes.

Fluid level alteration, poor nutrition, and some of the medical illness also leads to NMS.

Treatment incorporates cessation of the antipsychotics and the foundation of strong restorative consideration to treat lack of hydration and hyperthermia.

Tardive Dyskinesia

Tardive Dyskinesia (TD) is caused by prolonged use of Antipsychotics with involuntary movement. This is most generally brought on by the long haul utilization of antipsychotic medications. There is no treatment accessible. The side effect of TD incorporates automatic involuntary movement of the tongue, facial, and neck muscles, upper and lower lips. Projections of the tongue, lip smacking, flickering, frowning, and other over the top superfluous facial developments are trademark. Once TD has occurred, it is irreversible.

Agranulocytosis

A few antipsychotics produce agranulocytosis. This grows all of a sudden and is portrayed by:

- ☐ Fever
- ☐ Malaise
- ☐ Ulcerative sore throat
- ☐ Leucopenia

The medication must be stopped promptly if the WBC drops by half or to under 3,000.

Antidepressant Drugs

In spite of the fact that the mechanism of activity is not totally comprehended, antidepressants, in some way or other connect with the 2 neurotransmitters, norepinephrine and serotonin. Frequently used antidepressants are mentioned below.

Antidepressants Are Separated into 4 Gatherings

Table No. 5(g) 4: List of Antidepressants

Tricyclic and the related cyclic Antidepressants	☐ Imipramine	☐☐ 50–300mg/day
	☐ Trimipramine	☐☐ 50–600mg/day
	☐ Clomipramine	☐☐ 75–250mg/day
	☐ Amitriptyline	☐☐ 50–300
	☐ Doxepin	☐☐ 25–300
	☐ Nortriptyline	☐☐ 25–100
Selective serotonin reuptake inhibitors (SSRIs)	☐ Fluoxetine (Prozac)	☐☐ 20–80mg/day
	☐ Escitalopram (Lexapro)	☐☐ 10–30mg/day
	☐ Fluvoxamine (Luvox)	☐☐ 50–300mg/day
	☐ Citalopram (Celexa)	☐☐ 20–60mg/day
	☐ Sertraline (Zoloft)	☐☐ 50–200mg/day
	☐ Paroxetine (Paxil)	☐☐ 20–50mg/day
MAO inhibitors (MAOIs)	☐ Phenelzine	☐☐ 45–90mg/day
	☐ Tranylcypromine	☐☐ 30–60mg/day
	☐ Isocarboxazid	☐☐ 20–60mg/day
Other antidepressants	☐ Venlafaxine (Effexor)	☐☐ 75–225mg/day
	☐ Bupropion (wellbutrin)	☐☐ 150–450mg/day
	☐ Duloxetine (cymbalta)	☐☐ 30–120mg/day
	☐ Trazodone (desyrel)	☐☐ 150–600mg/day
	☐ Nefazodone (Serzone)	☐☐ 200–600mg/day

MAOIs have an existence-debilitating symptom; hypertensive emergency may happen if the patient ingests foods which contain tyramine (an amino corrosive) while taking MAOIs.

- ➢ Mature or aged cheeses
- ➢ Aged meats (sausage, pepperoni)
- ➢ Tofu
- ➢ Beers and microbrewery beer
- ➢ Sauerkraut, soy sauce, or soybean condiments
- ➢ Yogurt, sour cream, peanuts

MAOIs cannot be given in mix with different MAOIs, tricyclic antidepressants, Demerol, CNS depressants, and hypertensive or general analgesics. MAOIs are conceivably deadly in overdose and represent a potential danger for customers with discouragement who might consider suicide. SSRIs, venlafaxine, nefazodone, and bupropion are frequently better decisions for the individuals who are possibly self-destructive or very imprudent, in light of the fact that they convey no danger of deadly overdose as opposed to the cyclic mixes and the MAOIs. SSRIs are most effective medications for mild to moderate sadness.

The significant activities of antidepressants are with the monoamine neurotransmitter frameworks in the cerebrum, especially norepinephrine and serotonin. Norepinephrine, serotonin, and dopamine are expelled from the neurotransmitters after discharge by reuptake into presynaptic neurons. After reuptake, these 3 neurotransmitters are reloaded for consequent discharge or metabolized by the protein MAO.

The SSRIs block the reuptake of serotonin; the cyclic antidepressants and venlafaxine block the reuptake of norepinephrine primarily and block serotonin to some degree; and the MAOIs interfere with enzyme metabolism.

Mood Stabilizing Drugs

Mood stabilizing medications are utilized to treat bipolar disorder by settling the mood of the patients. These medications are especially given in the case of mania. Lithium is viewed as the main line specialist in the treatment of bipolar disorder. Lithium standardizes the reuptake of specific neurotransmitters, for example, serotonin, norepinephrine, acetylcholine, and dopamine. It additionally diminishes the release of norepinephrine through rivalry with calcium. Lithium delivers its effects intracellularly instead of inside neuronal neurotransmitters.

Lithium serum levels ought to be around 1.0 mEq/L. Levels under 0.5 mEq/L are occasionally helpful, and levels of more than 2 mEq/L are generally viewed as toxic. On the off chance that Lithium levels surpass 3.0 mEq/L, dialysis might be indicated. Valproic acid and topiramate are known to increase the levels on the inhibitory neurotransmitter GABA. Both are thought to balance out thought by repressing the kindling procedure.

Table No. 5(g) 5: Mood Stabilizing Drugs

Names	Usual Dosage(mg/day)
Lithium carbonate	900–1500 (Acute stage), 900–1500 (Maintenance)
Carbamazepine	600–1200
Sodium Vaporate	1000–3000
Lamotrigine	300–500
Gabapentin	900–1800

Anti-Anxiety Drugs (Anxiolytics)

To reduce the anxiety in patients with general anxiety disorder and other mental health disorders, Barbiturates like Phenobarbital, secobarbital and thiopentone are given as anti-anxiety drugs. Benzodiazepines intervene in the activities of the amino acid GABA, the major inhibitory neurotransmitter in the cerebrum. These anxiolytic drugs are used even during surgical procedures and while giving ECT.

Anti-Anxiety Drugs (Anxiolytics)

Table No. 5(g) 6: List of Anxiolytics

Diazepam	2–40mg/day
Lorazepam	2–6mg/day
Clonazepam	0.5–6mg/day
Alprazolam	0.25–1mg (in 3 divided dose)

Stimulants

The essential utilization of stimulants is in children with ADHD. Sometimes, even for adolescents and adults who have residual attention deficit disorder and narcolepsy, stimulants are given for therapeutic purpose. Stimulants usually act over amines and cause release of the neurotransmitters; they also help in blocking the reuptake of these neurotransmitters, to help convey electrical impulse in the brain.

Non-Pharmacological Therapies

In non-pharmacological therapy patients with psychological problems will be treated with psychological measurement, with or without medication. The non-pharmacological therapy includes psychotherapy, positive reframing, assertive training, Electro convulsion therapy.

Psychotherapy

Psychotherapy is treatment given to psychiatric patients having psychological problems by the mental health professionals to alleviate distressing symptoms. Psychotherapy also modifies the behavior pattern of the patients who have maladaptive behavior and it promotes personality growth.

The psychotherapy is based on the numbers of the persons; it can be given for the individual person as individual therapy, while group psychotherapy will be given to patients who have similar kind of problem. Patients and family both will be treated during family therapy. Another therapy is marital therapy, in which couples are treated with psychotherapy. Psychotherapy is of various types, as follows:

- ➤ Psychodynamic psychotherapy in which therapy is based on psychoanalytical theory by focusing on early life experiences and relationships, which will lead to problem being resolved.

- ➤ Behavior therapy is working based on learning theory, in which are covered relaxation therapy, systemic desensitization, graded exposure, flooding, shaping, modeling, token economy, and aversion therapy.

- ➤ Cognitive behavior therapy is based on principles of psychoanalysis, cognitive psychology and behavior psychology. In which the current problem of the patient will be resolved by correcting the negative thoughts.

- Interpersonal therapy is based on the interpersonal theory in which human behavior is shaped by 2 drives that are drive for satisfaction and drive for security.

- Humanistic therapy, in which the therapist facilitates the patient to understand him or herself. Therapist helps the patient to understand his or her self-worth.

- Milieu therapy provides good and conducive environment for the patient to acquire adaptive coping skill. In Milieu therapy overall life experience and its coping mechanism is taught by the therapist in non-threatening environment.

- Group therapy is given based on the problems of the patients. Therapists have important role in this to identify the problems of the patients who have similar problem and various problem solving methods used by everyone. Here, the therapist will help the patient and family to identify the support groups and self-help group.

- Family therapy and marital therapy focus on the problem of the whole family based on the interpersonal relationship within the family members and couples.

Electro Convulsion Therapy

Electroconvulsive therapy (ECT) is a procedure in which generalized seizures are induced by passing a small amount of electrical current through the brain by using electrodes in scalp regions. The clinical indication includes life-threatening events such as suicide and catatonia. Patients to whom this is administered are those who express violence, poor response or intolerance to the drugs, and during first trimester in the pregnant mothers who are having mental illness.

Psychosocial Therapy

Psychosocial interventions were defined as any intervention that emphasizes psychological or social factors rather than biological factors (Ruddy and House, 2005). This definition allows for the inclusion of psychological interventions and health education, as well as interventions with a focus on social aspects, such as social support. Interventions with a physiological component in addition to a psychosocial component are also considered.

Nursing Therapy

Mental health nurses need to face a lot of challenges during health care delivery by responding to the social demands, providing education, promoting and preventing mental illness. Mental health nurses are also responsible for identifying the vulnerable group or populations, risk factors for mental illness, early treatments and rehabilitations in institutions and community. They provide care through collaboration with client, family, multidisciplinary team of mental health professionals and Community health care workers.

Alternative Therapy

Complementary and Alternative Medicines (CAM) includes a broad range of non-medical materials used for treatment or prevention. CAM is one way of treating illness that has developed outside the mainstream of modern medicine. Many are traditional remedies that have developed in different cultures over centuries. They include herbal medicines, foods, nutritional supplements, such as vitamins and minerals, Yoga, prayers, meditation. All these treatments can be used on their own, or with conventional medicine. Many CAMs have been used for mental health problems, but there is little good evidence to support their use.

Preventive Approaches for the Individuals and Group to Stop Psychological Ill Health

To advance emotional well-being, and prevent the mental illness with dysfunctional behavior there is a need to make great environment and living conditions that will bolster psychological well-being and keep up a sound way of life. Health care system needs to concentrate more on preventing mental illness as in the case of existing projects which are followed to prevent and treat HIV, tuberculosis, maternal and child health problems, sexual and reproductive problems. As per the objective of the national mental health program, mental health services are supposed to be merged with general health services.

Goodyer & Altham, (1991) found that negative life events such as the death of a parent, parental separation or divorce, or any kind of psychological trauma (e.g., exposure to violence, natural disaster) play a major causal role in the development of internalizing disorders. Family characteristics may be at higher risk for these disorders either through genetic transmission or, as social learning theory would suggest, through social modeling and reinforcement.

Khrone and Hock (1991) conducted the study and found that over controlling or overprotective parenting practices contribute to childhood anxiety by negatively impacting children's ability to learn problem solving skills.

Hains and his colleagues **(Hains, 1992; Hains & Ellmann, 1994; Hains & Szyjakowski, 1990)** designed a school-based prevention program (Stress Inoculation Training I) to reduce negative emotional arousal and other psychological problems associated with stress.

Eggert and her colleagues found that school-based intervention programs are a solution to prevent suicide. Barrett, Rapee, Dadds, and Ryan suggest that compared to nonclinical parents, anxious parents may be the role model for their children to perceive threat in ambiguous situations and utilize avoidant solutions to solve social problems.

Prevention strategies can be effective in preventing and reducing severity of some mental illnesses, such as depression, schizophrenia, childhood disorder and post-traumatic stress disorder. Additionally, good prevention strategies can delay the onset of mental illness and support treatment outcomes while treatment is in progress. The preventive approaches are based on primary, secondary and tertiary preventions as follows.

Table No. 5(g) 7: Preventive Strategies

S. No.	Preventive Strategies	At Hospital	At Community
1	**Primary prevention** It means, taking action before behavioral health problems occur, rather than waiting to intervene after symptoms appear or incidents occur.	Health education towards general health and mental health and risk factors identification at hospitals.	Community health workers provide population-based education to prevent mental illness for risk group like family with mental illness, poor access to health care, pregnant adolescent, substance abusers, children with behavioral problems and destitute women and elders.
2	**Secondary prevention** It refers to reducing the frequency or severity of the mental disorder.	Here measures are used to limit the disease process through screening, early diagnosis and prompt treatment of mental disorder. Case management through supportive therapy, illness management, education about drug therapy, client and family psycho education about information on illness, principles of management and treatment, improvement towards medication compliance, stress management and coping skill.	Screening of mental disorders, early diagnosis and prompt treatment of mental disorder would be done through district mental health team and national mental health team. Case management through supportive therapy, illness management, education about drug therapy, client and family psycho education about information on illness, principles of management and treatment will be based on community-based rehabilitation program.

S. No.	Preventive Strategies	At Hospital	At Community
3	**Tertiary prevention** This aims to reduce long term disability through rehabilitation with the goal of getting back the pre-illness functional level	The task here is reconstruction of the client ego strengths through vocational rehabilitation, in which specialized services such as counseling and vocational training, development of adequate work tolerance, social skills, job finding, selecting job placement and adequate vocational follow-up services will be made available.	A multidisciplinary clinical team Approach (Assertive Community Treatment) of providing 24-hour intensive community services in the individual's natural setting that help individuals with serious mental illness live in the community. Following are some of the community care facilities for rehabilitation of chronic mentally ill. Residential facilities like Quarter way Homes, Half Way Homes. Nonresidential facilities like day care centers, ASHA, CHETANA, Richmond Fellowship etc.

Based on the proposal of **Gordon (1983, 1987),** the IOM (Institute of Medicine) report replaced the primary, secondary and tertiary preventive strategies to universal, selective, and indicated preventive strategies.

Universal preventive intervention targets the general public or a whole population group that has not been identified on the basis of individual risk. It includes prenatal care, childhood immunization, and school-based competence enhancement programs. Because universal programs are positive, proactive, and concentrate on independent risk status, participants feel minimum stigma and they may be more ready to accept and adapt with the training programs.

Selective preventive intervention targets individuals or subgroups (based on biological or social risk factors) whose risk of developing mental disorders is significantly higher than average. Examples of selective intervention programs include: home visitation and infant day care for low birth weight children, preschool programs for all children from poor neighborhoods, and support groups for children who have suffered losses/traumas.

Indicated preventive intervention targets individuals who are identified as having prodromal signs or symptoms or biological markers related to mental disorders, but who do not yet meet diagnostic criteria. Providing social skills or parent-child interaction training for children who have early behavioral problems are examples of indicated preventive interventions.

General Preventive Strategies Based on Universal, Selective and Indicated Preventive Strategies

The investigators, specialists, strategy and approach makers have built up a more sensible point of view on the fundamental power and breadth of programming to avoid psychopathology and elevate positive advancement to prevent emotional instability or mental illness. Following are some of the principles underlying preventive strategies:

- ☐ To make a prevention approach of mental issue as a general well-being need.
- ☐ Mental disorders have numerous determinants, preventive action should be a multipronged exertion.
- ☐ Effective prevention can decrease the danger of mental health problems.
- ☐ Implementation of strategies should be based on evidence. Successful projects and arrangements ought to be made broadly accessible.
- ☐ Knowledge on confirmation for adequacy needs further extension.
- ☐ Prevention should be based on the culture and available resources.

- ☐ Population-based results require human and money related speculations.
- ☐ Multidisciplinary, collaborative and team work will enhance the preventive strategy.
- ☐ Protecting human rights is a best way to prevent mental disorders.

Common Preventive Measures Based on Developmental Phases

Based on the universal, selective and indicative prevention, following are some of the common interventions in order to prevent mental illness.

- ☐ Proper evidence-based perinatal care needs to be provided to prevent postnatal depression and postnatal psychosis.
- ☐ Deprived women need to be supported in psychosocial aspects.
- ☐ Health visiting by family welfare personnel and reducing post natal depression.
- ☐ Encourage parent-child bonding and good parenting to prevent childhood behavioral problems.
- ☐ Parenting for children with persistent conduct disorders.
- ☐ Training of the teachers towards identification of learning disability in early childhood.
- ☐ Identify the children with dyslexia and educate the teachers towards management of children with dyslexia.
- ☐ School-based social and passionate administration expertise, improvement in learning projects to avoid conduct issues in childhood.
- ☐ Educating educators towards epilepsy and its administration.

- ☐ School-based instructive projects to diminish tormenting and kid misuse.
- ☐ School and school-based life aptitude administration and sex instruction for kids and young people.
- ☐ Screening system to recognize the behavioral issues in the schools and universities to counteract suicides.
- ☐ Conducting suicide counteractive action program in instructive establishment and corporate work zones.
- ☐ Early discovery of psychosis and early intercession for psychosis.
- ☐ Screening and brief intercession in liquor abuse.
- ☐ Workplace screening for melancholy and nervousness issue.
- ☐ Promoting well-being in the work place.
- ☐ Population level suicide mindfulness preparation and meditation.
- ☐ Bridge safety measures for suicide prevention.
- ☐ Collaborative care for depression in people with Type II diabetes, Carcinoma and HIV.
- ☐ Tackling the unexplained side effects.
- ☐ Regular psychological well-being screening for the individuals with liquor and other substance misuse, and individuals who are having hereditary risk like offspring of mentally sick and kin of mentally sick.
- ☐ Strengthening social backing amidst the emergency circumstances after a disaster.
- ☐ Enhance the backing towards elderly, which may forestall late onset psychosis and other emotional sickness.

Family Role in Prevention of Mental Illness

- ☐ Understanding each and everyone in the family and neighborhood.

- ☐ Development of harmonious relationship within family and society to maintain good environment at home and society. Enhancing the mother and child bonding from the childhood.

- ☐ Avoid over protectiveness to develop independencies in children.

- ☐ Educate the children towards assertiveness and positive thoughts and moral values in the basic life.

- ☐ The behavioral and educational techniques are used to help families in order to identify mental illness and cope with and handle the stress and difficulties of interacting with a mentally ill family member. The Government and Non-Governmental association will enhance this.

- ☐ Behavioral family management can be considered rehabilitative, that is tertiary preventive aspect, because it equips all members of the family, including the individual who has a mental disorder, with knowledge, skills, and supports to function better in daily life and to reach their own personal goals.

Role of Government and Non-Government as Stake Holders in Prevention of Mental Illness

- ☐ Government needs to create enabling environments that reduce stigma and discrimination, promote human rights, and improve the quality and quantity of a full range of services from education, health and social services through poverty alleviation initiatives and support people with mental and psychosocial disabilities to access the resources they need and to integrate into the community.[27]

- ☐ Academic institutions can generate the capacity of policy makers, planners and service providers from different sectors such as health, education and the judiciary in the area of mental health. Generate and synthesize research to improve policy for mental health.

- ☐ International agencies can advocate for the inclusion of mental health in national development and sectoral plans. Ensure that targeted projects to improve developmental outcomes address the needs of people with mental health conditions.

- ☐ Multilateral organizations can advocate for (i) the relocation of mental health issues in national agendas, (ii) the proper and necessary allocation of adequate resources to mental health, (iii) the ratification and implementation of Convention on the Rights of Persons with Disabilities, (iv) the recognition of people with mental and psychosocial disabilities as a vulnerable group, and (v) for mental health to be mainstreamed into sectoral policies.

Conclusion

Prevention of mental illness has a lot of profit, ranging from progress in individuals' well-being to optimistic economic and social changes. Prevention of these disorders is obviously one of the most effective ways to reduce the disease burden through the implementation of effective evidence-based interventions.

Key Points

Epidemiology: The division of medical science concerned with the occurrence, transmission, and control of epidemic towards mental health disorders. WHO projected that internationally over 450 million people suffer from mental disorders.

Mental illness: A state of ill health in which the person's mental health is disrupted so that their thinking, emotions or behavior are affected to an extent that it has an effect on their daily personal and social life.

Risk factors: The hereditary, behavioral, environmental factors, or other causes which increase the likelihood of developing a disease or disorder. Some of the chronological classifications of etiological factors are perpetuating factors, precipitating factors and predisposing factors.

Diagnostic evaluations: A type of evaluation with the purpose of discovering exact mental illness such as general physical examination along with history collection, neurological examination and mental status, mini mental status examination, laboratory and radiological investigations. Signs and symptoms of Mental disorder: A clinically significant behavioral or psychological condition or pattern that occurs in an individual and is associated with present distress (e.g., a painful symptom), disability (impairment in one or more important areas of functioning), or with a significantly increased risk of suffering death, pain, disability, or an important loss of freedom.

Treatment: The manner of handling or dealing with a person suffering with mental illness such as pharmacological treatment, non-pharmacological therapies (e.g. cognitive and behavioral therapy, electro convulsion therapy, psychosocial therapy, nursing therapy, alternative therapy.)

Interventions: Interventions are planned to cure or reduce the symptoms or effects of a mental health disorder. It includes psychotherapy such as individual/family/group psychotherapy or other evidence-informed practice offered by an appropriately trained and/or licensed mental health professional.

Early intervention: In which intervention helps to recognize warning signs for mental health problems and to take early action against factors that push individuals at risk. Early intervention can help people get better in less time and can prevent problems from becoming worse.

Cognitive/Behavioral Therapy: A combination of cognitive and behavioral therapies, this approach helps people change negative thought patterns, beliefs, and behaviors so they can manage symptoms and enjoy more productive, less stressful lives.

Behavioral Therapy: The behavioral therapy focuses on behavior – changing unwanted behaviors through rewards, reinforcements, and desensitization. Desensitization, or Exposure Therapy, is a process of confronting something that arouses anxiety, discomfort, or fear and overcoming the unwanted responses.

Prevention Strategies: Prevention strategies can delay the onset of mental illness and support treatment outcomes while treating mental illness. The preventive approaches are based on primary, secondary and tertiary prevention.

Assertive Community Treatment: A multidisciplinary clinical team approach of providing 24 – hour intensive community services in the individual's natural setting that help individuals with serious mental illness live in the community.

References

1. World Health Organization. Emotional wellness and advancement: Targeting individuals with psychological wellness conditions as a helpless gathering. WHO, Geneva. (2010).

2. World Health Organization. The World Health Report. Mental Health: New Understanding, New Hope. Geneva, World Health Organization, 2001.

3. WHO: Disease and harm local evaluations for 2004. Geneva, World Health Organization (http://www.who.int/healthinfo/global_burden_ malady/gauges provincial/en/index.html 22 May 2009). Multi-sectoral Activity Plan on the Prevention and Control of NCD in Nepal 2014–2020.

4. WHO Global NCD Action Plan 2013–2020 and Prevention of Mental Disorders, Effective inclusion and Policy Options, Summary Report, A Report of the World Health Organization, Department of Mental Health and Substance Abuse in a joint effort with the Prevention Research Center of the Universities of Nijmegen and Maastricht.

5. HU Wittchen et al. The size and weight of mental issue and different issue of the mind in Europe 2010. European Neuro psychopharmacology. 2011; 21: 655–679.

6. Sheila l Videbeck, Psychiatric–Mental Health Nursing, fifth edn. Wolters Kluwer Health Lippincott Williams and Wilkins, 2011.

7. Hosman C, Jane-Llopis E and Saxena S, eds. Anticipation of Mental Disorders: Effective and Policy Options. Oxford, Oxford University Press, 2005.

8. American psychiatric affiliation. Diagnostic and measurable manual of Mental Disorders. 4th edn. Washington: American psychiatric press, 2002.

9. World Health Organization. The ICD Classification of Mental and Behavioral Disorders: Clinical depiction and Diagnostic Guidelines, Geneva, 1992.

10. American Psychiatric Association. Rehearse Guidelines for Psychiatric Evaluation of grown-ups. American diary of psychiatry, 1995; 152(11): 67–70.

11. Stuart, GW Psychiatric Nursing fifth edn. St. Louis: Mosby Inc.; 2002.

12. Sadock, B and Sadock, V Kaplan and Sadocks Synopsis of Psychiatry. 7th edn. Philadelphia: Lippincott Williams & Wilkins, 2003.

13. American Psychiatric Association. The act of Electro Convulsive treatment: Recommendations for treatment, preparing, and privileging. 2nd edn. Washington DC: 2000.

14. Limandri, B What's more, Boyd, M. A. Identity and drive control issue. In Boyd, M. A. (ed), Psychiatric nursing: Contemporary practice. Second version. Philadelphia: Lippincott; 2002, pp. 502–55.

15. Liberman RP, Hilty DM, Drake RE and Tsang HWH: Prerequisites for Multidisciplinary Teamwork in Psychiatric Rehabilitation, Psychiatric Services, 2001.52: 1331–35.

16. Liberman RP, Kopelowicz A, Smith TE: Psychiatric recovery, in Comprehensive Textbook of Psychiatry, Seventh Edition. Baltimore, MD, Lippincott Williams and Wilkins, 1999; pp. 3218–3245.

17. Liberman RP, Blair KE, Glynn SM, et al.: Generalization of aptitudes preparing to the common habitat, in Current Status of Schizophrenia Treatment. Altered by Brenner HD, Boker W, Germer R, Toronto, ON, Hogrefe and Huber.2000; pp 175–192.

18. Martin Prince, Vikram Patel, Shekhar Saxena, Mario Maj, Joanna Maselko, Michael R Phillips, Atif Rahman. Lancet 2007; 370: 859–77, Published Online September 4, 2007 DOI: 10.1016/S01406736(07) 61238-0.

19. Barrett PM, Rapee RM, Dadds MR, and Ryan S. Family treatment of youth uneasiness: A controlled trial. Diary of Consulting and Clinical Psychology.1996; 64: 333–342.

20. Eggert LL, Hompson EA, Herting JR & Nicholas LJ. Reducing Suicide Potential among high-hazard youth: Tests of a school-base anticipation program. Suicide and Life-Threatening Behaviour.1995; 25: 276–296.

21. Fendrich, M, Warner, V, and Weissman, MM. Family hazard variables, parental dejection, and psychopathology in posterity. Formative Psychology. 1990; 26: 40–50.

22. Goodyer, IM, and Altham, PM. Lifetime exit occasions and late social and family misfortunes in restless and discouraged school-matured youngsters. Diary of Affective Disorders. 1991; 21: 219–228.

23. Hains, A A Correlation of subjective behavioral anxiety administration systems with youthful young men. Diary of Counseling and Development. 1992; 70: 600–605.

24. Hains, AA, and Ellman, SW Stress immunization preparing as a precaution mediation for secondary school young people. Diary of Cognitive Psychotherapy. 1994; 8: 219–232.

25. Hains, A A and Szyjakowski A psychological anxiety decrease mediation program for young people. Diary of Counseling Psychology. 1990; 37: 79–84.

26. Krohne, HW, and Hock, M (1991) Relationships between prohibitive mother-youngster associations and tension of the kid. Nervousness Research, 4, 109–124.

27. Eckman TA, Wirshing WC, Marder SrR, et al. Strategies for preparing patients in ailment self-administration: a controlled trial. AmJ Psychiatry 149: 1549–1555, 1992.

28. Mark T Greenberg Ph.D. Celene Domitrovich Ph.D. Brian Bumbarger. Anticipating MENTAL DISORDERS IN SCHOOL-AGE CHILDREN: A Review of the Effectiveness of

Prevention Programs, Prevention Research Center for the Promotion of Human Development, College of Health and Human Development, Pennsylvania State University. June, 2000 (changed).

29. Hogarty GE, Anderson CM, Reiss DJ: Family instruction, social abilities preparing and support treatment in aftercare treatment of schizophrenia. Curve Gen Psychiatry. 1986; 43: 633–642.

30. Dixon L, Adams C, Lucksted. An Update on family psycho instruction for schizophrenia. Schizophrenia Bulletin. 2000 26: 5–20.

31. Drake RE, Mercer-McFadden C, Mueser KT, et al.: Review of incorporated psychological well-being and substance misuse issue for patients with double issue. Schizophr. Bull 1998; 24: 589–608. Drake RE, Becker D, McHugo GJ, et al.: A randomized clinical trial of supponed vocation for internal city patients with serious mental issue. Curve Gen Psychiatry. 199956: 627–633.

32. Martin Knapp, David McDaid and Michael Parsonage (editors). Emotional well-being advancement and dysfunctional behavior counteractive action: The financial case. Personal Social Services Research Unit, London School of Economics and Political Science, April 2011. Report distributed by the Department of Health, London.

33. Petrou S, Cooper P, Murray L, Davidson LL Taken a toll viability of a preventive advising and bolster bundle for postnatal melancholy. Global Journal of Technology Assessment in Health Care.2006; 2: 443–453.

34. Paulson JF, Bazemore SD. Pre-birth and post birth anxiety in fathers and its relationship with maternal wretchedness:

a meta-analysis. Diary of the American Medical Association, 2010; 303(19): 1961 1969.

35. World Health Organization. Enhancing mother/tyke association to advance better psychosocial improvement in kids. Geneva, WHO. 1998. WHO/MSA/MHP/98.1.

36. Shochet IM et al. The viability of a general school-based project to anticipate immature dejection. Diary of Clinical Child Psychology, 2001; 30: 303–15.

37. Olds DL et al. Enhancing the life-course advancement of socially impeded moms: A randomized trial of medical caretaker home appearance. American Journal of Public Health, 1988; 78: 1436–1444.

38. Shochet IM et al. The adequacy of a widespread school-based project to counteract adolescent depression and discouragement. Diary of Clinical Child Psychology, 2001; 30: 303–15.

39. Zenere FJ third, Lazarus PJ The decay of youth self-destructive conduct in an urban, multicultural government funded educational system after the presentation of a suicide counteractive action and intercession program. Suicide and Life-Threatening Behavior, 1997; 27: 387–402.

40. Clarke GN et al. A randomized trial of a gathering intellectual mediation for avoiding despondency in juvenile posterity of discouraged guardians. Documents of General Psychiatry. 2001; 58: 1127–1134.

41. Danica Brown Liberman, BA Robert Paul Liberman Involving Families in recovery Through Behavioral Family management, psychservices, psychiatry online, org. 2003; 54(5).

42. World Health Organization. Psychological wellness and advancement: Targeting individuals with emotional well-being

conditions as a helpless gathering. WHO Press, Geneva, 2010. http://www.who.int/mental_health/approach/improvement/en/index.html and http://www.psychiatry.uct.ac.za/mhapp/

43. Anna K Forsman, Johanna Nordmyr and Kristian Wahlbeck. Psychosocial mediations for the advancement of emotional wellness and the counteractive action of sadness among more established grown-ups. Wellbeing Promotion International, 2011; Vol. 26 No. S1.

44. Duzgun Yildirim. Radiologic Imaging in Psychiatric Disorders in the Light of Recent Developments, Psychiatric Disorders – Worldwide Advances, Dr. Toru Uehara (Ed.), 2011. ISBN: 978-953-307-833-5, InTech.

Chapter VI

A Comprehensive Approach to the Prevention and Control of NCDs

Janarthanan B

The rapid rise of non-communicable diseases represents one of the major health challenges to global development in the coming century. This growing challenge threatens economic and social development as well as the lives and health of millions of people. Worldwide, non-communicable diseases (NCD) currently represent 43% of the burden of disease and are expected to be responsible for 60% of the disease burden and 73% of all deaths by 2020. Most of this increase will be accounted for by emerging non-communicable disease epidemics in developing countries. Effective prevention strategies for NCDs do exist. However, they require specific data on risk factors so that priorities can appropriately be set and targeted interventions developed and monitored. The WHO Global NCD Risk Factor Surveillance initiative directly responds to this need. (WHO Report, 2000 – A Global Strategy for prevention & Control of NCD)

To lessen the impact of NCDs on individuals and society, a comprehensive approach is needed that requires all sectors, including health, finance, foreign affairs, education, agriculture, planning and others, to work together to reduce the risks associated with NCDs, as well as promote the interventions to prevent and control them. An important way to reduce NCDs is to focus on lessening the risk factors associated with these diseases. Low-cost solutions exist to reduce the common modifiable risk factors (mainly tobacco use, unhealthy diet and physical inactivity, and the harmful use of alcohol) and map the epidemic of NCDs and their risk factors.

Other ways to reduce NCDs are high-impact essential NCD interventions that can be delivered through a primary health care approach to strengthen early detection and timely treatment. Evidence shows that such interventions are excellent economic investments because, if applied to patients early, they can reduce the need for more expensive treatment. These measures can be implemented at various resource levels. The greatest impact can be achieved by creating healthy public policies that promote NCD prevention and control and reorienting health systems to address the needs of people with such diseases.

Lower-income countries generally have lower capacity for the prevention and control of non-communicable diseases. High-income countries are nearly 4 times more likely to have NCD services covered by health insurance than low-income countries. Countries with inadequate health insurance coverage are unlikely to provide universal access to essential NCD interventions. (Alwan A, Maclean D, 2009)

Thus, should policy makers and communities mobilize "and make prevention and targeted treatment of such diseases a priority," sustainable measures can be implemented to stagnate (and eventually even reverse) this emerging global health threat. Potential measures currently being discussed by the World Health Organization and Food and Agriculture Organization include reducing the levels of salt in foods, limiting inappropriate marketing of unhealthy foods and non-alcoholic beverages to children, imposing controls on harmful alcohol use, raising taxes on tobacco, and curbing legislation to curb smoking in public places. (WHO Report, 2006).

The Need to Control the Emerging Epidemic of NCDs

Governments need to plan to control the emerging NCD epidemics. The economic burden associated with NCDs is increased by expensive modern medical and surgical treatment that is both labor-intensive and technologically sophisticated. Hence, there is an urgent need to prioritize resources for the prevention of non-communicable diseases in the first place. Prevention and control programs require specific goals and quantifiable outcomes to be reached within a defined timeframe. Assessment of progress towards these goals requires surveillance of NCDs and their risk factors.

Prevention through risk factor-focused interventions requires country-specific data on risk factors so that priorities can be appropriately set, targeted programs developed and interventions monitored. For surveillance to inform this process most effectively, data must be collected, analyzed and used in a regular and systematic way. Repeated collection of data on risk factors as surrogate measures of disease can be undertaken to monitor trends.

Focusing and Addressing the Common Risk Factors: An Initial Step in the Prevention and Control of NCDs

Risk factors can be encountered at all ages, and risk-associated behaviors may be adopted early in life. As a result, comprehensive, long-term strategies for control of NCDs must take a life course approach to prevention of risk factor exposure, commencing in early life and continuing with interventions for adults and the elderly. Four of the most prominent non-communicable diseases— cardiovascular disease, cancer, chronic respiratory disease and diabetes—are linked by common preventable risk factors related to lifestyle. These factors are tobacco use, unhealthy diet and physical inactivity.

Action to prevent these diseases should therefore focus on controlling the risk factors in an integrated manner. Intervention at the level of the family and community is essential for prevention because the causal risk factors are deeply entrenched in the social and cultural framework of the society. Addressing the major risk factors should be given the highest priority in the global strategy for the prevention and control of non-communicable diseases. Continuing surveillance of levels and patterns of risk factors is of fundamental importance to planning and evaluating these preventive activities.

Existing Information Pertaining to the Need of Prevention and Control of NCDs

Much is known about the prevention of non-communicable diseases. Experience clearly shows that they are to a great extent preventable through interventions against the major risk factors and their environmental, economic, social and behavioral determinants in the population. Countries can reverse the advance of these diseases if appropriate action is taken. Such action may be guided by the lessons learned from existing knowledge and experience, which are summarized below.

1. A comprehensive long-term strategy for control of non-communicable diseases must therefore necessarily include prevention of the emergence of risk factors in the first place.

2. In any population, most people have a moderate level of risk factors, and a minority have a high level. Taken together, those at moderate risk contribute more to the total burden of non-communicable diseases than those at high risk.

3. Review of studies has shown that, for substantial reductions in the levels of risk factors and in disease outcomes, delivery of interventions should be of appropriate intensity and sustained over extended periods of time. However, even modest changes in risk factor levels will have a substantial public health benefit.

4. The success of community-based interventions requires community participation, supportive policy decisions, intersectoral action, appropriate legislation, health care reforms, and collaboration with non-governmental organizations, industry and the private sector.

5. Decisions made outside the health sector often have a major bearing on elements that influence the risk factors. More health benefits in terms of prevention are achieved by

influencing public policies in domains such as trade, food and pharmaceutical production, agriculture, urban development, and taxation policies than by changes in health policy alone.

6. The long-term needs of people with non-communicable diseases are rarely dealt with success by the present organizational and financial arrangements of health care.

Various Approaches to Prevention of NCDs

In any population, the majority of people have a moderate level of exposure to NCD risk factors and a minority have a high level of exposure. An exposure in this context is either an external risk factor, such as tobacco use, or a physiological condition, such as raised blood pressure. When observed as a whole, the larger, moderate risk group contributes more to the total burden of NCDs than the minority group with higher risk. Comprehensive NCD prevention strategies must take this into account, and blend together 2 types of approaches,

Public health interventions aimed at reducing population level risk factor levels, and Medical interventions targeted specifically at high risk individuals. Both population-wide primary prevention approaches and individual health care strategies are needed to reduce NCDs and their impact. In countries that have achieved major declines in cardiovascular deaths, for example, declines are attributed to reduced NCD incidence rates combined with improved survival after cardiovascular events, due to dual prevention and treatment initiatives. **(Samb B et al, 2010)**

(i) Generating an information base for action

- Assess and monitor mortality attributable to NCD, and the level of exposure to risk factors and their determinants in the population.

- Devise a mechanism for surveillance information to contribute to policymaking, advocacy and evaluation of healthcare.

(ii) Establishing a national program for promotion of health and NCD prevention

- Form a national coalition of all stakeholders including governmental and non-governmental organization.
- Establish pilot prevention programs based on an integrated risk factor approach that may be extended territory-wide.
- Build capacity at the national and community level for the development, implementation and evaluation of integrated NCD programs.
- Promote research on issues related to prevention and management.

(iii) Tackling issues outside the health sector which influence NCD control

- Assess the impact of social and economic development on the burden of the major NCDs with a view to conducting a comprehensive, multidisciplinary analysis.
- Develop innovative mechanisms and processes to help coordinate government activity as it affects health across the various arms of government like coordinating the funds.
- Give priority to activities that place prevention high on the public agenda, and mobilize support for the necessary societal action.

(iv) Ensuring health sector reforms responsive to NCD challenge

- Develop cost-effective healthcare packages and evidence-based guidelines for the effective management of priority NCD W(e.g., Annual NCD screening package).
- Transform the role of healthcare management by vesting managers with responsibility not for institutions

(e.g., hospitals) but for the effective management of resources to promote and maintain the health of a defined population.

Key Commitments

In achieving health for all, new direction is given to health promotion by calling for uniformity in policies across all levels of governments, United Nations bodies, and other organizations, including the private sector. These similar policies across nations will strengthen compliance, transparency and accountability with international agreements and treaties that affect health. **(Source: WHO Global Strategy for Prevention & Control of NCD, WHO, 2000)**

The 4 key commitments which are necessary to promote health are as follows,

- The policies created related to the prevention and control of NCDs should be central to the global development agenda across different countries.

- It should remain as a core responsibility for all of governments

- The process of policy making should be the key focus of communities and civil society

- Policy creation should be made as a requirement for good corporate practice, because corporates serve as a major stakeholder.

The actions which are taken towards the prevention and control of NCDs necessitate sustained advocacy, strong political action and broad participation. All sectors and settings must act to:

- Advocate for health of the public, based on human rights and the imminent needs.

- Invest in sustainable policies, actions and infrastructure to address the basic determinants of health;

- Build capacity for policy development, leadership, health promotion practice, knowledge transfer, research and health literacy;
- Regulate and legislate to ensure a high level of protection and enable equal opportunity for health and well-being for all people; and
- Develop partnership and build alliance with public, private, non-governmental and international organizations and civil society to create sustainable actions, which would last for a long time.

Every country, regardless of the level of its human and financial resources, has the potential to make substantial improvements in NCD prevention and control. To offer a flexible and practical approach to assist ministries of health in balancing diverse needs and priorities, formulating strategies and implementing evidence-based interventions in NCD prevention and control, the WHO has provided a stepwise framework which includes 3 main planning steps and 3 implementation steps.

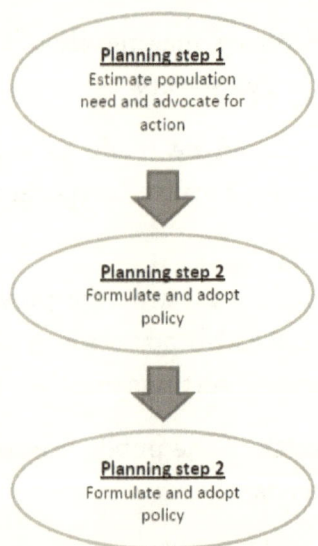

Fig. No.6.1: *The WHO stepwise framework for preventing chronic diseases*

Table No. 6.1: WHO Stepwise Framework

Policy Implementation Steps	Interventions for Individuals
Implementation Step: 1 (Core)	Interventions that are feasible to implement with existing resources in the short term
Implementation Step: 2 (Expanded)	Interventions that are possible to implement with a realistically projected increase in, or reallocation of, resources in the medium term
Implementation Step: 3 (Desirable)	Desirable Evidence-based interventions which are beyond the reach of existing resources

A Global Strategy for Prevention and Control of Non-Communicable Diseases – By WHO

The global strategy has 3 main objectives:

1. To map the emerging epidemics of non-communicable diseases and to analyze the latter's social, economic, behavioral and political determinants with particular reference to poor and disadvantaged populations, in order to provide guidance for policy, legislative and financial measures related to the development of an environment supportive of control.

2. To reduce the level of exposure of individuals and populations to the common risk factors for Non-communicable diseases, namely tobacco consumption, unhealthy diet and physical inactivity, and their determinants.

3. To strengthen health care for people with non-communicable diseases by developing norms and guidelines for cost-effective interventions, with priority given to cardiovascular diseases, cancer, diabetes and chronic respiratory diseases.

Components of Prevention and Control of NCDs

To achieve the above objectives, the following components require the support of the global community and WHO as a whole in order to give shape to a global strategy.

- Surveillance is essential to quantify and track non-communicable diseases and their determinants, and it provides the foundation for advocacy, national policy and global action.

- Promotion of health across the life course and prevention are the most important components for reducing the burden of premature mortality and disability due to such diseases, and are seen as the most feasible approach for many Member States.

- Health care innovations and health sector management that address needs arising from the epidemics are essential. Equally important is the provision of cost-effective and equitable interventions for the management of established non-communicable diseases.

WHO has the unique authority and the clear mandate to lead the development and implementation of the global strategy for the prevention and control of non-communicable diseases and thereby to create a better environment for world health in 2020 and beyond. As outlined below, implementation of the strategy will require action at every level, from global and regional organizations and individual communities.

WHO will focus on the 4 broad interrelated areas described below,

(**Source:** WHO report on Health Resource Financing, 2010)

- **Global partnerships:** WHO will take the lead in strengthening international partnerships for surveillance, prevention and control of non-communicable diseases.

- **Global networking:** A global network of national and regional programs for prevention and control of non-communicable diseases will be established in order to disseminate information, exchange experiences, and support regional and national initiatives.

- **Technical support:** WHO will support implementation of programs at national or any other appropriate level by:

- providing norms and standards, including definition of key indicators of non-communicable diseases and their determinants, diagnostic criteria, and classifications of the major diseases (cardiovascular diseases, cancer, diabetes and chronic respiratory diseases);

- providing technical support to countries in assessing the current situation, identifying strengths and constraints of existing activities, defining appropriate policies, building national capacity, and working to ensure effective programs;

- leading and coordinating surveillance in order to map the epidemic and measure the effectiveness of interventions;

- strengthening and establishing systems for surveillance, and providing technical support for monitoring and evaluating standard indicators of the major risk factors.

- preparing state-of-the-art guidance on development of prevention and control programs, incorporating recommendations based on the knowledge and experience gained on a global scale adapted to different national contexts.

- encouraging development of innovative organizational models for care of non-communicable diseases to ensure the improvement of preventive and clinical care by cost-effective use of available resources.

- foster the launching of pilot projects on prevention and health promotion based on integrated reduction of the 3 main risk factors **(Weingarten SR et al., 2002)**.

  tobacco use,

  unhealthy diet and

  physical inactivity.

The expected outcome is the creation of models in selected countries to demonstrate that community-based programs for risk factor reduction can be effectively implemented in low – and middle-income countries;

- conduct a critical review of the global burden of non-communicable diseases from the view-point of the poor in order to identify control policies that are particularly oriented to poorer populations in developing countries, taking into consideration the likely impact of globalization of trade and marketing on risk factors.

- help patients to manage their own conditions better by assessing and designing appropriate models for self-management education. Emphasis will be laid on diseases that affect women in particular, in order to promote women's health and gender equity.

Strategic support for research and development.

WHO, in close collaboration with other partners like Food & Agricultural Organization, will promote and support research in priority areas of prevention and control, including analytical, operational and behavioral research to facilitate program implementation and evaluation. Special attention will be given to innovative research on issues of poverty, gender, cost-effective care, and genetic approaches to prevention. WHO will strengthen the role of WHO collaborating centers in supporting implementation of the global prevention and control strategy, particularly in coordinating collaborative research. **(Renders CM et al, 2001)**.

National Strategic Framework

Implementation of the global strategy at country or any other appropriate level should be planned along the lines set out below and coordinated within the context of the national strategic framework. **(Lim S S, 2007)**.

Generating a local information base for action.

Assess and monitor mortality attributable to non-communicable diseases, and the level of exposure to risk factors and their determinants in the population. Devise a mechanism for surveillance information to contribute to policymaking, advocacy and evaluation of health care.

Establishing a program for promotion of health across the life course and prevention and control of non-communicable diseases.

Form a national coalition of all stakeholders; develop a national, regional or other appropriate level plan, define the strategies, and set realistic targets. Establish pilot (demonstration) prevention programs based on an integrated risk factor approach that may be extended countrywide. Build capacity at national and community levels for development, implementation and evaluation of integrated prevention programs. Promote research on issues related to prevention and management.

Tackling issues outside the health sector which influence prevention and control of Non-communicable diseases.

Assess the impact of social and economic development on the burden of the major non-communicable diseases with a view to conducting a comprehensive, multidisciplinary analysis. Develop innovative mechanisms and processes to help coordinate government activity as it affects health across the various arms of government. Accord priority to activities that place prevention high on the public agenda, and mobilize support for the necessary societal action.

Ensuring health sector reforms are responsive to the challenge.

Design cost-effective health care packages and draw up evidence-based guidelines for the effective management of the major non-communicable diseases. Transform the role of health care managers by entrusting managers with responsibility not for institutions (e.g. hospitals) but for the effective management of resources to promote and maintain the health of a defined population.

Multi-sectoral action

Experience has shown that community-based NCD programs both inform and support national action towards appropriate policy formulation, as well as legislative and institutional changes. Effective community-based NCD interventions require a number of combined elements at the national level: meaningful community participation and engagement, supportive policy prioritization and setting, multi-sectoral collaboration and active partnerships among national authorities, non-governmental organizations, academia and the private sector.

Decisions made outside the health sector often have a major bearing on factors that influence NCD-related risk. More prevention gains may be achieved by influencing public policies in domains such as trade, food and pharmaceutical production, agriculture, urban development, pricing, advertising, information and communication technology and taxation policies, than by changes that are restricted to health policy and health care alone.

Strengthening health care for people with NCDs

(**Source:** Global policy recommendations, WHO, 2010)

A major challenge in many countries is to promote access to essential standards of health care for people living with NCDs. Effectively managing specific NCDs requires well-functioning and equitable health systems that are capable of providing long-term care that is person centered, community-based and sustainable. The following approaches can be specifically considered by health policy makers in relation to NCDs:

- Ensure that national health strategies and plans are based on accurate situation analysis and include NCD prevention and control as part of the national health priorities.

- Strengthen political commitment to NCD prevention at all levels of government.

- Integrate the delivery of basic health care for NCD prevention and management into primary health care systems.

- Expand the package of essential NCD-related interventions available at the primary healthcare level by including a prioritized and realistic set of high-impact interventions to detect and treat common conditions.

- Address health system gaps, such as by strengthening surveillance systems, strengthening the capacity of the health workforce, and improving access to essential medicines and technology.

- Remove financial barriers to essential health care interventions, such as user fees, and reduce out-of-pocket payments. Consider financing mechanisms including the use of tobacco or alcohol taxation to increase revenues for primary health care.

Incorporating Research

The key research priority areas have been identified in 4 broad domains:

a. research to monitor NCDs and their impact on health and socio-economic development;

b. multi-sectoral and multidisciplinary research to understand and influence the social determinants of NCDs;

c. translational and health system research to a wider implementation of proven cost-effective interventions; and

d. research to enable affordability of high-cost but effective technologies in the context of various resource settings.

Key Points

Prevention and control of non-communicable diseases has become a major challenge for all the countries as the risk factors for these keep increasing. Hence monitoring and surveillance of risk factors is the first step in the prevention of NCDs. The various approaches to prevent non-communicable diseases are generating an information base for action, establishing a national program for promotion of health and NCD prevention, tackling issues outside the health sector which influence NCD control and ensuring health sector reforms responsive to NCD challenge.

References

1. Global strategy for the prevention and control of non-communicable diseases. Geneva, World Health Organization, 2000.

2. Alwan A, Maclean D. A review of non-communicable diseases in low – and middle-income countries. International Health, 2009, 1: 3–9.

3. A prioritized research agenda for the prevention and control of non-communicable diseases. Geneva, World Health Organization, 2010.

4. The Global Health Workforce Alliance: Reviewing progress, renewing commitments: the first progress report on the Kampala declaration and agenda for global action in priority countries. Geneva, The Global Health Workforce Alliance, 2011.

5. Samb B et al. Prevention and management of chronic disease: a litmus test for health-systems strengthening in low-income and middle-income countries. The Lancet, 2010, 376: 1785–1797.

6. Weingarten SR et al. Interventions used in disease management programs for patients with chronic illness-which ones work? Meta-analysis of published reports. BMJ, 2002, 325: 925.

7. Renders CM et al. Interventions to improve the management of diabetes in primary care, outpatient, and community settings: a systematic review. Diabetes Care, 2001, 24: 1821–1833.

8. Lim SS. Prevention of cardiovascular disease in high risk individuals in low-income and middle-income countries: health effects and costs. The Lancet, 2007, 370: 2054–2062.

9. The world health report 2010: Health system financing. Geneva, World Health Organization, 2010.

10. The world health report 2006: Working together for health. Geneva, World Health Organization, 2006.

11. Increasing access to health workers in remote and rural areas through improved retention. Global policy recommendations. Geneva, World Health Organization, 2010.

12. Global code of practice on the international recruitment of health personnel. Geneva, World Health Organization, 2010.

13. Outcome statement of the second global forum on human resources for health. Geneva, Global Health Workforce Alliance, 2011.

Chapter VII

Trajectory Model for Chronic Diseases

*Prof. (Dr.) Usha Ukande ** Mrs. Shweta Pattnaik

Introduction

Health and illness are part of the human experience. Unfortunately, most people have encountered or know someone who has been diagnosed with a chronic illness at some point in their lives. As nurses, we often encounter chronic illnesses when caring for patients. Nurses must learn how patients experience chronic illness, and what the best ways to care for those patients are. The transition and trajectory theories are important for nursing care because they frame a patient's experience with and progression through the stages of chronic illness. Chronic illnesses are serious diseases which could last the whole life of the concerned person affecting the person's mental, emotional and social well-being.

Trajectory means "a course of illness over time plus the actions taken by patients, families and health professionals to manage or shape the course." The term "trajectory" refers to the course of a chronic disease in its different stages and phases.

It is the description for a holistic, case accompanying nursing system, with one permanent caregiver that includes the patient's biography (his life story) and his social field in chronic and very serious courses of the disease. The patient is seen as an active partner in health, prevention, disease and rehabilitation. Hereby the involved nursing person supports the patient in his independence, self-help and self-determination, and helps to enable him to live an as much as possible "normal" life. She assists him to gain access to the resources of health and social facility benefits, she offers providing continuum and she accompanies him custodially during the whole case history. The model intends to transfer the "Case Management" into practice.

Historical Evolution of (Trajectory Model) Theory

The Trajectory model particularly considers the situation of people with chronic diseases. Its application is based on empirical research which has been carried out for a period of approximately 30 years in terms of grounded theory. Among other things job related praxis of nursing persons and their experience in nursing of patients with different chronic diseases as well as the subsequent practical application of this model to these patients (with Cancer, Cardio vascular diseases, HIV, AIDS, Diabetes mellitus) was observed during this research project.

Basic Concepts and Relationships

As nurses, we often encounter chronic illnesses when caring for patients. Nurses must learn how patients experience chronic illnesses and the best ways to care for those patients. The transition and trajectory theories are important for nursing care because they frame a patient's experience with and progression through the stages of chronic illness.

The trajectory theory refers to the **developmental stages** of illness. These include the physiological aspects of the disease as well as the effects a chronic illness can have on the emotional and psychological well-being. The theory allows for framing the patient and **family's experience of living with a chronic illness.** According to Corbin (1998) a trajectory **"refers not only to the illness/condition course, but to the actions taken by various participants to shape or control that course."** Therefore, it is imperative that nurses and other healthcare providers intervene effectively in the chronic illness trajectory to allow the patient to achieve the best health status possible. The **interventions** provided should not only be **treatments** but **education** and **emotional support** as well.

In this nursing model the patient is seen as an active member in health, prevention, disease and rehabilitation, and the nursing person supports the patient in his independence, self-help, self-determination, and helps to enable him to live an as much as possible "normal life".

Major Phenomena of Concern to Nursing: (Juliet Corbin and Anselm Strauss)

The Chronic Illness Trajectory Model formulated by Corbin and Strauss synthesizes the literature on chronicity to create a conceptual framework that gives meaning to chronic disease management. The model provides a guideline and philosophy for nursing practice by examining the patient's disease experience from multiple perspectives in order to provide holistic care. The Trajectory Model is constructed around the idea that chronic illness is dynamic and therefore requires phases to address the disease evolution (Corbin & Strauss, 1992). The framework offers a comprehensive theory in order to address the complexity of issues that arise in the context of chronic management over time **(Corbin, 1998)**.

The Trajectory Model

The trajectory theory has 8 stages:

1. PRE-TRAJECTORY
2. ONSET
3. CRISIS
4. ACUTE
5. STABLE
6. UNSTABLE

7. DOWNWARD

8. DYING

   1. **Initial or pre-trajectory phase:** The stage experienced prior to contact with medical care providers. Occurs before any signs and symptoms are present.

   2. **Trajectory onset phase:** Occurs with the first onset of signs and symptoms and includes the diagnostic period. Nature of onset may play an important role on impact of illness on a family.

   3. **The crisis phase:** is when a potentially life-threatening situation arises.

   4. **The acute phase:** follows the crisis phase and refers to the period when the patient's symptoms can be controlled by a prescribed regimen.

   5. **Stable phase:** this phase starts once symptoms are controlled.

   6. **Unstable phase:** when the patient's symptoms are not controlled by the previously adopted regimen.

   7. **Downward phase:** characterized by progressive deterioration in mental and physical status.

   8. **Dying phase:** refers to a period of weeks, days, or hours preceding death.

Application of Transition and Trajectory Theory in Nursing

Health and illness are part of the human experience. As nurses, we often encounter chronic illnesses when caring for patients. Success in a nursing career depends on our ability to learn how patients experience chronic illnesses and the best ways to care for those patients. The transition and trajectory theories are important for nursing care because they frame a patient's experience with and progression through the stages of chronic illness.

According to Corbin (1998) a trajectory "refers not only to the illness/condition course, but to the actions taken by various participants to shape or control that course." Therefore, it is imperative that nurses and other healthcare providers intervene effectively in the chronic illness trajectory to allow the patient to achieve the best health status possible. The interventions provided should not only be treatments but education and emotional support as well. This theory allows nurses to think of clients in a holistic manner—as a person going through life changes and transitions and reacting to those changes along a trajectory path. It allows nurses to visualize each unique client and to plan care in an individual manner.

The Nursing Process in Trajectory Framework

The Corbin and Strauss Chronic Illness Trajectory Framework consists of 6 steps:

1. Identifying the trajectory phase.
2. Identifying problems and establishing goals.
3. Establishing plans to meet goals.
4. Identifying factors that facilitate or hinder attainment of goals.
5. Implementing interventions.
6. Evaluating the effectiveness of interventions.

Theory Testing

The development and testing of theories for use in nursing research and practice is essential for advancement of the profession.

The Trajectory Theory of Chronic Illness Management is a middle-range nursing theory that has been proposed by **Corbin and Strauss (1991)**. Analysis and evaluation of this theory was performed using **Fawcett and Downs's (1992)** guidelines. Theory analysis makes this theory more understandable and helps to identify the strengths and weaknesses of the theory. **Results of the theory analysis and evaluation suggest that the Trajectory Theory has theoretical and social significance but that further theoretical work is necessary to enhance the internal consistency of the theory.**

Nursing Action That Direct Favorable Outcomes

The Trajectory Model denotes an illness course which often generates uncertainty in one's life. A sense of uncertainty felt by patients with chronic illness is often attributed to a major life transition. Transition Theory describes how people reconstruct their reality and resolve uncertainty when a defined reality becomes disrupted. The interconnectedness between Trajectory and Transition Theory is demonstrated by the shaping of one's transition to resolve uncertainty initiated by current reality. A patient experiencing a transition can lose a sense of self and become vulnerable when old norms no longer hold true due to illness limitations. In order to reduce the primacy of chronic illness, the patient must confront the disease circumstances and integrate the consequences into one's life to achieve normalization.

The nursing profession is called upon to facilitate reality modifications by reducing uncertainty which otherwise sustains a patient's health outcome as indeterminate. Offering the patient the opportunity to verbalize concerns and gather information can reduce the circular pattern of vulnerability contributing to further uncertainty. To manage transitions associated with chronic illness, the patient is required to bridge the gap between disrupted reality and current reality, in order to create new meaning and regain self-identity **(Selder, 1989).**

Conclusion

Trajectory model can be used as a management instrument for the professional care. It helps the nursing person to get familiar with the patient's perspective. Trajectory model has been applied in conditions like cancer, cardiovascular diseases, HIV, AIDS, diabetes mellitus and multiple sclerosis. Furthermore, the TM can be easily combined with other, already used nursing models in order to supplement these by aspects of the nursing of chronically sick persons. It pursues a holistic approach, it completely fits in the concept of the integrated health care and thus also in the structures of the care and case management. However, the required basic conditions must be guaranteed and made available by the health care system: enough workforces must be available, the length of service must be flexibly adapted to the patient's requirements and it must be worked actively on the inpatient and ambulatory integration. In our country, a difficulty consists in the conversion to make a nursing person responsible for the patient. Therefore, in terms of the integrated health care, a networking of institutions should take place in order to ensure a care continuum.

References

1. Corbin J, and Strauss A. A Nursing Model for Chronic Illness Management Based upon the Trajectory framework. Scholarly Inquiry for Nursing Practice, 1991, 5, 155–174.

2. Smeltzer SC. Use of the Trajectory Model of nursing in multiple sclerosi. Sch Inq Nurs Pract. 1991 Fall; 5(3): 219–34.

3. McCorkle R, Pasacreta JV. Enhancing caregiver outcomes in palliative care. Cancer Control. 2001 Jan-Feb; 8(1): 36–45. Available at http://www.moffitt.org/CCJRoot/v8n1/pdf/36.pdf. Accessed on 31/1/2011.

4. Kabinga M, Banda SS. A Conceptual Review of the Demands of chronic care and the Preparedness of Nurses Trained with the General Nursing Council of Zambia Curriculum. Medical Journal of Zambia, 2008; 35: 3.

Chapter VIII

A Survey Study to Determine the Risk Factors Associated with Chronic Diseases

*Shweta Pattnaik ** Dr. Usha Ukande

Background of the Study

India is undergoing rapid epidemiological transition as a consequence of social, economic and ongoing lifestyle changes. Chronic diseases have become a major public health problem. Chronic diseases account for 48% of the global disability (WHO 2011) and account for 60% of all deaths worldwide.

The latter half of the 20th century had brought in substantial progress in societal development, health, nutrition as well as life expectancy. Consequently, deaths from communicable diseases have decreased while those from NCDs have risen. This has been attributed to multiple health transitions such as demographic (population aging), epidemiological (change from communicable to non-communicable diseases) and nutritional (high caloric consumption and low physical activity levels) transitions. As a result, NCDs currently account for 53% of the total deaths and 44% of DALYs lost. Projections indicate a further increase to 67% of total deaths by 2030. CVD is the major contributor to this burden, attributable to 52% of NCD associated deaths and 29% of total deaths. **(Sailesh Mohan, Srinath Reddy, 2014)** Chronic diseases affect people with at least one quarter of deaths occurring in those under the age of 60 years and affect both men and women equally, making it a major concern in health.

Need of the Study

Chronic non-communicable diseases such as heart disease, cancer and diabetes are the biggest killers worldwide. Of the estimated 10·3 million deaths that occurred in India in 2004, 1·1 million (11%) were due to injuries and 5·2 million (50%) were due to chronic diseases (figure 1; web appendix pp 4–7). The chronic diseases discussed in this report caused an estimated 3·6 million (35%) deaths. Mortality rates for people with age-specific chronic diseases are estimated to be higher in India than in high-income countries. In 2004, the overall age standardized mortality rates for chronic diseases were 769 per 100000 men (56% higher than in high-income countries in 2004) and 602 per 100000 women (100% higher than in high-income countries in 2004). Cardiovascular diseases, especially coronary heart disease, are major contributors to the higher death rates in India, because Indians are more likely to develop coronary heart disease and have an earlier age of disease onset than people in high-income countries, and because the case fatality rate in India is higher than in high-income countries. **(Vikram Patel, Somnath Chatterji, 2011)**

While the global Chronic Disease Lifestyle burden is enormous, common risk factors related to chronic diseases are largely modifiable and actions can be taken to reduce the relevant morbidity and mortality.

The present study aimed to prepare evidence-based guidelines and strategies for prevention of chronic diseases and promotion of health of people living with chronic diseases basically aiming at prevention of Cardiovascular diseases, Diabetes Mellitus and Chronic Kidney Disease.

Objectives

- To assess the distribution of chronic diseases (Cardio Vascular Disease, Diabetes Mellitus, and Chronic Kidney Disease) among the patients admitted in hospitals from Jan 2012–Dec 2012.

- To assess the common risk factors associated with chronic diseases (Cardio Vascular Disease, Diabetes Mellitus, and Chronic Kidney Disease).

Research Methodology

The study was conducted in 4 regions of India, i.e., East, West, North and South.

- **Research Design:** A non-experimental survey design was used in the study.
- **Population:** Diagnosed cases of CVD, DM and CKD either from Inpatient Department or Outpatient Department of the hospital.
- **Sampling Technique:** Purposive sampling technique.
- **Sample Size:** Total 5000 samples were used wherein 1250 samples were to be collected from each region.
- **Setting:** One Private and one Government Hospital not less than 300 bedded capacity.

Data Collection Procedure

PART – 1: To assess the distribution of chronic diseases

1. The setting for data collection was one Private and one Government Hospital not less than 300 bedded capacity
2. The first page of the tool consists of hospital description where the percentage of chronic diseases will be calculated against the total number of patients admitted in the hospital. This will give a worldwide distribution of chronic diseases in a particular region.
3. This data was collected from the Record Department after taking permission from the hospital authority.

PART – 2: To assess the common risk factors associated with chronic diseases.

1. A total of 1250 samples were supposed to be collected from each region.
2. Samples would be diagnosed cases of CVD, DM and CKD either from Inpatient Department or Outpatient Department of the hospital.
3. The data was collection by asking questions to the samples from the given questionnaire.

Tool

- **Section-I:** Socio Demographic data
- **Section-II:** Associated risk factors which has subdivisions as
    - ✓ II a (Cardiovascular Diseases)
    - ✓ II b (Diabetes Mellitus)
    - ✓ II c (Chronic Kidney Disease)

Findings

- **Section-I: Socio Demographic data**

    The data suggests that majority of the samples, i.e., 521(57.5%) belong to the group of 41–60years Chronic diseases were found to be most prevalent among males, i.e., 543(60%). Primary education 350(38.6%) is more even though living in urban areas (60.7%). Maximum belong to Hindu religion 563(62.2%). Unemployment (65.5%) was seen in majority of the samples. Maximum families were nuclear (74.4%) and 409(45.1%) had an average family income of <5000 per month. 859(94.9%) were married and majority 429(47.4%) of them had 1–2 children.

It was found that more than half of the samples, i.e., 519(57.3%) and 396(56.1%) were Non-vegetarian and weighed between 41–60kgs respectively. In regard to height and BMI it was found to be 326(46.2%) and 575(63.5%) respectively. Talking about habits 303(33.4%) are currently consuming alcohol and are smoking. Very few percentage of the samples, i.e., 282(31.2%) are suffering from dental diseases.

Most of the families' 479(53%) priority for seeking care was the government hospital. Alternative therapies 807(89.2%) were not in use even in South region. The number of samples who did not receive any information from the nurse was more, i.e., 717(79.3%).

- **Section-II(a): Associated Risk Factors related to Cardiovascular diseases**

The findings revealed that majority 678(74.9%) of the samples had the onset of CVD for <5years and no associated diseases were found with it. The samples 576(63.6%) suffering from CVDs were on regular medication. Larger samples 555(61.3%) have no family history of CVD. Maximum 653(72.1%) of them were moderate workers.

Half of the samples 468(51.7%) did not have any problem in falling asleep. Majority 623(68.8%) did not show any presence of disturbed thoughts and 627(69.2%) had a normal appetite. The last cholesterol level in samples 329(36.3%) was found between 151–200mg and for 296 (32.6%) it was <150mg. Weight in maximum samples 516(57%) before disease occurred was between 41–60 kgs and Fast food was a preference for 513(56.6%).

The onset of hypertension was <5 years in maximum samples, i.e. 615(67.9%), and 593(65.5%) were on regular medication intake. Out of total 476 women it was found that 147(30.8%) attained menopause at the age of 41–45 years.

- **Section-II(b): Associated Risk Factors related to Diabetes Mellitus**

  Hereditary factor was seen in majority of samples, i.e. 456(60.6%) suffering with DM. For majority of the samples 436(57.9%) the age of diagnosis of DM was between 41–60 years. The waist size of 51–60cm was found in maximum samples, i.e. 302(40.1%). The blood glucose level was between 101–150 mg/dl for 327(43.4%). Out of 752 samples only 182(24.3%) had pre-existing cardiac diseases and 266(35.4%) suffered from hypertension.

  Maximum samples 724(96.2%) did not undergo any surgery of pancreas gland. For 361 diabetic females only 22(6.1%) and 20(5.6%) had a history of DM during pregnancy and PCOD respectively. The range of cholesterol for 360(47.8%) samples was 151–200 mg/dl.

  Maximum samples (82.8%) preferred homemade food in DM. Majority 476(63.2%) did not suffer from any stress or tension.

- **Section-II(c): Associated Risk Factors related to Chronic Kidney Disease**

  Majority of the samples 228(54.8%) were found to be in the age group of 21–40 years. Only a few, 45(10.8%) out of 416 had an obstruction in the urinary bladder. The problem of recurrent urinary stone, hematuria was found in 136(32.7%) samples and history of UTI was just found in 167(40%) of the samples. Maximum did not complain of any injury to kidneys, i.e. 400(96.1%). Only 63(15.2%) and 38(9%) had severe dehydration and excessive blood loss (anemia).

  In total out of 416, 329(79%) samples underwent dialysis and 263(63.5%) had a duration of < 5years. Urine output per day was between 501–1000 ml for majority of the samples, i.e. 206(49.5%). Daily salt intake for 302(72.5%) was <10gm. There was no history of any digestive tract related diseases/surgeries for maximum samples, i.e. 355(85.3%) whereas 61(14.7%) suffered from some digestive tract disorders. Majority of CKD samples 378(90.8%) had no plan for kidney transplantation whereas 39(9.2%) planned for the same.

Hospital Description

West Region

S. No	Name of Hospital	No. of Patients Admitted	CVD (f)	DM (f)	CKD (f)
	PRIVATE HOSPITAL				
1.	Choithram Hospital & Research Centre, Indore (M.P.)	11725	653	607	399

North Region

S. No	Name of Hospital	No. of patients admitted	CVD (f)	DM (f)	CKD (f)
1.	Govt. Hospital, Hoshiarpur (Punjab)	21838	14587	5771	1480
2.	SPN Hospital, Mukerian (Punjab)	22718	13408	4811	4499

South Region

S. No	Name of Hospital	No. of patients admitted	CVD (f)	DM (f)	CKD (f)
	GOVERNMENT HOSPITAL				
1.	General Hospital, Trivandrum	27148	2111	803	594
2.	Deva Raj Urs Hospital Karnataka	3143	1043	1107	993
3.	Govt. Hospital, Nagarcovil	161640	17653	15062	10773

S. No	Name of Hospital	No. of patients admitted	CVD (f)	DM (f)	CKD (f)
	PRIVATE HOSPITAL				
1.	Holy Cross Hospital,	29426	2541	5050	422
2.	Dr. Jeya Shekharan's Hospital, Nagarcoil	4905	1380	1078	360
3.	Narayana Health Hospital, Karnataka	25845	9389	745	427

Conclusion: Planning and Strategies for Prevention of Chronic Diseases

It is vital that the increasing importance of chronic diseases is anticipated, understood and acted upon urgently. This requires a new approach by national leaders who are in a position to strengthen chronic disease prevention and control efforts. As a first step, it is essential to communicate the latest and most accurate knowledge and information to front-line health professionals and the public at large.

This Can Be Achieved with the Help of Lifestyle Modification Package Which Includes

- Awareness programs.
- Community Health Camps.
- Assessment of the risk factors.
- In-service education for staff nurses.
- Health education to patients.
- Government support in terms of manpower and finance.
- Providing training and arranging trainers to educate people in each region so that the village areas are covered.
- Continuous education for 2–3 years, then feedback should be taken about the present situation and then again reassessment.

- Health checkup to be made mandatory for all people after 30–35 years emphasizing on different lab investigations.

- Information and awareness of chronic diseases to be imparted to college students.

- Sharing experiences of the clients suffering from these diseases to everyone through videos.

- Lastly, sending the report of the findings of this research study to the Government will help them to form new policies and strategies to overcome the problem.

References

1. Sailesh Mohan, Srinath Reddy, Swiss Re, Centre for global dialogue Chronic Diseases in India: Burden And Implications, 30 Jan 2014.cgd.swissre.com.

2. Vikram Patel, Somnath Chatterji, Dan Chisholm et al. India: Towards Universal Health Coverage 3: Chronic diseases and injuries in India, Lancet 2011; 377: 413–28, Published Online January 12, 2011 DOI: 10.1016/S0140-6736(10) 61188-9.

3. Leeder S, Raymond S, Greenberg H, Liu H, Esson K. A race against time: the challenge of cardiovascular disease in developing countries. New York: Trustees of Columbia University, 2004.

4. Prabhakaran D, Yusuf S, Mehta S, et al. Two-year outcomes in patients admitted with non-ST elevation acute coronary syndrome: results of the OASIS registry 1 and 2. Indian Heart J 2005; 57: 217–25.

5. Xavier D, Pais P, Devereaux PJ, et al. Treatment and outcomes of acute coronary syndromes in India (CREATE): a prospective analysis of registry data. Lancet 2008; 371: 1435–42.

www.ingramcontent.com/pod-product-compliance
Lightning Source LLC
Chambersburg PA
CBHW020719180526
45163CB00001B/40